# Healthwise® Handbook

- Better Care, Lower Costs
- First Aid and Emergencies
- Common Health Problems
- Living Better with Chronic Disease
- Staying Healthy

## A Self-Care Guide
for You and Your Family

**17th Edition**

Donald W. Kemper, MPH

Katy E. Magee, Editor

Steven L. Schneider, MD, Medical Editor

A. Patrice Burgess, MD, Medical Editor

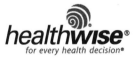

*healthwise*®
*for every health decision*®

Healthwise
P.O. Box 1989
Boise, Idaho 83701

First edition 1976
Seventeenth edition 2006

17hwhb/1st/5-06
ISBN 1-932921-22-2

Printed in the United States of America

Printed on recycled paper

## About Healthwise

Healthwise is a nonprofit organization. Our mission is to help people make better health decisions. People use our handbooks, online content, and nurse call center resources 70 million times a year for help with their health decisions. To learn more about Healthwise, please visit www.healthwise.org.

## About This Book

No book can replace the need for doctors—and no doctor can replace the need for people to care for themselves. This new edition of the *Healthwise® Handbook* will help people deal with common health problems, partner with their doctors, live better with chronic disease, stay healthy, and avoid unnecessary costs. With clearer language, full-color format, all-new illustrations, and a simpler organization, the book is easier to use and easier to understand than ever.

 The new book also makes it easier to reach decision-focused, action-oriented content in the Healthwise® Knowledgebase. Each time you see the "Go to Web" icon, you will find instructions about how to reach content that can help you make a decision, master a skill, or learn more about your health through a quiz or other tool.

If your doctor gives you advice that conflicts with this book, please follow your doctor's advice. Because your doctor knows your specific history and needs, his or her advice may be the best for you. Likewise, if you follow the book's self-care tips but do not get positive results, be sure to consult your doctor.

This book is only a guide. We cannot guarantee that it will work for you in every case. Nor will the authors or publishers accept responsibility for any problems that may occur from following its guidelines. Remember to use your common sense and good judgment.

We wish you the best of health!

Donald W. Kemper

# Table of Contents

## Living Better With Chronic Disease

## Staying Healthy

# Acknowledgements

For Healthwise, the 17th edition of the *Healthwise Handbook* arrives after three decades of helping people make better health decisions. While this edition departs from past editions in myriad ways, it's also a recommitment to that simple mission.

Many, many people on the Healthwise staff have contributed to this edition of the book—some in ways they may not even be aware of. With others, it's a little more obvious. Special thanks go to Katy Magee, for editing the book and driving the shape, scope, and style of its content; Andrea Blum, for steering the book through the earliest stages of design all the way to final production; Steve Schneider, MD, and Patrice Burgess, MD, for thoughtful medical guidance from start to finish; Terrie Britton and John Kubisiak, for their layout, design, and typesetting expertise; Jo-Ann Kachigian, Michele Cronen, and Terrina Vail, for careful (yet speedy!) copyediting and proofreading; Marilyn Allen, for her help with all manner of tasks large and small; Kourtney Funke, for her work on the cover design and print-to-Web icon; Steve Graepel, for guiding the development of the new illustrations; Dave Foster and Mark Audas, for their help with the print-to-Web strategy; and Don Kemper, for his ever-evolving yet steadfast vision of what the book should be.

Special acknowledgement goes to Michael Linkinhoker, MA, CMI, at Link Studio, for creating the book's beautiful illustrations.

We also thank the following health professionals for the clinical wisdom and experience they shared in reviewing the book:

| | |
|---|---|
| Randall D. Burr, MD | Joy Melnikow, MD |
| Colin H. Chalk, MD | Charles M. Myer III, MD |
| Heather O. Chambliss, PhD | Theresa O'Young, PharmD |
| Arden G. Christen, DDS | Caroline S. Rhoads, MD |
| Lisa Cooper-Patrick, MD | Ruth Schneider, RD |
| Alan C. Dalkin, MD | Avery L. Seifert, MD |
| Seymour Diamond, MD | Michael J. Sexton, MD |
| William M. Green, MD | Peter Shalit, MD |
| Carol L. Karp, MD | Brent T. Shoji, MD |
| Robert B. Keller, MD | R. Steven Tharratt, MD |
| Robert A. Kloner, MD | Arvydas D. Vanagunas, MD |

This edition of the *Healthwise Handbook* stands on the broad shoulders of the sixteen that came before it—and the hundreds of health professionals, educators, writers, editors, and others who have ensured that Healthwise content has gotten better and better over the past 30 years. Your work has given millions of people a better chance at better health. This book is dedicated to you.

# Better Care, Lower Costs

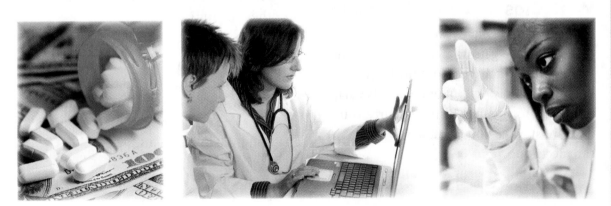

# Better Care at Lower Costs

Good health care doesn't just happen. You have to do your part. Taking an active role in your health care is the best way to make sure you get great care and reduce costs at the same time.

This chapter is a practical guide to getting the care you need—no more and certainly no less—and getting it for the best price. It covers the five areas where you can have the biggest impact on both the cost and quality of your care:

◆ Working closely with your doctor.

◆ Being smart about medicines.

◆ Saving the emergency room for emergencies.

◆ Using medical tests wisely.

◆ Considering all your options before you decide on treatment.

With just a little effort in these five areas, you can:

◆ Reduce your health care costs today and in the future.

◆ Make sure you get the care that's the best choice for you.

◆ Avoid medical errors by being involved in your own care and avoiding care that you don't need.

## Work Closely With Your Doctor

A strong partnership between you and your doctor is key to getting great care and reducing costs. A doctor who not only knows your medical history but understands what's important to you may be the resource you need most when you face a major health care decision.

## Wellness: The Best Way to Save

The best way to reduce health care costs is to stay healthy. Healthy lifestyle choices and preventive care ("wellness" visits, screening tests, immunizations) can help you avoid high-cost problems. Staying well also helps you avoid the medical errors that can come with treating health problems.

To learn how to start living healthier today, see page 299.

**1. Use your doctor as a teacher and coach.** Some patients just want their doctors to tell them what to do. They don't want to know the whys and the hows. Some of the time, that's fine. But if you really want to get care that best meets your needs, be a patient *and* a student.

◆ Don't just ask your doctor what you should do. Ask why. Your doctor is in a unique position to help you understand your care.

◆ Always ask if you have options. Which seem best for you? What are their pros and cons? What effects might your choice have in the short term and over the long run?

◆ Benefit from your doctor's experience with other patients. While every patient's situation is unique, your doctor has probably helped other patients work through the same questions and decisions that you have to deal with.

**2. Tell your doctor that you care about cost.** A doctor's main focus is to help you get better, not to save you money. But your doctor may be able to help with both if you speak up.

Don't expect your doctor to know the exact cost of a drug or test or treatment. There are so many things that determine the cost of care—your health plan's arrangement with your doctor, how your plan bills for care, where you get the care, and others. But your doctor can give you an idea of how the cost of one choice compares to another.

**3. Prepare for every doctor visit.** This helps your doctor give you better care and helps both of you make the most of the visit.

◆ Be ready to say what your main symptoms are, when they started, and what you have done to treat them so far. It may help to write these things down beforehand.

◆ Write down the three questions that you most want to have answered. If the doctor does not bring them up, don't be afraid to ask.

◆ Bring a list of any medicines, vitamins, and herbal supplements that you are taking.

◆ Bring copies of recent test results if the tests were done by a different doctor.

**4. Take an active role in every visit or call.** Pay attention. Ask questions if you don't understand something. Write down the diagnosis, the treatment plan, and any guidelines for self-care and follow-up visits or calls. Be honest and direct about what you do or do not plan to do.

## Smart Money Tips for Medicines

If you and your doctor have decided that you need prescription medicine, these three tips can help you get it at a lower cost:

◆ Choose generic medicines instead of brand names when you can. (Generics are the same medicine without the brand.)

◆ If there is no generic option, know whether your health plan makes you pay more for one brand name than another. Many plans do, using a list called a drug formulary.

◆ Compare prices and shop smart.

### Generics and Brand Names

All drugs have a generic name, also known as the scientific name. Many also have one or more brand names. For example, Viagra is a brand name for the generic drug sildenafil. The generic name for Prozac is fluoxetine.

For years after a new drug is created, patent laws prevent other companies from making the same drug. But once the patent expires, other drug companies can make and sell the drug. They just can't sell it by its brand name. So they use the generic name.

A generic drug has the same active ingredients as its brand-name version and almost always costs less. In many cases, generics are less than half the cost of the brands.

### Are generics really as good as brand-name drugs?

◆ Yes. Generics are very carefully tested to make sure they have the same ingredients, same effects, and same safety profile as the brands. The medicines may look or taste slightly different.

◆ For a few medicines, the body does not respond to the generic drug in quite the same way as it does the brand-name drug. These generics are rated "B." The "B" rating does not mean that the generic is not as good or that you can't use it. It does mean that you should talk to your doctor or pharmacist before you switch from the brand to the generic (or vice versa). A pharmacist can tell you whether a drug is rated "B."

That's it. The safety and quality of FDA-approved generics are the same as brands. Generics just cost less. If you want to save money, always ask your doctor or pharmacist, "Is there a generic I can take?"

## Medicines and Your Health Plan

Most health plans use a **drug formulary** to help control costs. A formulary is simply a list of preferred prescription medicines. The plan will pay more of the cost of drugs on the list than it will for other drugs that treat the same health problem.

The formulary may put drugs into three groups, or "tiers," based on how much your health plan will pay and how much you have to pay.

◆ **Group 1: Generic drugs.** These are usually drugs that have been in use for a long time, have proven benefits, and cost less to make and sell. You pay the least for drugs in this group.

◆ **Group 2: Brand-name drugs that are on the formulary.** For the same health problem, there often are competing drugs from different companies. Your health plan may put one drug on the formulary instead of the others if the drug company agrees to reduce the price. You still pay more for the "formulary" brand-name

drug than for the generic, but it costs less than the competing brand-name drugs that are not on the formulary.

◆ **Group 3: Brand-name drugs that are not on the formulary.** These drugs cost more because your health plan does not have an agreement with the drug company to reduce the price. When the health plan pays more, so do you. Your other choice is to switch to a generic or a brand-name drug that is on the formulary.

The difference in cost to you between these three groups can be huge. If your doctor prescribes a medicine, make sure you know how much you will have to pay and whether a different choice would save you money without giving up quality.

Sometimes there are good reasons to use a brand-name drug that's not on the formulary instead of one that is. The drug may have a dosing schedule that works better for you. Or it may have fewer or different side effects. You can still get the drug, but you'll have to pay more for it than for the one that's on the formulary.

But in most cases, there probably is a medicine on the list that will work just as well. Keeping medicine costs low is partly up to you.

◆ Know how your health plan pays for medicines.

◆ If your doctor prescribes a medicine that is not on your health plan's preferred list, ask if there is a medicine on the list that will cost you less and work just as well.

◆ If a drug you need is not on the list, call your health plan and ask about it. This is your right as a consumer and a member of that plan.

## Smart Shopping for Medicines

If you pay for medicines out of your own pocket or through a health savings account (HSA), you have even more to gain from careful spending.

**1. Compare prices.** The speed and convenience of a local pharmacy helps in emergencies or if you're in a rush. But for medicines you take on a regular basis, mail-order or online pharmacies may be cheaper. They may be more convenient too, sending the medicines right to your mailbox.

If you order online, look for Web sites that have the VIPPS (Verified Internet Pharmacy Practice Sites) seal from the National Association of Boards of Pharmacy. This means the site has met state and federal requirements.

**2. Ask your doctor for free samples** if you are trying a new medicine. This can let you try out the medicine for a couple of weeks without buying a full prescription.

But beware—often the samples doctors get are for newer, more expensive drugs. If you don't switch to a cheaper drug later, you may be paying more than you need to.

**3. Buy in bulk.** Once you know you will be using a medicine for a long time, you can often save money and time by ordering a large supply (90 days' worth, for example). Ask your doctor to write a prescription that covers a few months.

**4. Ask your doctor about pill splitting.** You can buy some pills at twice the dose you need (100 mg instead of 50 mg, for instance) for the same or nearly the same cost as the lower dose. By splitting the larger dose, you can get two doses for the price of one. To split the dose, you cut the pill in half. It is best to use a pill splitter for this, which is a small tool that helps make a clean cut. (You can buy one at most drugstores.)

It is not safe to split all medicines this way. Capsules and time-release pills should never be split. With many medicines, the dose needs to be extremely precise. So be sure to check with your doctor about whether splitting your pills is safe.

**5. Find out about discounts and patient assistance programs.** Some drug companies offer free or discounted drugs for people who need help paying for medicine. Your doctor may need to contact them on your behalf. To learn more about these programs, look online at RxAssist (www.rxassist.org) or at the Partnership for Prescription Assistance (www.pparx.org).

Help may also be available through your state, your community, or the Veterans Administration (for veterans and their families). Some pharmacies and organizations, such as AARP, may offer discounts for older adults.

## Save the Emergency Room for Emergencies

Hospital emergency rooms (ERs) are set up to focus on medical emergencies. They are not set up to focus on routine health care. If you go to the ER for a problem that is not an emergency:

◆ It will cost a lot more than it would at your doctor's office or a "walk-in" clinic (see page 6). A trip to the ER for an earache, for example, may cost three or four times as much as it would at your doctor's office.

◆ You will probably spend a lot more time there than you would at a walk-in clinic or doctor's office.

◆ You will get care from a doctor who has probably never seen you before. It's always best to get as much of your care as you can from a doctor who knows and understands you.

Go to the ER if you think you are having a medical emergency. That's what the ER is for. Otherwise, call your doctor's office first, or go to a walk-in clinic. It will save you money and time.

### How do you know when it's an emergency?

There are few clear rules about what is an emergency and what isn't. Most doctors would agree on a short list of problems that should always be treated as emergencies—chest pain that could be a heart attack, not being able to breathe, severe and uncontrolled bleeding, stroke symptoms, and a few others.

Most health problems are *not* emergencies. You may want to take care of the problem right away because you feel sick or uncomfortable, but nothing bad is going to happen to you if you wait a bit. Then again, you don't always know that for sure. Some problems that seem minor can become serious if you ignore them. And it may be even harder to know what to do when a child is sick.

One good question to ask yourself is, "Am I thinking about going to the ER because it's *convenient* or because it's *necessary*?" If you are choosing the ER because you can get in without an appointment, keep in mind the high price you will pay for that convenience. And you may have other options.

You can always call your doctor's office or a nurse line for help. You can also look for information about your problem in this book or at the Web site on the back cover to help you decide what to do.

## What's a "Walk-in" Clinic?

Walk-in clinics are often called "minor emergency," "urgent care," or "immediate care" centers. They deal with all kinds of health problems and are often open in the evenings and on weekends. You do not need an appointment.

These types of clinics can be a great option when:

◆ You can't or don't want to wait for an appointment at your doctor's office.

◆ You don't need the level of care an ER provides.

Care at a walk-in clinic costs a lot less than care for the same problem at an ER. And if it turns out you are having a true medical emergency, a walk-in clinic will send you to the ER.

Unless you have a walk-in clinic in your neighborhood or already know where one is, it may be hard to find one when you need it. So, at your next doctor visit, ask your doctor to recommend one. Check with your health plan to see if it offers better coverage at some clinics than others.

## What if a problem happens on a weekend or at night?

If you think you are having a medical emergency, go to the ER.

If you don't think the problem is an emergency:

◆ Look up your problem in this book or at the Web site on the back cover, and read the information about when to call a doctor. See if there is home treatment you can try.

◆ Call your doctor's office and see if there is a number to call for after-hours service.

◆ Call a nurse line for advice. The nurse can help you decide whether you need to get help now or whether it is safe to wait.

◆ Go to a walk-in clinic (if one is open).

◆ Go to the ER if you feel the problem cannot wait until your doctor's office or a walk-in clinic is open.

## Smart Money Tips for Medical Tests

Medical tests are expensive. If you need a test, do your part to make sure that you do not have to repeat it. The tips below can make a big difference:

**1. Follow instructions about how to prepare.** Are you supposed to stop eating the night before? Not drink alcohol? Stop taking medicines, or take a special medicine? Get written instructions from your doctor or nurse, and follow them. This reduces the chance of error and the need to repeat the test, which saves you money.

Before you have a medical test, look it up at the Web site on the back cover so you know more about the test and what you need to do.

**2. Keep a copy of the results.** Get a copy of the full test results, even if they're normal. Do not assume that no news is good news. If you do not hear from your doctor, call to get your written test results. This helps in three ways:

◆ It makes sure you have the results if you later need to compare them to past or future tests.

◆ You have a backup record in case you see a different doctor who does not get your test results from your previous doctor. If you can provide a copy, he or she may not have to repeat the test.

◆ Having the results helps you better understand what's going on with your health.

**3. Do not check into the hospital just for tests unless you have to.** Sometimes a hospital stay is necessary, but often the point is just to better control what you eat, drink, and do before the test.

Talk to your doctor. He or she may be fine with you having the tests as an outpatient (which means not staying in the hospital overnight) as long as you agree to follow instructions for before and after the test. If it is safe for you to do those things at home instead of at the hospital, you may greatly lower the cost of the testing.

**4. Don't have tests more often than you need to.** If you have a health problem that requires frequent tests and you are worried about the cost, tell your doctor. Maybe you can go a little longer between tests. Maybe you can have a less costly test some of the time and the more expensive one less often.

**5. Ask about options, and shop around.** The cost of some testing can vary widely without any difference in how reliable the results are. For expensive tests, it may pay to compare the costs of your best options.

## Smart Decisions: Know Your Options

Good health decisions can help you reduce costs and get better care. A good decision takes into account:

◆ The benefits of each option.

◆ The risks of each option.

◆ The costs of each option.

◆ Your own needs and wants.

**1. Always ask why.** Too much care can be just as bad as—or worse than—too little. Most medicines can have side effects. Medical tests can give false results that lead to the wrong care. Surgery almost always has risks. And anytime you get care, there is a chance of error.

When your doctor suggests or orders a medicine, surgery, a test, or any other kind of care, ask why you need it and what would happen if you waited. If you don't need it now, you might want to wait.

But also remember that there can be costs to doing nothing. The "wait and see" option is not always the best. If you don't get care when you need it and a health problem gets worse, you may face higher costs than you would have if you had taken care of the problem sooner.

Asking why can help you and your doctor make the decision that's right for you.

**2. Know the pros and cons.** Every treatment choice has pros and cons. It's up to you to know what they are. Your doctor can be a big help here, as can the Web site on the back cover.

Partner with your doctor to help you understand what a decision might mean for you now and in the long run.

Remember, the goal is to get the care you need, no more and no less, and to get it at the lowest cost you can.

**3. Think about your needs and wants.** People value things differently. When you have a health care decision to make, you have to balance issues like:

◆ The desire for better health versus the risks of treatment.

◆ The certainty of doing something versus the uncertainty of waiting (the known versus the unknown).

◆ Convenience versus cost.

You are the only person who knows what mix is right for you. You may be willing to pay more if you can get the problem taken care of quickly. You may be willing to go through a very risky surgery if it could cure a serious health problem. Or you may be willing to put up with some pain if it means you can avoid a treatment with bad side effects or high cost.

For many decisions, these issues are just as important as the medical facts. They are part of what makes a decision right for *you*. They affect whether you get the care you want at a cost that seems reasonable to you.

## Surgery Decisions

Surgery tends to come with high costs and risks. When the choice to have surgery is not clear, good decisions are especially important.

Before you have surgery for anything other than an urgent, life-threatening problem, make sure you get answers to these key questions:

◆ How might surgery help you?

◆ What results would you have to get from the surgery for you to consider it a success? How likely are those results?

◆ What could go wrong if you have surgery?

◆ How long would it take to recover from surgery? How much time off would you have to take? What kind of rehab would you need?

◆ What happens in the short term if you don't have surgery? What might happen over the long run if you don't have it?

◆ Are there other treatments you could try first?

◆ Can the problem come back after surgery?

◆ If you need surgery, where should you have it? How can you reduce the chance of an error?

You will probably have other questions unique to your health problem and situation. The Web site on the back cover has tools that can help you work through these decisions.

# First Aid and Emergencies

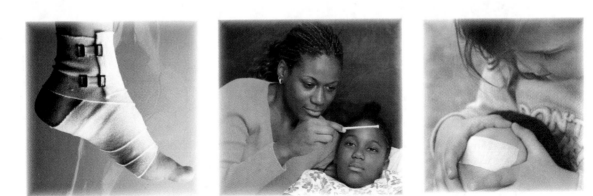

# Abdominal Injury

## When to Call a Doctor

**Call 911 if:**

◆ The person has severe belly pain after an injury.

◆ The belly is swollen and hard all over, or pressing anywhere on the belly causes severe pain.

◆ The person faints.

◆ The person vomits blood or what looks like coffee grounds.

◆ The person passes maroon or bloody stools, or there is a lot of blood in the toilet.

**Call a doctor if:**

◆ There is any bleeding from the rectum or in the stools, blood in the urine, or unexpected vaginal bleeding.

◆ The injury causes nausea, vomiting, heartburn, or loss of appetite.

◆ You have constant mild or moderate pain that gets worse or does not improve after 12 hours.

For a cut or puncture to the belly, also see Cuts and Punctures on page 29.

A blow to the belly (abdomen) can cause severe bruising and bleeding inside the body. Such injuries are often caused by car, bike, sledding, or skiing accidents, when the person is thrown into an object or to the ground.

If there is internal bleeding or organ damage, the person may go into shock (see page 47). This can be life-threatening.

## Home Treatment

◆ Have the person lie down with the feet higher than the heart. Loosen the person's clothing, and cover him or her with a blanket for warmth.

◆ Do not give the person anything to eat or drink until a medical evaluation has been done and you are sure the person is okay.

◆ Watch the person for the next couple of days. Signs of serious internal bleeding may not show up right away.

# Bites From Animals and Humans

## When to Call a Doctor

- The wound is severe and may need stitches, or it is on your face, hand, or foot, or over a joint. If the wound needs stitches, you should get them within 6 to 8 hours. See page 30.

- The bite or scratch is from a bat or other wild animal.

- The bite is from a human or a cat. These bites get infected quickly and easily.

- The bite is from a dog, cat, or ferret that foams at the mouth, acts strangely, or attacked for no clear reason. Also call the local animal control or public health office.

- You can't find the owner of a pet that bit you, or the owner can't confirm that the pet's rabies vaccine is up to date.

- You lose feeling or movement below the wound.

- You have signs of infection. These may include increased pain, swelling, warmth, or redness; red streaks leading from the wound; pus; and fever.

- You have not had a tetanus shot in the past 5 years or don't know when your last shot was. If you need a shot, you should get it within 2 days.

Infection and scarring are the main concerns with bites and scratches that break the skin. You can also get tetanus if your shots are not up to date. See page 326.

After an animal bite, you may want to know if you need a rabies shot. Rabies is quite rare, but it is deadly if you are not vaccinated soon after a bite from an infected animal.

- The main carriers of rabies in North America are bats, raccoons, skunks, and foxes.

- Vaccinated pets, such as dogs, cats, and ferrets, rarely have rabies.

- Many stray animals have not been vaccinated.

## Home Treatment

- Let the wound bleed freely for up to 5 minutes, unless the bleeding is heavy.

If you are bleeding a lot, see Stopping Severe Bleeding on page 17.

- Scrub the wound with soap and water. Do not use alcohol, iodine, or any other cleansers.

- Call the local animal control or public health office for advice on what to do. In general:

  - If a pet dog, cat, or ferret bites you, find out whether the animal has a current rabies vaccine. A healthy pet that does not have a current vaccine should be confined and watched for up to 10 days by a veterinarian.

  - If a wild animal bites or scratches you, the animal control or public health office can tell you whether you need to worry about rabies.

# Bites and Stings—Insects, Spiders, and Ticks

## When to Call a Doctor

### Call 911 if:

◆ You have signs of a severe allergic reaction soon after a bite or sting. These may include:

  ❖ Wheezing or trouble breathing.

  ❖ Swelling around the lips, tongue, or face.

  ❖ Severe swelling around the bite or sting (for example, your entire arm or leg is swollen).

  ❖ Fainting or other signs of shock. See page 47.

◆ You have just been bitten or stung by something that caused a serious reaction in the past.

### Call a doctor if:

◆ You get a spreading skin rash, itching, a feeling of warmth, or hives.

◆ You get a blister at the site of a spider bite, or the skin around it changes color.

◆ A black widow, brown recluse, or hobo spider bites you.

◆ Symptoms are not better in 2 to 3 days.

◆ You have signs of infection. These may include increased pain, swelling, warmth, or redness; red streaks leading from the bite; pus; and fever.

◆ A tick is attached to you and you cannot remove the whole tick.

◆ You were recently exposed to ticks and have a spreading red rash. The rash may or may not be in the bite area and may or may not occur with flu-like symptoms, such as fever, headache, body aches, and fatigue.

◆ You want to talk about allergy kits or allergy shots because you have had a serious allergic reaction in the past.

## Insects and Spiders

Bites and stings from insects (bees, wasps, yellow jackets) and spiders usually cause pain, swelling, redness, and itching at the site of the sting or bite. In some people, especially children, the redness and swelling may be worse and last up to a few days.

A few people have severe allergic reactions that affect the whole body. This type of reaction can be deadly. If you have had a severe allergic reaction to a past sting or bite, you may want to keep an allergy kit with an epinephrine syringe (such as EpiPen) with you at all times. Ask your doctor or pharmacist how and when to use it.

**Spider bites** are rarely serious. But any bite can be serious if it causes a person to have an allergic reaction.

A single bite from a poisonous spider, such as a black widow, brown recluse, or hobo spider, may cause a severe reaction and needs medical care right away.

◆ A bite from a female black widow spider may cause chills, fever, nausea, and severe belly cramps.

◆ A bite from a brown recluse or hobo spider causes intense pain, and you may get a blister that turns into a large, open sore. The bite may also cause nausea, vomiting, headaches, and chills.

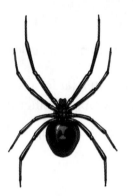

Black widow spiders can be up to 2 inches across and are shiny black with a red or yellow hourglass mark on their undersides.

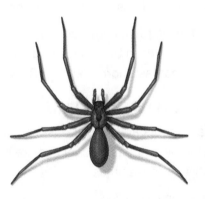

Brown recluse (fiddler) spiders are smaller than black widows and have long legs. They are brown with a violin-shaped mark on their heads.

## Ticks

Ticks are small bugs that bite into the skin and feed on blood. They live in bird feathers and animal fur. Tick bites occur more often from early spring to late summer.

◆ Most ticks do not carry diseases, and most tick bites do not cause serious health problems. Still, it is best to remove a tick as soon as you find one.

◆ Many of the diseases that ticks may pass to humans (such as Lyme disease, Rocky Mountain spotted fever, relapsing fever, and Colorado tick fever) have the same flu-like symptoms: fever, headache, body aches, and fatigue.

◆ Sometimes a rash or sore may occur with the flu-like symptoms. A red rash that gets bigger is a classic early sign of Lyme disease. It may appear 1 day to 1 month after a tick bite.

## Home Treatment

### For insect and spider bites and stings:

◆ Remove a bee stinger by scraping or flicking it out. Do not squeeze it; you may release more venom into the skin. If you can't see the stinger, assume it's not there.

◆ If a black widow, brown recluse, or hobo spider bites you, put ice on the bite and call a doctor. Do not use a tourniquet.

◆ Put ice or a cold pack on the bite or sting. For some people, a paste of baking soda or unseasoned meat tenderizer mixed with a little water helps relieve pain and decrease the reaction.

◆ Take an antihistamine (such as Benadryl or Chlor-Trimeton) to relieve pain, swelling, and itching. Calamine lotion or hydrocortisone cream may also help.

◆ Wash the area with soap and water.

◆ Trim your fingernails so you don't scratch too hard.

◆ Do not break any blisters that develop. They could get infected.

**More**

**For ticks:**

◆ Check your body often for ticks when you are out in the woods. Closely check your clothes, skin, and scalp when you get home. Check your pets for ticks too. The sooner you remove ticks, the less likely they are to spread infection.

◆ If you find a tick, try to remove it. Use tweezers to gently pull on it as close to the skin (where its mouth is) as you can get. Fine-tipped tweezers may work best. Pull straight out, and try not to crush the tick's body. Do not try to "unscrew" the tick.

◆ Do not try to burn off the tick or smother it with petroleum jelly, nail polish, gasoline, or rubbing alcohol.

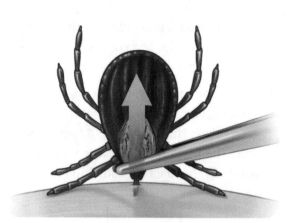

Use tweezers to pull the tick straight out.

◆ Save the tick in a jar for tests in case you get flu-like symptoms after the bite.

◆ Wash the area with soap and water.

# Mosquitoes and West Nile Virus

West Nile virus is an infection spread to humans by mosquitoes. Most people who get the virus do not get sick.

When symptoms do occur, they appear 3 to 14 days after the bite and include fever, headache, body aches, and sometimes a skin rash. This is called West Nile fever. It is usually a mild illness.

Rarely, West Nile virus may affect the brain, causing serious illness that can lead to long-lasting problems or even death. Older adults are most likely to have serious illness from the West Nile virus.

### When to Call a Doctor

Call a doctor if you were exposed to mosquitoes in the past 2 weeks and have any of these symptoms:

◆ Fever, headache, stiff neck, and confusion.

◆ Muscle weakness or loss of movement.

◆ Mild fever, rash, body aches, or swollen lymph nodes in the neck, armpits, or groin that last more than 2 or 3 days.

### How to Avoid West Nile Virus

◆ Stay indoors at dawn, at dusk, and in the early evening. Mosquitoes are most active at these times.

◆ Wear long-sleeved shirts and pants made of thick fabric.

◆ Use an insect repellent that contains DEET, picaridin, or oil of lemon eucalyptus. For the best protection, apply and reapply as the label says.

◆ Don't keep open containers of water near your home. Mosquitoes can breed in even a small amount of standing water.

# Bleeding Emergencies

## When to Call a Doctor

**Call 911 if:**

◆ You have severe bleeding that you cannot stop.

◆ You are bleeding and you faint or feel lightheaded.

◆ You vomit a lot of blood. Bloody vomit may look like coffee grounds.

◆ You pass maroon or bloody stools, or there is a lot of blood in the toilet.

◆ You are pregnant and have severe vaginal bleeding (bleeding that soaks more than 2 pads or 2 super tampons in a 2-hour period).

## Stopping Severe Bleeding From a Wound

◆ Raise the area that is bleeding.

◆ Wash your hands well with soap and water. Put on medical gloves or place several layers of fabric or plastic bags between your hands and the wound.

◆ Remove any objects you can see on the surface of the wound. Do not try to clean out the wound.

◆ Press firmly on the wound with a clean cloth or the cleanest material you can find. If there is an object deep in the wound, put pressure around the object but not directly over it. Do not try to remove the object.

◆ Apply steady pressure for a full 15 minutes. Do not lift your hands to see if bleeding has stopped before 15 minutes are up. **If bleeding from a large or deep wound has not slowed down or stopped after 15 minutes, call 911** and continue to put pressure on the wound. If blood soaks through the cloth, put another cloth on top of the first one.

◆ If bleeding slows down after 15 minutes but a little bleeding starts again once you release the pressure, put direct pressure on the wound for another 15 minutes. For light bleeding, you can apply pressure for up to three 15-minute periods (total of 45 minutes). If any bleeding that is more than just oozing continues after 45 minutes of direct pressure, call a doctor.

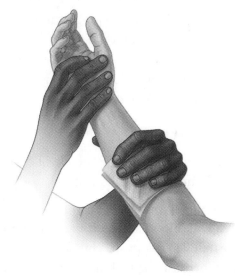

Elevate the area and apply pressure with a clean cloth.

# Blood Under a Nail

## When to Call a Doctor

- The pain is severe, and you do not want to drain the blood from the nail yourself.

- You drained the blood from under the nail, but your finger or toe still hurts a lot.

- You have diabetes, blood flow problems, or a weakened immune system (from HIV, steroid use, cancer treatment, or organ transplant) and need help with blood under a nail.

- You have signs of infection. These may include increased pain, swelling, warmth, or redness; red streaks leading from the nail; pus draining from the hole; and fever.

- You need help removing a nail that has torn or separated from the nail bed.

When a fingernail or toenail gets banged or smashed, blood may build up under the nail. The pressure can hurt a lot. Ice and acetaminophen (Tylenol) or ibuprofen (Advil, Motrin) may help with the pain and swelling.

If the pain is severe and throbbing, the only way to relieve it is to make a hole in the nail to drain the blood. Do not try this unless you have severe pain. If you have diabetes, blood flow problems, or a weakened immune system, don't try it at all.

**To drain the blood:**

- Straighten a paper clip. Then heat the tip in a flame until it is red-hot.

- Place the tip of the paper clip over the area with blood and let it melt through the nail. Do not push. This should not hurt, because the nail has no nerves. Go slowly and reheat the clip as needed. A thick nail may take a few tries.

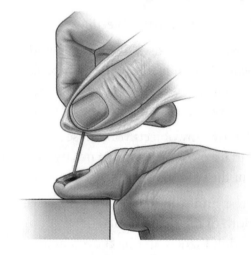

- As soon as there is a hole, blood will drain out and the pain should go away. If the pain does not go away, you may have a more serious injury, such as a broken bone or a deep cut. In this case, you should see a doctor.

- Soak the finger or toe twice a day for 10 minutes in warm, soapy water. Apply an antibiotic ointment and a bandage.

- If the pressure builds up again in a few days, repeat the process. Use the same hole.

# Breathing Emergencies

## When to Call a Doctor

### Call 911 if:

◆ The person stops breathing for longer than 15 to 20 seconds.

◆ An adult or older child has severe trouble breathing. A person with this problem may:

  ❖ Have chest tightness so severe that the person is worried he or she can't keep breathing.

  ❖ Be so short of breath that he or she can't speak.

  ❖ Gasp for breath or have severe wheezing.

  ❖ Feel very anxious, afraid, or restless.

  ❖ Respond slowly or have trouble waking up or staying awake.

◆ A child has severe trouble breathing. Look for these signs:

  ❖ Breathing very fast.

  ❖ Drooling or grunting with each breath.

  ❖ Not being able to speak, cry, or make sounds.

  ❖ Using the neck, chest, and belly muscles to breathe. The skin may "suck in" between the ribs with each breath, and the child may need to sit up and lean forward or tilt the nose up.

  ❖ Flaring the nostrils with each breath.

  ❖ Having a gray, blotchy, or blue color to the skin. Look for color changes in the nail beds, lips, and earlobes.

For less severe breathing problems, see When to Call a Doctor on page 107.

## Rescue Breathing and CPR

Doing CPR the wrong way or on a person whose heart is still beating can cause serious harm. Do not do CPR unless:

1. An adult is not breathing normally (may be gasping for breath), or a child is not breathing at all.

2. The person does not breathe or move in response to rescue breaths.

3. No one with more training in CPR than you is present. If you are the only one there, do the best you can.

The chart on the next page has the basic steps for CPR. Use it for quick reference. The rest of this topic explains each step in more detail and with pictures.

**More** ▶

## CPR Basics

| What to do | Recommendations for: | | |
| --- | --- | --- | --- |
| | **Adults and older children (age 9 and up)** | **Young children (ages 1 to 8)** | **Babies younger than 1 year** |
| If the person is not breathing, start rescue breaths. | Give 2 breaths. | Give 2 breaths. | Give 2 breaths. |
| If the person does not breathe or move after you give 2 rescue breaths, find the spot to do chest compressions. | Place two fingers on the spot where the ribs come together. Put the heel of your other hand just above your fingers on the breastbone. | Place two fingers on the spot where the ribs come together. Put the heel of your other hand just above your fingers on the breastbone. | Place two fingers on the breastbone just below the nipple line. |
| How do you give chest compressions? | Use the heel of one hand with the other hand stacked on top of it. Lace your fingers together. | Use the heel of one hand. If you need more force for a larger child, use both hands as you would for an adult. | Use two fingers. |
| How fast should you do compressions? | Do 100 compressions per minute (between 1 and 2 per second). | Do 100 compressions per minute (between 1 and 2 per second). | Do 100 compressions per minute (between 1 and 2 per second). |
| How far down should you press the chest? | Press chest down 1.5 to 2 inches. | Press chest down 1/3 to 1/2 its depth. | Press chest down 1/3 to 1/2 its depth. |
| How many compressions and breaths do you give? | **30 compressions, 2 breaths.** Repeat this 30/2 cycle until help arrives or person breathes on his or her own. | **30 compressions, 2 breaths.** Repeat this 30/2 cycle until help arrives or child breathes on his or her own. | **30 compressions, 2 breaths.** Repeat this 30/2 cycle until help arrives or baby breathes on his or her own. |

### Step 1: Check to see if the person is conscious.

Tap or gently shake the person and shout, "Are you okay?" But do not shake someone who might have a neck or back injury. That could make the injury worse.

If the person does not respond, follow these steps.

◆ For a person age 9 or older, **call 911**.

◆ For a child under 9 who is not breathing, give 2 breaths and 30 chest compressions, 5 times in a row (about 2 minutes). If the child is still not breathing, **call 911**.

## Step 2: Check for breathing for 5 to 10 seconds.

◆ Kneel next to the person with your head close to his or her head.

◆ Look to see if the person's chest rises and falls.

◆ Listen for breathing sounds.

◆ Put your cheek near the person's mouth and nose to feel whether air is moving out.

◆ If an adult is not breathing normally or if a child is not breathing at all, roll the person onto his or her back. If you think the person might have a neck or back injury, gently roll the person's head, neck, and shoulders together as a unit.

## Step 3: Start rescue breaths.

◆ Put your hand on the person's forehead, and pinch the person's nostrils shut with your thumb and finger. Use your other hand to tilt the chin up to keep the airway open.

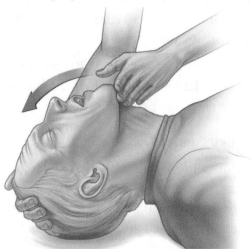

Tilt the chin up to open the airway.

◆ Take a normal breath (not a deep one), and place your mouth over the person's mouth, making a tight seal. For a baby, place your mouth over the baby's mouth and nose. Blow into the person's mouth for 1 second, and watch to see if the person's chest rises.

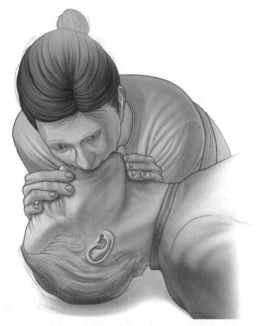

When you give a breath, watch to see if the chest rises.

◆ If the chest does not rise, tilt the person's head again, and give another breath.

◆ Between rescue breaths, remove your mouth from the person's mouth and take a normal breath. Let his or her chest fall, and feel the air escape.

◆ If the person is still not breathing normally after 2 rescue breaths, start chest compressions.

**More** ➤

21

## Step 4: Start chest compressions.

### For an adult or child older than 1 year:

◆ Kneel next to the person. Use your fingers to locate the end of the person's breastbone, where the ribs come together. Place two fingers at the tip of the breastbone.

◆ Place the heel of the other hand right above your fingers (on the side closest to the person's face).

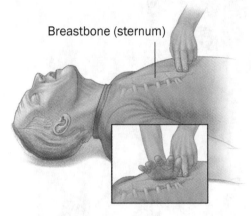

Breastbone (sternum)

Place two fingers at the tip of the breastbone. Then put the heel of the other hand right above your fingers.

◆ For adults and larger children, use both hands to give compressions. Stack your other hand on top of the one that you just put in position. Lace the fingers of both hands together, and raise your fingers so they do not touch the chest.

◆ For smaller children, use the heel of one hand to give compressions.

◆ Straighten your arms, lock your elbows, and center your shoulders directly over your hands.

◆ Press down in a steady rhythm, using your body weight. The force from each thrust should go straight down onto the breastbone, pressing it down 1.5 to 2 inches for an adult or from one-third to one-half of the chest's depth for a child.

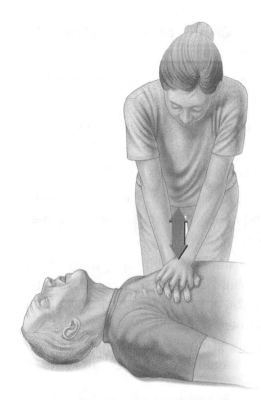

Keep your shoulders directly over your hands with your elbows straight as you push on the chest.

◆ **Give 30 compressions. Push hard and push fast** (at a rate of 100 compressions per minute). After 30 compressions, give 2 rescue breaths.

◆ Keep repeating the cycle of 30 compressions and 2 breaths until help arrives or the person is breathing normally.

### For a baby under 1 year:

◆ Picture a line connecting the nipples, and place two fingers on the baby's breastbone just below that line. Press the chest one-third to one-half of the way down.

◆ **Give 30 compressions** (at a rate of 100 compressions per minute). After 30 chest compressions, give 2 rescue breaths.

◆ Keep giving chest compressions and rescue breaths until help arrives or the baby is breathing normally.

# Breathing Too Fast

## When to Call a Doctor

◆ You cannot get your breathing under control.

◆ You often have problems with fast breathing and anxiety (see page 80).

When you breathe very fast and deep (hyperventilate), the carbon dioxide level in your blood can drop too low. This can cause:

◆ Numbness or tingling in your hands and feet or around your mouth or tongue.

◆ Anxiety and a fast, pounding heartbeat.

◆ A feeling that you cannot get enough air.

◆ Lightheadedness or fainting.

◆ Muscle cramps or spasms, often in the hands.

◆ Chest pain.

## Home Treatment

◆ Sit down and focus on slowing your breathing. Try breathing through pursed lips or through your nose. Try for 1 breath every 5 seconds.

◆ Try a relaxation technique. See page 320.

◆ Hold a paper bag over your nose and mouth, and take 6 to 12 easy, natural breaths. Keep doing this on and off for 5 to 15 minutes. Do not breathe continuously into the bag. Do not use this technique at all if you have heart or lung problems or if you are at an altitude above 6,000 feet.

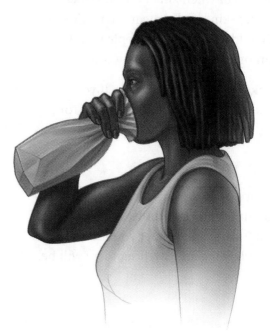

Breathing into a paper bag on and off for a few minutes may help slow your breathing.

# Bruises

## When to Call a Doctor

- The pain is severe.

- You can't use or move the bruised body part.

- You have signs of infection. These may include increased pain, swelling, warmth, or redness; red streaks leading from the bruise; and fever.

- You suddenly start to bruise easily, or you have lots of bruises for no clear reason.

- After a blow to the eye:

  - You have blood in the colored part of your eye or blood in the white part of your eye.

  - You have vision changes.

  - You can't move your eye normally in all directions.

  - You have severe pain.

Bruises occur when small blood vessels under the skin break or tear after a bump or fall. Older adults and people who take aspirin or blood thinners may bruise easily.

A **black eye** is a type of bruise. If you get a black eye, use the home treatment for a bruise, and check the eye for blood.

## Home Treatment

- Put ice or cold packs on the bruise for 10 minutes several times a day for the first 2 days. The sooner you use ice, the less bleeding and swelling there will be.

- Take ibuprofen (Advil, Motrin) or naproxen (Aleve) for pain and swelling.

- Keep the bruised area above the level of your heart when you can. (For example, if you bruise your foot, prop it up on a pillow when you are sitting or lying down.) This helps keep the swelling down.

- Rest the area so you don't hurt it more.

- If the area still hurts after 2 days, put a warm towel or heating pad on it.

# Burns

## When to Call a Doctor

- ◆ The burn is deeper than a blistering burn. (A blistering burn is a second-degree burn.)

- ◆ You have severe pain.

- ◆ You are not sure how serious the burn is.

- ◆ You have a burn worse than a mild sunburn on your face, ears, eyes, hands, feet, genitals, or a joint.

- ◆ The burn encircles an arm or leg, or it covers more than 25 percent of any body part.

- ◆ Pain from the burn lasts longer than 48 hours.

- ◆ You have signs of infection. These may include increased pain, swelling, warmth, or redness; red streaks leading from the burn; pus; and fever.

- ◆ A child younger than 5, an older adult, or a person with a weakened immune system or a chronic health problem (such as cancer, heart disease, or diabetes) is burned.

- ◆ There is a chance the burn was caused on purpose.

The degree of a burn is based on how deep it is, not on how much pain it causes.

- ◆ A **first-degree burn** involves only the outer layer of skin. The skin is dry and painful and hurts when you touch it. A mild sunburn is a first-degree burn.

- ◆ A **second-degree burn** involves several layers of skin. The skin may be swollen, puffy, weepy, or blistered.

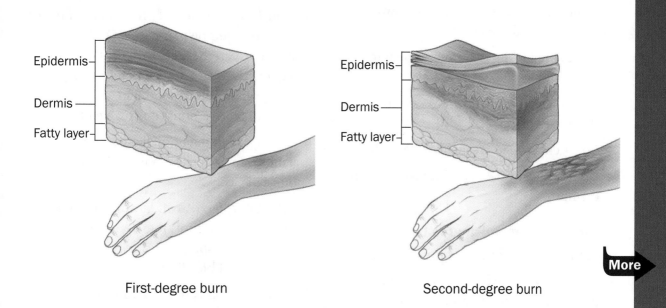

First-degree burn        Second-degree burn

**More**

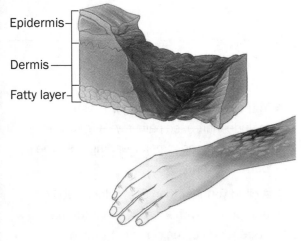

Epidermis

Dermis

Fatty layer

Third-degree burn

◆ A **third-degree burn** involves all layers of skin and may include tissue beneath the skin. The skin is dry, pale white or charred black, and swollen. It sometimes breaks open. This kind of burn destroys the nerves, so it may not hurt except on the edges.

◆ A **fourth-degree burn** extends through the skin to muscle and bone.

## Home Treatment

### For third-degree and fourth-degree burns:

These burns need medical care right away. Call a doctor, and then:

◆ Make sure the fire that caused the burn has been put out.

◆ Have the person lie down to prevent shock (see page 47).

◆ Cover the burned area with a clean sheet.

◆ Do not put any ice, salve, or medicine on the burn.

### For first- and second-degree burns:

You can treat most of these burns at home.

◆ Run cool water over the burn until the pain stops (15 to 30 minutes). Do not use ice or ice water, because it may further damage the skin.

◆ Remove rings, jewelry, or clothing from the burned limb. Swelling may make these items hard to remove later. And if they are left on, they may damage nerves or blood vessels.

◆ Clean the burn with mild soap and water.

◆ Use an antibiotic ointment such as Bacitracin, Polysporin, or Silvadene. Do not use butter, grease, or oil. They increase the risk of infection and do not help the burn heal.

◆ If the skin breaks open, use a bandage. Otherwise, don't cover the burn unless clothing rubs on it. If you need to cover the burn:

   ❖ Use a nonstick gauze pad. Make sure the tape is well away from the burn.

   ❖ Do not wrap tape all the way around a hand, arm, or leg.

   ❖ Keep the bandage clean and dry. If it gets wet, replace it.

   ❖ Remove the bandage once a day, clean the burn, and put on a new bandage.

◆ If blisters form, do not break them. If they break on their own, use water and mild soap to clean the area. Don't cut off the flap over a blister; it's a natural bandage. Apply an antibiotic ointment, and cover the burn with a nonstick gauze pad.

◆ Do not touch the burned area with your hands or any unclean objects. Burns get infected easily.

◆ Take ibuprofen (Advil, Motrin) or aceta-minophen (Tylenol) to help relieve pain. Do not take aspirin—it can increase swelling and bleeding.

◆ After 2 to 3 days, use aloe to soothe the burn.

# Chemical Burns

Burns can occur when a harmful chemical, such as a cleaning product, gasoline, or turpentine, splashes into an eye or onto the skin. Fumes can also burn the eyes, the skin, and the airways and lungs.

A burned eye may be red and watery and may be sensitive to light. If the damage is severe, the eye may look white.

Chemically burned skin may be red, blistered, or blackened. It depends on how strong the chemical was.

## Home Treatment

◆ Call Poison Control for specific advice. Have the chemical's container or label nearby.

◆ Right away, flush your eye or skin with a lot of water. Use a cold shower for skin burns. For eye burns, fill a sink or bowl with water, put your face in the water, and open and close your eyelids with your fingers to force the water to all parts of the eye. Or rinse your eye under a faucet or shower. A sink with a sprayer also works well.

◆ Keep rinsing with water for 30 minutes or until the pain stops, whichever takes longer.

# Choking

Choking is usually caused by food or an object stuck in the windpipe. A person who is choking cannot talk, cough, or breathe, and may turn gray or blue. The Heimlich maneuver can help get the food or object out.

**WARNING:** Do not try the Heimlich maneuver unless you are sure the person is choking.

## If a person older than 1 year is choking

◆ Stand behind the person, and wrap your arms around his or her waist. If the person is standing, place one of your feet between his or her legs so you can support the person if he or she faints.

◆ Make a fist with one hand. Place the thumb side of your fist against the person's belly, just above the belly button but well below the breastbone.

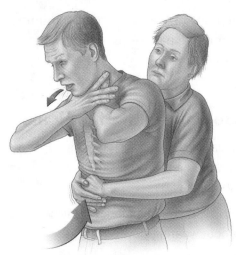

Give quick upward thrusts.

◆ Grasp your fist with your other hand. Give a quick upward thrust into the belly. This may cause the object to pop out. You may need to use more force for a large person and less for a child or small adult.

◆ Repeat thrusts until the object pops out or the person faints.

**Call 911 if the person faints. Then:**

◆ Start CPR if you know how. See page 19.

◆ Each time you open the airway during CPR, look for an object in the mouth. If you see an object, remove it.

◆ Do not do any more Heimlich thrusts.

◆ Keep doing CPR until the person is breathing on his or her own or until help arrives.

## If you are choking

If you choke while you are alone, use your fists to do thrusts on yourself. Or lean over the back of a chair and press hard to pop out the object.

## If a baby younger than 1 year is choking

◆ Put the baby facedown on your forearm so the baby's head is lower than his or her chest. Support the baby's head in your palm, against your thigh. Do not cover the baby's mouth or twist his or her neck.

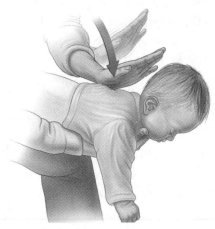

Give up to 4 firm thumps between the baby's shoulder blades.

◆ Use the heel of one hand to give up to 4 firm thumps (back blows) between the baby's shoulder blades.

◆ If the object does not pop out, support the baby's head and turn him or her faceup on your thigh. The baby's head should point toward the floor.

◆ Place two or three fingers on the lower part of the baby's breastbone, and give up to 5 upward thrusts.

◆ Look for an object in the baby's mouth. If you can see one, remove it. Then give 2 rescue breaths. To give rescue breaths:

❖ Place one hand on the baby's forehead, and tilt the baby's chin up to keep the airway open. Then place your mouth over the baby's mouth and nose and slowly blow air in until the baby's chest rises. Between breaths, remove your mouth, take a breath, and watch for the baby's chest to fall.

◆ If the object does not come out with these steps, **call 911**.

◆ Continue with back blows, chest thrusts, looking for the object, and rescue breaths until the baby coughs up the object and starts breathing on his or her own, or until help arrives.

# Cuts and Punctures

## When to Call a Doctor

**Call 911 if:**

◆ The person faints or has other signs of shock (see page 47), even if the bleeding has stopped.

◆ A large or deep cut continues to bleed through bandages after 15 minutes of direct pressure.

**Call a doctor if:**

◆ The skin near the wound is blue, white, or cold.

◆ You have numbness, tingling, or loss of feeling or movement below the wound.

◆ You have a puncture wound to the head, neck, chest, or belly, unless you are sure it is minor.

◆ You cannot remove an object from the wound, or you think part of the object may still be in the wound.

◆ A cut has removed all the layers of skin.

◆ Bleeding is under control but has not stopped after 45 minutes of direct pressure.

◆ The cut needs stitches. See page 30. Stitches usually need to be done within 6 to 8 hours.

◆ A deep puncture to the foot occurred through a shoe.

◆ A cat or human bite punctured the skin.

◆ You have not had a tetanus shot in the past 5 years or don't know when your last shot was. If you need a shot, you should get it within 2 days.

◆ You have signs of infection. These may include increased pain, swelling, warmth, or redness; red streaks leading from the wound; pus; and fever.

**More**

## Cuts

When you get a cut, the first steps are to stop the bleeding and decide whether to see a doctor. Bleeding from a minor cut will usually stop on its own or after you apply a little pressure.

If the cut is bleeding heavily or spurting blood, you need to stop the bleeding before you do anything else. Raise the area and apply firm pressure with a clean cloth for at least 15 minutes. See Stopping Severe Bleeding on page 17.

## Home Treatment

◆ Wash the cut well with soap and water. Do not use any other cleanser.

◆ If you think the cut may need stitches (on this page), see a doctor right away. If the cut does not need stitches, proceed with home treatment.

◆ Bandage the cut if it is large or in an area that may get dirty or irritated.

❖ Use antibiotic ointment, such as Bacitracin or Polysporin, to keep the cut from sticking to the bandage.

❖ Use an adhesive strip (such as a Band-Aid) to put pressure on the cut and protect it. Always put the bandage across a cut rather than lengthwise. Butterfly bandages can help hold the edges of the cut together.

❖ Replace the bandage once a day and anytime it gets wet or dirty.

## Punctures

Punctures are caused by sharp, pointed objects (nails, tacks, knives, needles, teeth) that go through the skin. Puncture wounds get infected easily because they are hard to clean and are a warm, moist place for bacteria to grow.

## Do You Need Stitches?

For best results, cuts that need stitches should get them within 6 to 8 hours. Stitches can help some cuts heal with less scarring.

After you have washed the cut and the bleeding has stopped, pinch the sides of the cut together. If it looks better that way, you may want to get stitches. If you think you need stitches, do not use an antibiotic ointment until after a doctor has looked at the cut.

If the cut does not need stitches, you can clean and bandage it at home.

You may need stitches for:

◆ Deep cuts (more than ¼ inch deep) that have jagged edges or gape open.

◆ Deep cuts on a joint, such as an elbow, knuckle, or knee.

◆ Deep cuts on the hands or fingers.

◆ Cuts on the face, eyelids, or lips.

◆ Cuts in any area where you are worried about scarring.

◆ Cuts that go down to the muscle or bone.

◆ Cuts that keep bleeding after you have applied direct pressure for 15 minutes.

## Home Treatment

◆ If the object that caused the wound is small, such as a tack or a sewing needle, remove it. Be careful not to break it off in the wound. If the object is large or caused a deep wound, leave it in place and call a doctor right away.

◆ Let the wound bleed freely for up to 5 minutes to clean itself out, unless you are losing a lot of blood or the blood is squirting out. If bleeding is heavy, raise the area and apply firm pressure for at least 15 minutes. If there is an object in the wound, press around it, not directly on it. See Stopping Severe Bleeding on page 17.

◆ Clean the wound with soap and water twice a day. Do not use any other cleansers.

◆ Put antibiotic ointment on the wound, and cover it with a nonstick bandage. Replace the bandage when you clean the wound and whenever the bandage gets wet or dirty.

◆ Watch for signs of infection. If the wound closes, an infection under the skin may be hidden for several days.

# Dehydration

## When to Call a Doctor

**Call 911** if there are signs of severe dehydration. These include:

◆ Sunken eyes, no tears, and a dry mouth and tongue.

◆ Sunken soft spot on a baby's head.

◆ Little or no urine for 8 hours.

◆ Skin that sags when you pinch it.

◆ Feeling very dizzy when you move from lying down to sitting up.

◆ Fast breathing and heartbeat.

◆ Not acting alert, or having trouble waking up.

**Call a doctor if:**

◆ You are sick to your stomach and cannot hold down even small sips of fluid.

◆ Symptoms of mild dehydration (dry mouth, dark urine, not much urine) get worse even with home treatment.

One of these topics may be helpful as well:

❖ Diarrhea, Age 11 and Younger, page 136

❖ Diarrhea, Age 12 and Older, page 138

❖ Vomiting, Age 3 and Younger, page 258

❖ Vomiting and Nausea, Age 4 and Older, page 260

Dehydration means that your body has lost too much fluid. When you stop drinking water or lose a lot of fluids through diarrhea, vomiting, sweating, or exercise, your body's cells take fluid from the blood and other tissues. Severe dehydration can be life-threatening.

**More**

*Dehydration*

Dehydration is harmful for everyone, but it is most dangerous for babies, small children, and older adults. Watch closely for its early signs anytime you have high fever, vomiting, or diarrhea. The early symptoms are:

- A dry, sticky mouth.

- Dark, yellow urine, and not much of it.

- Having no energy, or acting fussy or edgy.

## Home Treatment

### Age 12 years and up

- To stop vomiting or diarrhea, do not eat any solid foods for several hours or until you feel better. During the first 24 hours, take frequent, small sips of water or a rehydration drink.

- Once the vomiting or diarrhea is controlled, drink water, weak broth, or sports drinks a sip at a time until your stomach can handle larger amounts. Drinking too much fluid too soon can make you vomit again.

- If vomiting or diarrhea lasts longer than 24 hours, sip a rehydration drink to replace lost fluids and minerals. See page 33.

### Age 1 through 11 years

- Treat diarrhea or vomiting promptly. See Diarrhea on page 137 and Vomiting on pages 259 and 261.

- Make sure your child is drinking often. Frequent, small amounts work best.

- Give your child a rehydration drink. See page 33.

- Let your child drink as much as he or she wants. Let him or her drink extra fluids or suck on Popsicles.

- Cereals mixed with water can also help.

### Babies younger than 1 year

- Treat diarrhea or vomiting promptly. See Diarrhea on page 137 and Vomiting on page 259.

- Give your baby a rehydration drink. See page 33.

- Feed your baby more often than usual, whether you breast-feed or use a bottle.

- If your baby has started eating cereal, you may replace lost fluids with cereal.

## If You Exercise or Work in the Heat

- Drink water before, during, and after exercise or work.

- Use a sports drink if you will be working or exercising for more than an hour and will be sweating a lot.

- Don't take salt tablets. Most people already have enough salt in their diets. Use sports drinks instead.

- Avoid caffeine. It makes you urinate more often, which makes you dehydrate faster.

- Do not drink alcohol.

- Wear one layer of lightweight, light-colored clothing. Change into dry clothing if your clothes get soaked with sweat.

- If you start to feel dehydrated, stop what you are doing. Try to find a cool spot to rest in, and drink plenty of fluids.

## Rehydration Drinks

Diarrhea, vomiting, and sweating can cause you to lose large amounts of water and important minerals called electrolytes. If you are too sick to eat for a few days, you also lose nutrients.

Rehydration drinks (Pedialyte, Rehydralyte) and sports drinks (Gatorade, Powerade) replace fluids and electrolytes in amounts your body can use. These drinks won't make diarrhea or vomiting go away faster, but they will help prevent serious dehydration.

Plain water replaces fluids only and has no nutrition. If you have diarrhea, your body may not absorb the water anyway.

**For children under 12 years**, use rehydration drinks you can buy at a pharmacy or grocery store. The amount you should give depends on the child's weight. Ask your doctor for advice. Do not give sports drinks to babies and young children who are dehydrated.

**For people over 12**, you can make a cheap drink at home. Measure everything exactly. Small changes can make the drink less effective or even harmful. Mix:

◆ 1 quart water

◆ ½ teaspoon baking soda

◆ ½ teaspoon table salt *or* ¼ teaspoon salt substitute

◆ 3 to 4 tablespoons sugar

# Object in the Ear

## When to Call a Doctor

◆ You cannot remove the insect or object, or it does not fall out on its own within 24 hours.

◆ Pain, fever, swelling, bleeding, or drainage develops.

◆ You feel dizzy or have any new hearing problems.

Children sometimes place food or other small objects in their ears. A piece of cotton from a swab or cotton ball may get stuck in the ear canal. An insect may crawl into the ear.

These objects usually cause only mild symptoms, such as slight pain or strange noises in the ear. But if an object stays in the ear too long, it can lead to infection.

## Home Treatment

◆ Do not try to kill an insect in your ear. Pull the ear up and back, and let the sun or a bright light shine into it. The insect may crawl out toward the light.

◆ If the insect does not crawl out, fill the ear canal with warm mineral, olive, or baby oil. The insect may float out.

◆ To remove an object other than an insect from the ear, tilt the head to the side and shake it gently. (Never shake a baby.) Gently pulling the ear up and back may help the object fall out.

◆ If you can see the object, try to remove it gently with tweezers. Don't try this if the person will not hold very still or if the object is in the ear so far that you can't see the tips of the tweezers. Use care not to push the object farther in.

# Electrical Shocks and Burns

Sometimes when you touch a light switch or outlet, you get a small shock. It may tingle for a few minutes. But if the shock does not cause skin damage or other problems, you don't need to worry.

A shock that burns your skin is more serious. Electrical burns may look minor at first, with the damage not showing up for several days. You may have burns where the current entered and left your body.

Electricity can cause severe damage inside your body, including internal burns and heart rhythm problems. It can cause your throat and lungs to swell quickly, making it hard for you to breathe.

### For a minor burn

Rinse the burn with water, and apply a nonstick bandage.

## If someone has been electrocuted or struck by lightning

- ◆ **Call 911.**
- ◆ Do not approach the person until you are sure the area is safe. If you feel tingling in your lower body, turn around and hop to a safe place.
- ◆ Unplug or turn off the power if you can.
- ◆ If you can't turn off the power, try to remove the person from the electrical source if you can do it safely.
  - ❖ Do not touch the person with your hands until you have removed him or her from the electrical source.
  - ❖ Stand on a dry, nonmetal surface, like a rubber doormat or a pile of papers or books. Make sure you are not standing in or near water.
  - ❖ Use a dry piece of wood, like a broom handle, to push the person away from the electrical source. Do not use anything wet or made of metal.
- ◆ Once the power is off or you have removed the person from the source, check for breathing and a heartbeat. If needed (and if you know how), start rescue breathing and CPR while you wait for help to arrive. See page 19.

# Object in the Eye

## When to Call a Doctor

**Call 911** if the eyeball seems to be punctured.

**Call a doctor if:**

◆ The object is over the colored part of the eye or is stuck in the eye. Do not try to remove the object.

◆ There is blood over or in front of the colored part of the eye.

◆ You can't remove an object from the eye.

◆ You have removed the object but:

❖ The pain is severe or does not go away.

❖ It feels like there is still something in your eye.

❖ Light hurts your eye.

❖ Your vision is blurred.

Your cornea may be scratched. Keep your eye closed as often as you can until you visit the doctor.

---

A speck of dirt or a small object in the eye will often wash out with your tears. If the object does not come out, it may scratch the surface of the eye (the cornea). Most corneal scratches will heal on their own in 1 to 2 days.

If an object is thrown forcefully into the eye (from a machine, for example), it may puncture the eyeball. This needs emergency care.

Always wear safety glasses or other protective eyewear when you work with machines or tools, mow the lawn, or ride a bike or motorcycle.

## Home Treatment

◆ Wash your hands before you touch the eye.

◆ Do not rub the eye. You might scratch the cornea.

◆ Do not try to remove an object that is over the colored part of the eye or stuck in the white of the eye. Try flushing it out with water or saline.

◆ If the object is at the side of the eye or on the lower lid, moisten a cotton swab or the tip of a twisted piece of tissue and touch the end to the object. The object should cling to the swab or tissue. Your eye may be a little irritated afterward.

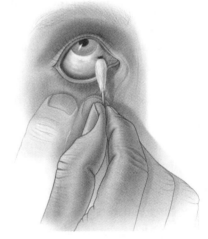

Use a moist cotton swab.

◆ Gently wash the eye with cool water. An eyedropper helps.

◆ Never use tweezers, toothpicks, or other hard items to remove an object from the eye.

# Frostbite

## When to Call a Doctor

◆ The skin is white or blue, and hard, rubbery, and cold. These are signs of severe frostbite. You need careful rewarming and antibiotics to prevent permanent tissue damage and infection.

◆ Blisters form. Do not break them. The risk of infection is very high.

◆ You have signs of infection. These may include increased pain, swelling, warmth, or redness; red streaks leading from the area; pus; and fever.

Frostbite is freezing of the skin and, if it is severe, the tissues beneath it. Frostbite is most likely to occur on the feet, hands, ears, nose, and face.

How severe the frostbite is depends on how long you were in the cold and how cold it was. Wind and damp air can make things worse.

With mild frostbite (sometimes called frostnip):

◆ The skin may be pale or red and may tingle or burn.

◆ If you rewarm the area soon, it will probably not blister or get worse.

As frostbite gets worse:

◆ The skin may feel hard, frozen, and numb. Later you may feel burning, throbbing, or shooting pain.

◆ Blisters may form as the skin warms. In severe cases, blisters may appear as small bloody spots under the skin.

◆ The tissue beneath the skin may freeze and harden.

◆ At its worst, the skin may turn dry, black, and rubbery. You may also have deep, aching joint pain.

## Home Treatment

◆ Get inside, or at least take shelter from the wind.

◆ Check for signs of hypothermia (see page 41), such as violent shivering, clumsy movement and speech, and confusion. Treat those before treating frostbite.

◆ Protect the frozen body part from further cold.

◆ To warm small areas (ears, face, nose, fingers, toes), breathe on them or tuck them inside warm clothing next to bare skin.

◆ Do not rub or massage the frozen area. This can further damage the skin and tissue beneath it. Do not walk on frostbitten feet unless you have no choice.

◆ Keep the area warm, and prop it up above the level of your heart. Wrap it with blankets or soft clothing to prevent bruising. If possible, soak it in warm water ($104°F$ to $108°F$) for 15 to 30 minutes.

◆ If blisters form, do not break them.

◆ Take ibuprofen (Advil, Motrin) or acetaminophen (Tylenol) for pain.

# Head Injury

Most bumps on the head are minor and heal as easily as bumps anywhere else.

Minor cuts on the head often bleed a lot because the blood vessels of the scalp are so close to the skin's surface. In these cases, the injury may look worse than it is. (In children, though, blood loss from a scalp injury may be enough to cause shock.)

But a head injury may also be worse than it looks. An injury that doesn't bleed on the outside may still have caused dangerous bleeding and swelling inside the skull. The more force involved in the injury, the more likely it is serious.

Anyone who has had a head injury should be watched carefully for 24 hours for signs of a serious problem.

## Home Treatment

◆ If the person is unconscious, assume he or she has a spinal injury. Do not move the person without first protecting the neck from movement. See page 49.

◆ If there is bleeding, put firm pressure directly over the wound with a clean cloth for 15 minutes. If the blood soaks through, put another cloth over the first one. See page 17.

◆ Check for injuries to other parts of the body. The panic from seeing a head injury may cause you to miss other injuries that need attention.

More

◆ Use ice or cold packs to reduce the swelling. A "goose egg" may appear anyway, but ice will help ease the pain.

◆ For the first 24 hours after a head injury, watch the person closely for signs of a severe head injury. Every 2 hours, check for the symptoms listed in When to Call a Doctor.

◆ The person should avoid contact sports until cleared by a doctor.

## Protect Children From Head Injuries

◆ Make sure all family members wear their seat belts every time they are in the car. Use child car seats. See page 333.

◆ Make sure your child wears a properly fitted helmet when biking, skating, snowboarding, riding a scooter, and doing other activities like these. Parents can set a good example by wearing helmets of their own.

◆ Teach your children never to dive into shallow or unfamiliar water.

◆ If you keep guns in your home, store them unloaded and locked up. Store and lock ammunition in a separate place.

# Heart Attack

## Signs of a Heart Attack

◆ Chest pain or pressure. This is the most common symptom. But some people—especially women, older adults, and people with diabetes—may not have chest pain during a heart attack.

◆ Sweating

◆ Shortness of breath

◆ Nausea or vomiting

◆ Pain or discomfort in the upper back, upper belly, neck, jaw, or arms

◆ Feeling dizzy or lightheaded

◆ Fast or uneven heartbeat

The symptoms of a heart attack usually last longer than 5 minutes and do not go away with rest.

## When to Call a Doctor

**Call 911** if you think you may be having a heart attack. Do not wait to see if you will feel better. After calling 911, chew and swallow one adult aspirin (unless you are allergic to it).

If an ambulance is not an option, have someone drive you to the hospital. Do not drive yourself unless you have no choice.

**Call a doctor** if you have mild chest pain that does not stop or keeps coming back, and there is no obvious cause. See Chest Pain on page 119.

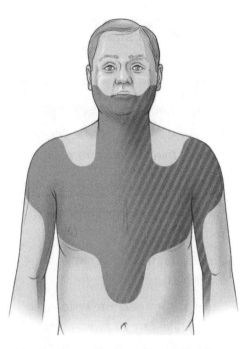

A heart attack occurs when one or more of the coronary arteries are blocked and blood cannot flow through. The coronary arteries carry blood to the heart (see the image on page 275). They can get blocked when plaque inside the artery breaks open and a blood clot forms.

Many people mistake a heart attack for another problem, such as heartburn or a pulled muscle. It is important to recognize the signals your body sends during the early stages of a heart attack and get help. Quick treatment may reduce the damage caused by a heart attack and may save your life.

A heart attack may cause discomfort in any of the shaded areas as well as the upper back.

# Heat Sickness

## When to Call a Doctor

**Call 911 if:**

◆ Body temperature reaches 102.3°F and keeps rising.

◆ A person has signs of heat stroke, such as:

❖ Confusion, fainting, or seizure.

❖ Skin that is red, hot, and dry, even in the armpits. The person may have stopped sweating or may be sweating a lot.

**Call a doctor** if you still have symptoms of heat exhaustion (headache, fatigue, dizziness, or nausea) after you have cooled off.

**Heat sickness** occurs when your body does not stay cool enough in hot temperatures.

**Heat exhaustion** usually occurs when you are sweating a lot and do not drink enough to replace lost fluids. It often happens when you are working or exercising in hot weather.

**Heat stroke** can quickly follow if you don't correct the problem. It occurs when your body cannot control its own temperature and your temperature keeps rising, often to 105°F or higher. This can lead to death.

More

| Symptoms of heat exhaustion | Symptoms of heat stroke |
|---|---|
| ◆ Sweating a lot | ◆ Sweating may be heavy or may have stopped |
| ◆ Skin is cool, moist, pale, or red | ◆ Skin is red, hot, and dry, even in the armpits |
| ◆ Fatigue, weakness, headache, dizziness, or nausea | ◆ Confusion, fainting, or seizure |

## Home Treatment

◆ Have the person stop and rest.

◆ Help the person get out of the sun to a cool spot and drink lots of cool water, a little at a time. If the person is nauseated or dizzy, have him or her lie down.

◆ Take the person's temperature. If it is over 102.3°F (or if you don't have a thermometer but think the person may have a high fever), call for help and try to lower the temperature quickly:

   ❖ Remove the person's clothing.

   ❖ Apply cool (not cold) water to the person's whole body. Then fan the person.

   ❖ Put ice packs on the groin, neck, and armpits.

   ❖ Do not put the person in an ice-water bath.

   ❖ Once the temperature is down to 102°F, take care to avoid overcooling. Stop cooling the person once body temperature is back to normal or the person's skin feels the same temperature as yours.

   ❖ Do not use aspirin or acetaminophen (Tylenol) to reduce the temperature.

◆ Watch for signs of heat stroke (confusion or unconsciousness; red, hot, dry skin).

◆ If the person stops breathing, start rescue breathing. See page 19.

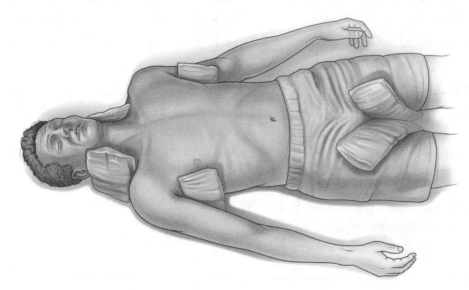

Put ice packs on the groin, neck, and armpits.

# Hypothermia

## When to Call a Doctor

**Call 911** if a person is very confused, stumbles a lot, or faints, and you suspect hypothermia.

### Call a doctor if:

◆ The person's temperature is still below 96°F after 2 hours of warming.

◆ The victim is a child or an older adult. It is a good idea to call even if the symptoms seem mild.

Hypothermia is below-normal body temperature that happens when the body loses heat faster than it can produce heat. It is an emergency that can quickly lead to death.

It does not have to be that cold for a person to get hypothermia.

◆ You can get it at temperatures of 50°F or even higher in wet and windy weather.

◆ It can happen in water that is 60°F to 70°F.

◆ Frail and inactive people can get hypothermia indoors if they are not dressed warmly enough.

Do not ignore early warning signs. Often a hiker or skier will lose a lot of heat before you notice something is wrong. If someone starts to shiver fiercely, stumble, or respond strangely to questions, suspect hypothermia and warm the person quickly.

## Home Treatment

The goal of home or "in-the-field" treatment is to stop heat loss and safely rewarm the person.

◆ Get the person out of the cold and wind.

◆ Remove cold, wet clothes first, and give the person dry or wool clothing to wear. Or, warm the person with your own body heat by wrapping a blanket or sleeping bag around both of you.

◆ Give the person warm fluids and high-energy foods, such as candy. Do not give food or drink if the person is confused or has fainted. Do not give the person alcohol or caffeine.

◆ If home treatment is not working and you cannot get help, put the person in a warm (100°F to 105°F) bath. This can cause shock or heart attack, so do it only as a last resort.

| Early warning signs | Advanced warning signs |
|---|---|
| ◆ Shivering | ◆ A cold belly |
| ◆ Cold, pale skin | ◆ Stiff, hard muscles. Shivering may stop if the person's temperature drops below 90°F. |
| ◆ Lack of interest or concern | |
| ◆ Poor judgment | ◆ Slow pulse and breathing |
| ◆ Clumsy movement and speech | ◆ Weakness or drowsiness |
| | ◆ Confusion |

More

## Stay Warm

Protect yourself whenever you plan to be out in cold weather.

◆ Dress warmly, and wear windproof, waterproof clothing. Wear fabrics that stay warm even when wet, such as wool or polypropylene.

◆ Wear a warm hat.

◆ Keep your hands and feet dry.

◆ Head for shelter if you get wet or cold.

◆ Eat well before you go out, and carry extra food.

◆ Do not drink alcohol while in the cold. It makes your body lose heat faster.

Older or less active people should keep indoor temperatures above 65°F and dress warmly.

# Object in the Nose

## When to Call a Doctor

◆ A disc battery is stuck in the nose. The moist tissue in the nose can cause the battery to release harmful chemicals, often in less than an hour.

◆ You cannot remove the object after several tries.

◆ Removing the object causes a severe nosebleed. See page 43.

Children sometimes put small objects, like beads, popcorn, or small batteries, up their noses. If the child does not tell you about it, your first clue may be a smelly, green or yellow discharge from just one nostril. The nose may also be tender and swollen.

## Home Treatment

◆ Have the child pinch the other nostril closed and try to blow the object out.

◆ If you can see the object, try to remove it with blunt-nosed tweezers. Hold the child's head still, and use care not to push the object farther in. If the child resists, do not try tweezers. Minor bleeding from the nostril is not serious.

◆ **Unless you think the object is a disc battery**, spray a nasal decongestant like Neo-Synephrine in the nostril to reduce the swelling.

# Nosebleeds

## When to Call a Doctor

◆ Your nose is still bleeding after 30 minutes of pinching it.

◆ Blood runs down the back of your throat even when you pinch your nose.

◆ Your nose looks or feels broken.

◆ You get lots of nosebleeds—four or more a week, for instance.

◆ You take blood thinners (such as warfarin or Coumadin) or high doses of aspirin and have more than one nosebleed in a day.

Most nosebleeds are not serious. You may get one because of dry air or high altitude, an injury to the nose, or medicines (especially aspirin). Blowing or picking your nose can also cause a nosebleed.

People who have allergy problems may get nosebleeds a lot because the inside of the nose is irritated. Allergy medicines may help with this, but they can make the problem worse if you use them too often. Talk to your doctor about how best to use these medicines.

## Home Treatment

◆ Sit up straight and tip your head slightly forward. Tilting your head back may cause blood to run down your throat, which may make you vomit.

◆ Blow your nose gently to remove any blood clots. Pinch your nose shut with your thumb and index finger for 10 minutes.

◆ After 10 minutes, check to see if your nose is still bleeding. If it is, pinch it shut for 10 more minutes. Most nosebleeds will stop after 10 to 30 minutes of doing this.

◆ Do not blow your nose for at least 12 hours after the bleeding has stopped.

◆ If your nose is very dry, breathe moist air for a while (such as in the shower). Then put a little petroleum jelly on the inside of your nose. A saline nasal spray may also help. See page 234.

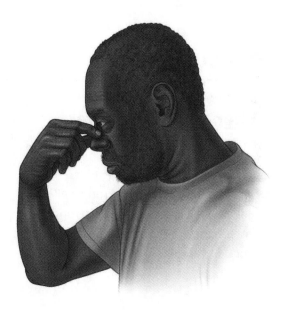

To stop a nosebleed, tip your head forward and pinch your nose shut.

# Poisoning

**Call 911 or Poison Control for any poisoning.** Have the poison's container or label nearby so you can describe it. The medical staff will tell you what to do.

Do not use syrup of ipecac or activated charcoal unless Poison Control staff tells you to.

Kids will swallow just about anything. When in doubt, assume the worst. Always believe a child who says that he or she has swallowed poison, no matter what the substance is.

## Common Household Poisons

Make sure you keep these kinds of items out of the reach of children and pets:

- Drugs and vitamins
- Makeup, nail polish, and perfumes
- Bleach, drain cleaners, and toilet bowl cleaners
- Dishwasher detergent
- Arts and crafts products like glue and paint
- Plant food and bug killer
- Some house plants
- Windshield washer fluid and antifreeze
- Batteries
- Mothballs

For more tips on how to protect your child from poisons, see page 332.

# Scrapes

## When to Call a Doctor

- The scrape is still bleeding after 30 minutes of pressure.
- You cannot clean the scrape well because it is too large, deep, or painful, or because dirt and other matter is stuck under the skin.
- You have not had a tetanus shot in the past 5 years or don't know when you last had one. If you need a shot, you should get it within 2 days.
- You have signs of infection. These may include increased pain, swelling, warmth, or redness; red streaks leading from the scrape; pus; and fever.

## Home Treatment

◆ Good home treatment may help reduce scarring and prevent infection.

◆ Scrapes are usually very dirty. Remove large pieces of dirt and gravel with tweezers. Then scrub well with soap and water and a washcloth. Scrubbing may cause some minor bleeding. Using a water sprayer from a sink is a good way to wash a scrape.

◆ Apply steady pressure with a clean cloth to stop any bleeding.

◆ Use ice or a cold pack to reduce swelling and bruising.

◆ If the scrape is large or in an area where clothing may rub on it, apply an antibiotic ointment (such as Bacitracin or Polysporin) and cover the scrape with a nonstick bandage. Change the bandage once a day and anytime it gets wet.

# Seizures

## When to Call a Doctor

If you think your child has had a fever seizure, see page 161.

### Call 911 if:

◆ A person having a seizure stops breathing for longer than 30 seconds.

◆ A seizure lasts longer than 3 minutes.

◆ More than one seizure occurs within 24 hours.

◆ A seizure occurs with any signs of stroke. These may include sudden numbness, paralysis, or weakness; new problems with walking or balance; sudden vision changes; sudden problems speaking to or understanding others; and sudden, severe headache.

◆ A seizure occurs with signs of serious illness, such as fever, severe headache, stiff neck, trouble breathing, or an unexplained rash.

◆ A seizure follows a head injury.

◆ A seizure occurs after using illegal drugs or drinking a lot of alcohol.

◆ A pregnant woman has a seizure.

◆ A person with diabetes has a seizure.

### Call a doctor if:

◆ You have a seizure and have not been diagnosed with epilepsy.

◆ You have been diagnosed with epilepsy and notice a change in your seizures.

**More**

The brain controls how the body moves by sending electrical signals through the nerves to the muscles. You can have a seizure if the normal signals from the brain change.

♦ Your whole body may stiffen or jerk violently, or you may have only slight shaking of a hand or other body part.

♦ You may briefly lose touch with your surroundings and appear to stare into space.

♦ You may or may not faint.

♦ You may not remember the seizure afterward.

A single seizure usually lasts less than 3 minutes and is not followed by a second one.

Any normally healthy person can have a single seizure under certain conditions. For instance, being hit in the head may cause a seizure. But a seizure may also be a sign of a more serious problem, so see a doctor to find the cause.

A quickly rising fever is a common cause of seizures in children. Fever seizures are scary but usually harmless. To learn more, see Fever Seizures on page 161.

## Home Treatment

No matter what causes the seizure, there are things you can do to help a person during and after a seizure.

### During a seizure:

♦ Protect the person from injury. If you can, keep him or her from falling. Try to move furniture or other objects out of the way.

♦ Don't force your fingers or anything else into the person's mouth.

♦ Don't try to hold down or move the person.

♦ Try to stay calm.

♦ Pay close attention to what the person is doing so you can describe the seizure to doctors.

♦ Time the seizure if you can.

### After a seizure:

♦ Check for injuries.

♦ Turn the person onto his or her side once he or she is more relaxed.

♦ If the person has trouble breathing, use your finger to gently clear the mouth of any vomit or saliva.

♦ Loosen tight clothing around the person's neck and waist.

♦ Provide a safe area where the person can rest.

♦ Do not give the person anything to eat or drink until he or she is fully awake and alert.

♦ Stay with the person until he or she is awake and aware of the surroundings. Most people will be sleepy or confused after a seizure.

# Shock

## When to Call a Doctor

**Call 911** if you think someone is in shock. Signs of shock include:

◆ Weakness, dizziness, and fainting.

◆ Cool, pale, clammy skin.

◆ Weak, fast pulse.

◆ Shallow, fast breathing.

◆ Low blood pressure.

◆ Extreme thirst, nausea, or vomiting.

◆ Confusion or anxiety.

Shock may develop as a result of sudden illness, injury, or bleeding. When the body cannot get enough blood to the vital organs, it goes into shock. Sometimes even a mild injury will lead to shock.

Prompt home treatment of shock can save the person's life.

## Home Treatment

◆ **Call 911.**

◆ Have the person lie down. If there is an injury to the head, neck, or chest, keep the legs flat. Otherwise, raise the person's legs at least 12 inches.

◆ If the person vomits, roll him or her to one side to let fluids drain from the mouth. Use care if there could be an injury to the back or neck. See page 49.

◆ Stop any bleeding (see page 17) and splint any broken bones (see page 52).

◆ Keep the person warm but not hot. Put a blanket under the person, and cover him or her with a sheet or blanket, depending on the weather. If the person is in a hot place, try to keep the person cool.

◆ Take the person's pulse in case medical staff on the phone need to know what it is. See page 48. Take it again if the person's condition changes.

◆ Try to keep the person calm.

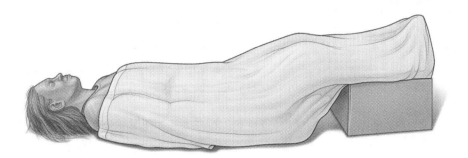

Raise the legs, and keep the person warm but not hot.

More

# Taking a Pulse

Your pulse is the rate at which your heart beats. It is measured in beats per minute.

As the heart pumps blood through the arteries to the rest of the body, you can feel a throbbing wherever the arteries come close to the skin's surface. Most of the time, you can take a pulse at the wrist, neck, or groin.

◆ Place two fingers gently against the wrist to find the heartbeat. Do not use your thumb. Or find the heartbeat in the neck, on either side of the windpipe. Press gently with two fingers.

◆ Count the beats for 30 seconds. Then double the result to know beats per minute.

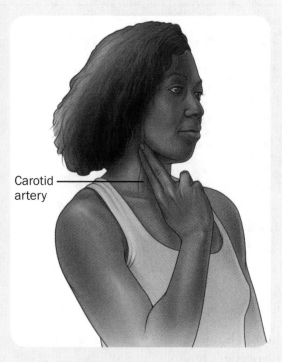

Carotid artery

Taking a pulse at the neck

### Resting pulse

To get a resting pulse, take the pulse after you have been resting quietly for at least 10 minutes. Certain illnesses can raise your pulse, so it helps to know what your resting pulse rate is when you are well. The pulse rate rises about 10 beats per minute for every degree of fever.

Normal resting pulse:

◆ Up to age 12 months: 100–160 beats/minute

◆ 1 to 6 years: 65–140 beats/minute

◆ 7 to 10 years: 60–110 beats/minute

◆ 11 years and up: 50–100 beats/minute

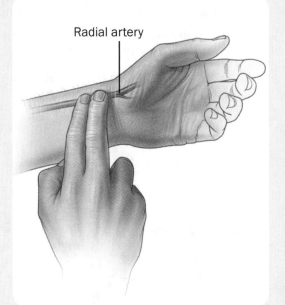

Radial artery

Taking a pulse at the wrist

# Spinal Injury

Any accident, injury, or fall that affects the back or neck can damage the spine. It is important to keep the spine from moving and transport the person the right way to prevent permanent loss of movement and feeling (paralysis).

If you suspect a spinal injury:

◆ Do not move the person unless there is an immediate threat to life, such as fire. Do not drag victims from car accidents unless you have no choice.

◆ If you must move the person to safety, try to move the head, neck, and shoulders together as a unit.

◆ If the person was hurt in a diving accident, do not pull him or her from the water. Float the person faceup in the water until help arrives. The water will act as a splint and keep the person's spine from moving.

# Splinters

## Home Treatment

To remove a splinter:

◆ Try Scotch tape first. Put a piece of tape over the splinter, and pull it up.

◆ If that doesn't work, grip the end of the splinter with tweezers, and try to gently pull it out.

◆ If the splinter is not sticking out where you can reach it, clean a needle with alcohol and make a small hole in the skin over the end of the splinter. Then lift the splinter with the tip of the needle until you can grab it with the tweezers.

◆ After you have removed the splinter, wash the area with soap and water. Use a bandage if the wound is in an area that might get dirty. Otherwise, leave the wound open to the air.

# Strains, Sprains, and Broken Bones

## When to Call a Doctor

◆ A bone is poking through the skin.

◆ The hurt limb or joint looks odd, is a strange shape, or is out of its normal position.

◆ The skin over the site of an injury is broken.

◆ You have signs of nerve or blood vessel damage, such as:

❖ Numbness, tingling, or a pins-and-needles feeling.

❖ Skin that is pale, white, or blue, or feels colder than the skin on the limb that is not hurt.

❖ Not being able to move the limb normally because of weakness, not just pain.

◆ You cannot bear weight on or straighten a hurt limb, or a joint wobbles or feels unstable.

◆ You have severe pain.

◆ You have a lot of swelling within 30 minutes of the injury.

◆ Swelling and pain do not improve after 2 days of home treatment.

◆ You have signs of infection after an injury. These may include increased pain, swelling, warmth, and redness; red streaks leading from the area; and fever.

A **strain** is caused by overstretching or tearing a muscle or tendon. Tendons connect muscle and bone.

A **sprain** is an injury to the ligaments or soft tissues around a joint. Ligaments connect one bone to another.

A broken bone is called a **fracture**.

A **dislocation** occurs when one end of a bone is pulled or pushed out of its normal position.

All of these injuries cause pain and swelling. Unless a broken bone is obvious, it may be hard to tell whether you have a strain, sprain, break, or dislocation. Rapid swelling often means you have a more serious injury.

## Stress Fractures

A stress fracture is a weak spot or small crack in a bone caused by overuse. For example, stress fractures in the small bones of the foot may occur during heavy training for basketball, running, and other sports.

The usual sign of a stress fracture is pain in one spot that keeps coming back or will not go away. The pain may get better while you exercise but will be worse before and after activity. There may not be any swelling you can see.

Stress fractures need 2 to 4 months of rest to heal.

You can treat most minor strains and sprains at home. Bad sprains, broken bones, and dislocations need medical care. Do home treatment while you wait to see your doctor.

## Home Treatment

The first steps in home treatment are usually the same no matter what the injury. They are known as "RICE," which stands for rest, ice, compression, and elevation. Start the RICE process right away.

### 1. Rest (**R**ICE)

◆ Do not put weight on the injury for at least 24 to 48 hours.

◆ Use crutches for a badly sprained knee or ankle.

◆ Support a sprained wrist, elbow, or shoulder with a sling. See page 52.

◆ Rest a sprained finger by taping it to the healthy finger next to it. This works for toes too. Always put padding between the two fingers or toes that you tape together. See page 52.

### 2. Ice (R**I**CE)

◆ Put ice or cold packs on the injury right away to reduce pain and swelling and help it heal. For the first 48 to 72 hours, use ice for 10 to 15 minutes at a time once an hour (or as often as you can).

For hard-to-reach injuries, a cold pack or a bag of frozen vegetables works better than ice. See Ice and Cold Packs on page 243.

◆ Heat feels nice, but it does more harm than good if you use it too soon. You may use heat (warm towel, heating pad) after 48 to 72 hours of cold treatments if the swelling is gone. Some experts say to switch back and forth between heat and cold.

### 3. Compression (RI**C**E)

◆ Wrap the injured area with an elastic (Ace) bandage or compression sleeve to reduce swelling. Do not wrap it too tightly. If the area below it feels numb, tingles, or feels cool, loosen the wrap.

◆ A tightly wrapped sprain may fool you into thinking you can keep using the joint. With or without a wrap, the joint needs total rest for 1 to 2 days.

### 4. Elevation (RIC**E**)

◆ Prop up the injured area on pillows whenever you use ice and anytime you are sitting or lying down.

◆ Try to keep the injury at or above the level of your heart to help reduce swelling and bruising.

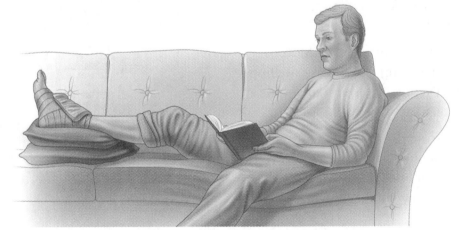

RICE: Rest, ice, compress (wrap), and elevate

**More** ➤

## Other Tips

You may prevent further damage and feel better faster if you follow these tips after you get hurt:

◆ Splint an arm, leg, finger, or toe that you think is broken until you can see your doctor. See Splinting on this page. You can also use a sling to protect an injured arm or shoulder until you see a doctor. Do not put an arm sling on a baby.

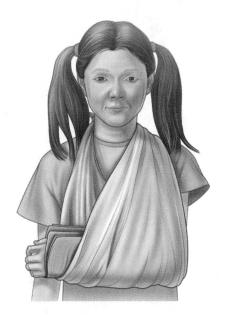

A homemade sling can protect an injured arm until you see a doctor.

◆ Remove all rings, watches, and bracelets from a hurt finger or hand right away. Swelling may make it hard to remove these items later.

◆ Take aspirin, ibuprofen (Advil, Motrin), or naproxen (Aleve) to help ease swelling and pain. Do not give aspirin to anyone younger than 20.

◆ Start gentle exercise as soon as the initial pain and swelling have gone away. If you have a broken bone or a severe sprain, your doctor may put the limb in a cast.

# Splinting

**These splinting methods are for short-term first aid only. Your doctor will give you a splint or cast that is right for your injury.**

If you think a bone is broken, you can splint it so that it doesn't move. This prevents further injury until you can see a doctor. Splinting may also help after a snakebite while you wait for help to arrive.

There are two ways to splint a limb:

**Method 1:** Tie the injured limb to a stiff object, such as rolled-up newspapers or magazines, a stick, or a cane. You can use a rope, a belt, or anything else that will work as a tie. Do not tie too tightly. Place the splint so the hurt limb cannot bend. Try to splint from a joint above the suspected break to a joint below it. For example, splint a broken forearm from above the elbow to below the wrist.

**Method 2:** Tape a broken finger or toe to the next finger or toe, with padding between them. Tie a hurt arm across the chest to keep it from moving.

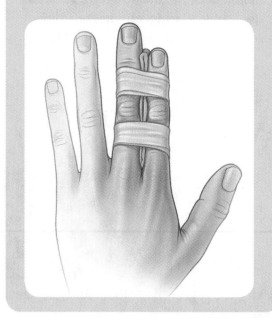

# Stroke

## Signs of Stroke

- New weakness, numbness, or loss of movement in your face, arm, or leg, especially on only one side of your body.

- Sudden blurred or decreased vision that does not clear when you blink.

- Trouble speaking or understanding simple statements.

- Sudden, severe headache that is different from any past headache.

- Severe dizziness, loss of balance, or loss of coordination, especially if another warning sign is present at the same time.

## When to Call a Doctor

**Call 911** if you think you may be having a stroke. If an ambulance is not an option, have someone drive you to the hospital. Do not drive yourself unless you have no choice.

**Call a doctor** if symptoms were definitely there and then went away after a few minutes. This could be a sign that a stroke may soon occur.

A stroke occurs when a blood vessel to the brain bursts or is blocked by a blood clot. Within minutes, the nerve cells in that part of the brain die. As a result, the part of the body controlled by those cells cannot work properly.

The effects of a stroke may range from mild to severe. They may get better, or they may last the rest of your life. A stroke can affect vision, speech, behavior, thought processes, and your ability to move. Sometimes it can cause a coma or death.

Get help as soon as you notice stroke symptoms. Quick treatment may reduce the damage in your brain so that you have fewer problems after the stroke.

## What's a TIA?

TIAs—transient ischemic attacks—are often called "mini-strokes" because their symptoms are like those of a stroke. The difference is that TIA symptoms usually go away within 10 to 20 minutes. (Rarely, they may last up to 24 hours.)

A TIA is a warning that you may soon have a stroke. It can occur months before a stroke occurs. You may have one or more TIAs before you finally have a stroke.

# Suicide

## When to Call a Doctor

**Call 911** if you or someone you know is about to attempt or is attempting suicide.

**Call a doctor, your local suicide hotline, or the national suicide hotline** at 1-800-784-2433 (1-800-SUICIDE) if:

◆ You are thinking about suicide.

◆ You think or know that someone has made suicide plans.

If you are very depressed or feel hopeless, you may sometimes think of taking your own life. Occasional, fleeting thoughts of death are normal. But if thoughts of suicide continue, or if you have made suicide plans, you need help today.

People who are thinking about suicide are often unsure whether they want to live or die. With help and compassion, they may choose to live.

## Warning Signs of Suicide

◆ Saying that you are going to kill yourself. Most people who commit suicide tell someone about it.

◆ Past suicide attempt. Failed attempts are often followed by a completed attempt.

◆ Giving away your favorite things.

◆ Being preoccupied or obsessed with death. A suicidal person may talk, read, draw, or write about death.

◆ Feeling depressed and socially isolated. A suicidal person may stop seeing or calling friends and stop doing his or her normal activities.

## Home Treatment

### For yourself

◆ Do not use alcohol or illegal drugs. They may make you more likely to do things you would not do when sober.

◆ Talk about your thoughts with someone you trust—a friend or family member, a clergy member, or a doctor. Or call a suicide hotline.

◆ If you think you are in a moment of crisis, ask someone you trust to stay with you until the crisis has passed or until you can get help.

### If you are worried about someone else

◆ Do not ignore warning signs, thinking that the person will "snap out of it."

◆ Talk about the problem as openly as you can. Show understanding and compassion. Do not argue with or challenge the person.

◆ Encourage the person to get professional help today. Do what you can to make it happen. Help the person set up the appointment, and make sure the person has a way to get there. Follow up to find out how the treatment is going.

◆ Use common sense and a direct approach to find out if the suicide risk is high. Ask the person:
  ❖ Do you feel there is no other way?
  ❖ Do you have a suicide plan?
  ❖ How and when do you plan to do it?

◆ If you think the risk is high, do not leave. Stay with the person until the crisis has passed or until you can get help.

# Sunburn

## When to Call a Doctor

**Call 911** if you have signs of heat stroke, such as confusion, fainting, or skin that is red, hot, and dry.

**Call a doctor if:**

◆ You have symptoms of heat exhaustion (dizziness, nausea, headache) even though you have cooled off.

◆ Symptoms of mild dehydration (dry mouth, dark urine, not much urine) get worse even with home treatment.

◆ You have severe blistering (more than half of the affected body part).

◆ You have severe pain with fever, or you feel very sick.

◆ You have a fever of 102°F or higher.

A sunburn is usually a minor (first-degree) burn to the skin's outer surface. Unless a sunburn is severe, it's usually something you can treat at home. Bad sunburns can be serious in babies, small children, and older adults.

## Home Treatment

◆ Drink plenty of water, and watch for signs of dehydration (especially in babies or children). See page 31. Also watch for signs of heat sickness. See page 39.

◆ Take a cool bath or use a cool, wet cloth to soothe the skin. Take acetaminophen (Tylenol) or aspirin for pain or mild fever. Do not give aspirin to anyone younger than 20.

◆ Use a moisturizing lotion to help with itching. There is nothing you can do to prevent peeling. It's part of the healing process.

**More**

55

## Don't Get Sunburned

Anytime you are going to be outdoors for more than 15 minutes:

◆ Wear light-colored, loose-fitting, long-sleeved clothes, and a broad-brimmed hat to shade your face. Wear sunglasses that have UV protection. Look for clothing with UV protection.

◆ Use a sunscreen with SPF 15 or higher. (Older adults should use a sunscreen with SPF 30 or higher.) Use one labeled "broad spectrum."

❖ Apply sunscreen at least 30 minutes before you will be in the sun.

❖ Put sunscreen on all skin that will be exposed, including the nose, ears, neck, scalp, and lips.

❖ Reapply sunscreen at least every 2 to 3 hours, and more often if you are swimming or sweating a lot.

◆ Avoid the sun between 10 a.m. and 4 p.m., when the burning rays are strongest. Seek shade whenever you can.

**For Your Kids**

The sun can be very hard on a child's tender skin. And repeated sunburns increase the risk for skin cancer later in life (see page 235).

◆ Teach your children safe sun habits early. Have them wear hats and sunscreen.

◆ Use a sunscreen with SPF 30 or higher on babies and children.

◆ Keep babies younger than 6 months out of the sun.

# Tooth Injury

## When to Call a Dentist

◆ You knock out a permanent tooth. The dentist may be able to reimplant it. This works best within 30 minutes of the injury. (After 2 hours, it probably won't work.) Pick up the tooth at its top, not by the root. Place the tooth in a small container of milk to take to your dentist. Use tap water if you don't have milk.

◆ You chip a permanent tooth. A blow that was hard enough to chip a tooth may have moved several teeth out of place or broken the bone that holds the tooth in place. Also, a chipped tooth can be repaired.

◆ A baby tooth gets knocked out. Make an appointment within 2 weeks. Baby teeth need to come out anyway, but your child may need a spacer until the permanent tooth comes in.

# Unconsciousness

## When to Call a Doctor

**Call 911** if a person is unconscious for more than a few seconds.

**Call a doctor if:**

◆ There is any bleeding from the rectum or in the stools, blood in the urine, or unexpected vaginal bleeding.

◆ A person faints for a second or two and is now awake.

◆ A person faints for a second or two after a head injury and is now awake. Also see Head Injury on page 37.

◆ A person with diabetes faints, even if he or she is now awake. This could be a low or high blood sugar emergency.

◆ Fainting has occurred more than once.

A person who is unconscious is completely unaware of what's going on and cannot make purposeful movements.

When you faint, you lose consciousness briefly—usually only a few seconds. This is most often caused by a brief drop in blood flow to the brain. When you fall or lie down, blood flow improves and you "wake up." Stress or injury can also make you faint.

Fainting is usually not a cause for concern. But if it happens often, there may be a problem.

Staying unconscious for more than a few seconds usually is a sign of a serious problem. There are many reasons why this might happen. These include stroke, epilepsy, very low or very high blood sugar, head injury, not being able to breathe, alcohol or drug overdose, shock, bleeding, heartbeat problems, and heart attack.

## Home Treatment

◆ Make sure the person can breathe. If the person is not breathing, start rescue breathing. See page 19. If the person does not respond to rescue breaths, call for help, and start CPR.

◆ Lay the person on his or her side.

◆ Look for a medical alert bracelet, necklace, or card that says the person has a problem like epilepsy, diabetes, or a drug allergy.

◆ Treat any injuries.

◆ Do not give the person anything to eat or drink.

# Common Health Problems

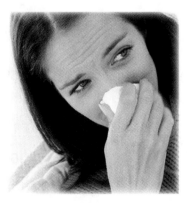
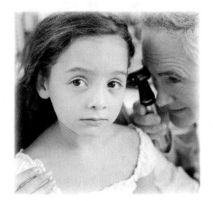
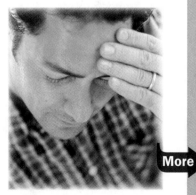

More

# Symptom Guides

Look on the left side of the chart to find the symptoms that most closely match yours. Then look on the right to see examples of what can cause those symptoms and where to go to learn more. The charts do not include all possible causes for each symptom.

| Skin Problems | |
|---|---|
| **Symptoms** | **Possible Causes** |
| Raised, red, itchy welts or fluid-filled bumps after an insect bite or taking a drug | Allergy, p. 76 <br> Hives, p. 194 <br> Insect or spider bite, p. 14 |
| Red, painful, swollen bump under the skin | Boils, p. 102 |
| Red, flaky, itchy skin | Dry skin, p. 142 <br> Atopic dermatitis, p. 83 <br> Fungal infection, p. 169 <br> Psoriasis, p. 224 <br> Also see Rashes, p. 225. |
| Crusty, honey-colored rash, most often between the nose and upper lip | Impetigo, p. 195 |
| Rash that develops after wearing new jewelry or clothing, being exposed to poisonous plants, eating a new food, or taking a new drug | Allergy, p. 76 <br> Also see Rashes, p. 225. |
| Red, itchy, blistered rash | Poison ivy, oak, or sumac, p. 226 <br> Chickenpox, p. 121 |
| Painful blisters in a band around one side of the body | Shingles, p. 122 |
| Change in the shape, size, or color of a mole, or a persistently irritated mole; a sore that does not heal | Skin cancer, p. 235 |
| Cracked, blistered, itchy, peeling skin between the toes | Athlete's foot (see Fungal Infections, p. 169) |
| Red, itchy, weeping rash on the groin or thighs | Jock itch (see Fungal Infections, p. 169) |
| Scaly, itchy, bald spots or sores on the scalp | Ringworm (see Fungal Infections, p. 169) <br> Also see Hair Loss, p. 174. |
| Flaky, silvery patches of skin, especially on the knees, elbows, or scalp | Psoriasis, p. 224 |
| Sandpapery skin rash with sore throat and a "raspberry" tongue | Scarlet fever (see Sore Throat, p. 239) |
| Sores on the lip or in the mouth | Canker sores, p. 115 <br> Cold sores, p. 123 |

## Headaches

| If Headache Occurs: | Possible Causes |
|---|---|
| Suddenly (like an explosion), and is very severe | Bleeding in the brain. **This may be an emergency.** |
| Right when you wake up | Tension headache, p. 176<br>Allergies, p. 76<br>Sinusitis, p. 232<br>Neck pain, p. 211<br>TM disorder, p. 199 |
| In jaw area or in both temples | TM disorder, p. 199<br>Tension headache, p. 176 |
| Each afternoon or evening; after hours of desk work; with sore neck and shoulders | Tension headache, p. 176<br>Neck pain, p. 211 |
| On one side of the head, with vision problems or runny nose | Migraine headache, p. 177<br>Cluster headache, p. 178 |
| After a blow to the head | Head injury, p. 37 |
| After exposure to chemicals (paint, varnish, insect spray, smoke) | Chemical headache. Get into fresh air. Drink water to flush poisons. Call a doctor if headache does not get better. |
| With fever, runny nose, or sore throat | Flu, p. 165<br>Sore throat, p. 239<br>Cold, p. 124<br>Sinusitis, p. 232 |
| With fever, stiff neck, nausea, and vomiting | Encephalitis or meningitis, p. 161 |
| With runny nose, watery eyes, and sneezing | Allergies, p. 76 |
| With fever and pain in the cheekbones or over the eyes | Sinusitis, p. 232 |
| When you drink less caffeine than usual | Caffeine withdrawal. Cut back slowly. See p. 177. |
| After a stressful event | Tension headache, p. 176 |
| At the same time during the menstrual cycle | Premenstrual syndrome, p. 219<br>Migraine headache, p. 177 |
| With new medicine | Drug allergy. Call your doctor. |
| With severe eye pain | Acute closed-angle glaucoma, p. 172. **This may be an emergency.** |
| With dizziness and vomiting, and everyone in the household feels the same | Carbon monoxide poisoning. **This may be an emergency.** |

## Eye and Vision Problems

| Symptoms | Possible Causes |
|---|---|
| Sudden vision loss that does not clear | Stroke, p. 53<br>Closed-angle glaucoma, p. 172<br>**You may need urgent care.** |
| Sudden onset of severe eye pain, blurred vision, reddened eyeball, or halos around lights | Object in the eye, p. 35<br>Chemical burn, p. 27<br>Closed-angle glaucoma, p. 172<br>**You may need urgent care.** |
| Sudden increase in floaters (dark spots, specks, or lines); new flashes of light that do not go away; shadow or "curtain" across your field of vision | Retinal detachment. **You may need urgent care.** (If you have had a few floaters or flashes for a while, mention it at your next eye exam.) |
| Red, itchy, watery eyes | Allergies, p. 76. Think about allergy to eye care products, makeup, or smoke.<br>Contact lens problem, p. 154 |
| Discharge or crust from eye; red, swollen eyelids; sandy feeling | Pinkeye, p. 151<br>Contact lens problem, p. 154<br>Blepharitis (eyelid inflammation) |
| Pimple or swelling on eyelid | Stye, p. 244 |
| Pain in the eye | Object in the eye, p. 35<br>Contact lens problem, p. 154<br>Pinkeye, p. 151<br>Chemicals or fumes, p. 27<br>Migraine or cluster headache, p. 177<br>Sinusitis, p. 232 |
| Red spot or blood on white of eye | Blood in the eye, p. 154 |
| Dry, scratchy eyes | Dry eyes, p. 153<br>Allergies, p. 76 |
| Eye twitches | Stress or fatigue. Call a doctor if twitching affects other face muscles or lasts longer than a week. |
| Black eye | Bruises, p. 24. |
| Gradual loss of side vision; tunnel vision | Glaucoma, p. 172 |
| Gradual onset of cloudy, filmy, or fuzzy vision or halos around lights | Cataract, p. 118 |

## Ear and Hearing Problems

| Symptoms | Possible Causes |
|---|---|
| Earache and fever; pulling at ears by babies and small children, especially with constant crying | Ear infection, p. 143<br>Object in the ear, p. 33 |
| Pain when you chew; headache | TM disorder, p. 199 |
| Pain when you wiggle your ear or chew; itching or burning in ear | Swimmer's ear, p. 143 |
| Discharge from ear | Swimmer's ear, p. 143<br>Eardrum rupture, p. 144 |
| Feeling of fullness in ear, with runny or stuffy nose, cough, fever | Cold, p. 124<br>Ear infection, p. 143 |
| Feeling of something moving or "bumping around" in ear | Object in the ear, p. 33 |
| Hearing loss; not paying attention | Hearing loss, p. 180<br>Earwax, p. 147<br>Fluid in the ear, p. 145 |
| Ringing or noise in the ears | Tinnitus, p. 181 |

## Nose and Throat Problems

| Symptoms | Possible Causes |
|---|---|
| Stuffy or runny nose with watery eyes, sneezing | Allergies, p. 76<br>Cold, p. 124 |
| Cold symptoms with fever, headache, severe body aches, fatigue | Flu, p. 165 |
| Thick green, yellow, or gray nasal discharge with fever and facial pain | Sinusitis, p. 232 |
| Bloody nose | See Nosebleeds, p. 43. |
| Foul odor from nose; swollen, painful nasal tissue | Object in the nose, p. 42<br>Sinusitis, p. 232 |
| Sore throat | See Sore Throat, p. 239. |
| Sore throat with white spots on tonsils, swollen lymph nodes, fever of 101°F or higher | Strep throat, p. 240 |
| Swollen tonsils, sore throat, fever | Tonsillitis, p. 239 |
| Swollen lymph nodes in the neck | See Swollen Lymph Nodes, p. 245.<br>Tonsillitis, p. 239 |
| Hoarseness, loss of voice | Laryngitis, p. 203 |

# Chest, Heart, and Lung Problems

| Symptoms | Possible Causes |
| --- | --- |
| Wheezing or fast, shallow, or troubled breathing | Allergies, p. 76<br>Asthma, p. 266<br>Bronchitis, p. 108<br>COPD, p. 271<br>Also see Breathing Problems, p. 107. |
| Cough, fever, yellow-green or rust-colored sputum, and trouble breathing | Bronchitis, p. 108<br>Pneumonia, p. 216 |
| Chest pain or pressure with sweating or quick pulse | **Call 911**. Possible heart attack. See p. 38.<br>Also see Chest Pain, p. 119. |
| Shortness of breath and coughing | Asthma, p. 266<br>Bronchitis, p. 108<br>COPD, p. 271<br>Heart failure, p. 291<br>Also see Breathing Problems, p. 107. |
| Burning, pain, or discomfort behind or below the breastbone | Heartburn, p. 183<br>Also see Chest Pain, p. 119. |
| Coughing | See Cough, p. 132. |
| Pounding or racing heartbeat; heart skipping or missing a beat | Heart palpitations, p. 181<br>Anxiety, p. 80 |
| Chest pain when you cough or breathe deeply | Pneumonia, p. 216<br>Pleurisy<br>Also see Chest Pain, p. 119. |
| Pain when you press on the chest | Strained chest muscles, p. 121<br>Costochondritis, p. 121<br>Also see Chest Pain, p. 119. |

# Digestive Problems

| Symptoms | Possible Causes |
|---|---|
| Belly pain (may be in a certain spot or all over) | See Abdominal Pain, p. 68. |
| Increasing pain in the lower right belly, with fever, nausea, and vomiting | Appendicitis, p. 69<br>Also see Abdominal Pain, p. 68.<br>**You may need urgent care.** |
| Feeling sick to your stomach; vomiting (throwing up) | Vomiting and nausea, p. 260<br>Drug reaction<br>Food poisoning, p. 167 |
| Frequent, watery stools | Diarrhea, p. 138<br>Food poisoning, p. 167<br>Irritable bowel syndrome, p. 197 |
| Stools are dry and hard to pass | Constipation, p. 130<br>Irritable bowel syndrome, p. 197 |
| Bloody or black, tarry stools | Ulcer, p. 249<br>Diarrhea, p. 138<br>Rectal problem, p. 187<br>**Also see Bleeding Emergencies, p. 17.** |
| Pain during bowel movements; bright red blood on surface of stool or on toilet paper | Hemorrhoids or other rectal problem, p. 187<br>Constipation, p. 130 |
| Painless lump or swelling in groin that comes and goes | Hernia, p. 189 |
| Burning or discomfort behind or below breastbone or in upper belly | Heartburn, p. 183<br>Ulcer, p. 249<br>Also see Chest Pain, p. 119. |
| Bloating and gas with diarrhea, constipation, or both | Irritable bowel syndrome, p. 197 |
| Women only: Lower belly cramps, bloating, diarrhea or constipation just before or during menstrual period | Menstrual cramps, p. 209<br>Also see Abdominal Pain, p. 68. |

## Urinary Problems

| Symptoms | Possible Causes |
| --- | --- |
| Pain or burning when you urinate | Urinary tract infection, p. 251<br>Prostatitis, p. 223<br>Sexually transmitted disease, p. 229<br>Kidney stone, p. 200 |
| Trouble urinating or weak urine stream (males) | Prostate enlargement, p. 222<br>Prostatitis, p. 223 |
| Leaking urine or loss of bladder control | Bladder control problem, p. 100<br>Prostate enlargement, p. 222<br>Prostatitis, p. 223 |
| Blood in urine<br>(Eating beets, blackberries, or foods with red food coloring can briefly turn your urine pink or red. Some medicines can also change the urine's color.) | Urinary tract infection, p. 251<br>Kidney stone, p. 200<br>Groin injury<br>Very hard exercise (such as running a marathon) |

# Abdominal Pain

## When to Call a Doctor

Bellyaches are very common and not often serious. Use the guide below to help you decide when you need to spend your time and money on a doctor visit and when you can take care of the problem yourself.

**Call 911 if:**

◆ You have belly pain and you faint.

◆ You have pain in your upper belly with chest pain or pressure, especially if it occurs with any other symptoms of a heart attack. See page 38.

◆ You have severe pain after a blow or injury to the belly. See page 12.

**Call your doctor if:**

◆ You have new, severe belly pain for several hours or more.

◆ You have steady or increasing pain in just one area of your belly for more than 4 hours.

◆ You have pain throughout the belly or cramping pain that has lasted longer than 24 hours and is not getting better.

◆ You are dehydrated and cannot keep down fluids. See page 31.

◆ Pain gets worse when you move or cough and does not feel like a pulled muscle.

◆ Any new belly pain lasts longer than 3 days.

If you did not find your symptoms here, check the index or the Digestive Problems chart on page 66.

Abdominal pain—pain in the belly—is very common. You can get clues about the cause of pain and how serious the problem may be by asking:

◆ **How bad is the pain?** People usually need to see a doctor when severe belly pain comes on suddenly and continues, or when new or different pain gets worse over several hours or days.

◆ **Does it hurt all over or just in one spot?**

❖ When your belly hurts all over and you cannot point to a specific spot that hurts, there is usually no reason to worry. This type of pain is very common and will usually go away on its own. Heartburn, stomach flu, food poisoning, and other common illnesses can cause this type of bellyache.

❖ When your belly hurts in just one spot, it can be a sign of a more serious problem. This is especially true if the pain is bad, starts suddenly and does not go away, or gets worse when you move or cough. It may be a sign of a problem such as appendicitis, pancreatitis, diverticulitis, an ovarian cyst, or gallbladder disease.

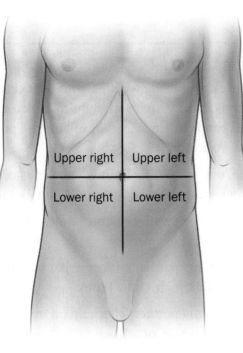

Upper right | Upper left
Lower right | Lower left

If you have belly pain, your doctor may ask you where it hurts. Lower right? Upper left? All over?

## Home Treatment

Most of the time, belly pain goes away on its own. The best home treatment may depend on what other symptoms you have, such as diarrhea or vomiting. Be sure to review the home treatment for any other symptoms you have. Use the index to find what you need, or check the Digestive Problems chart on page 66.

If you have mild belly pain without other symptoms, these tips might help:

◆ Rest until you feel better.

◆ Drink plenty of fluids to avoid dehydration (see page 31). Taking many small sips may be easier on your stomach than drinking a lot at once.

◆ Do not eat solid foods until the pain starts to go away. Then try several small meals instead of two or three large ones. Eat mild foods, such as rice, dry toast, crackers, bananas, and applesauce. Avoid spicy foods, alcohol, caffeine, and fruits other than bananas until 48 hours after all symptoms have gone away.

## Appendicitis

The appendix is a small sac attached to the large intestine. (See the picture on page 171.) If the appendix gets blocked, it can swell and get infected. This is called appendicitis.

Symptoms include:

◆ Pain that begins around the belly button or a little higher and then gets worse and moves to the lower right part of your belly. (See the picture on this page.) The pain is steady and gets worse when you walk or cough.

◆ Loss of appetite, nausea, vomiting, and constipation.

◆ Fever and chills.

◆ A hard, swollen belly.

Call your doctor if you have these symptoms. You may need to have your appendix taken out right away. If not, it could burst and spread infection all through your belly.

# Abuse and Violence

## When to Call a Doctor

**Call 911 if:**

◆ You or someone you know is in danger right now.

◆ You or someone in your family has just been physically or sexually abused or has been the victim of violence. Abuse is a crime no matter who does it.

**Call a counselor or doctor if:**

◆ You are worried about violence or abuse in your own relationship or that of a family member or friend.

◆ You need help controlling your anger, or someone in your family needs help. Also see Anger and Hostility on page 79.

◆ You suspect abuse, neglect, or maltreatment of a child, or a child reports this kind of treatment to you. You may also call local child protective services or the police.

Anger and disagreement are normal parts of healthy relationships. Threats and violence are not normal or healthy.

Abuse is an all-too-common problem. It often starts with threats, name-calling, and slamming doors or breaking dishes. It then gets worse with pushing, hitting, and other violent acts. Every year thousands of people are hurt or killed by their partners, spouses, or other family members.

## Signs of Abuse

If you are not sure whether your relationship is abusive, there are signs to look for. This can be the first step in solving the problem. Ask yourself:

◆ Does my partner limit where I can go, what I can do, and whom I can talk to?

◆ Does my partner call me names or tell me that I'm crazy?

◆ Does my partner criticize what I do and say, or criticize how I look?

◆ Does my partner "check up on me" at work, home, or school?

◆ Does my partner hit, shove, slap, kick, punch, or choke me?

◆ Does my partner blame me for the abuse he or she commits?

◆ Does my partner force me to have sex?

◆ Does my partner hurt my pets or destroy things that are special to me?

◆ Does my partner threaten to hurt or kill me?

If you answered yes to any of these questions, or if your partner could answer yes, you may be in an abusive relationship.

## What You Can Do

Physical, verbal, or sexual abuse is never acceptable. There is no excuse for it. No one deserves to be abused.

◆ Know that there are people who can help you—friends, family, neighbors, police, health professionals, social workers, clergy. Talk to someone you trust. Do not feel that you have to hide what's going on. Everyone has the right to be in a safe relationship.

◆ Be alert to warning signs, such as threats or heavy drinking. This may help you avoid danger.

◆ If you can, make sure there are no guns or weapons in the house.

◆ Have a plan for how to leave your house and where to stay in case of an emergency. Put some money aside if you can, or at least make sure you will be able to get to your money after you leave. Do not tell the person who has been abusing you about your plan. Your local YMCA, YWCA, police, hospital, or clinic can tell you about shelters and safe homes near you. Or call the National Domestic Violence Hotline toll-free at 1-800-799-7233.

## Preventing Violence Starts at Home

Violence is a learned behavior. It's important to teach your children that violence is not a healthy solution to conflict. Disagreeing is fine. Verbal or physical abuse is not.

Help your children learn that it's not okay to hurt people or to let other people hurt them. And model that behavior yourself. Try discipline techniques such as the "time-out" method that don't involve spanking or hitting your child. If you need help with discipline, take a course or read books on parenting skills, or talk to a counselor.

# Acne

## When to Call a Doctor

◆ Acne has not improved after 6 to 8 weeks of home treatment.

◆ Your skin is very red or purple, or you have hard bumps under your skin.

◆ Your pimples are large and hard or filled with fluid.

◆ Scars or marks form as acne heals.

◆ You get acne after starting a new medicine.

◆ Acne occurs with other symptoms, such as facial hair growth in women, or bone and muscle pain.

Acne is a skin problem that occurs when oil and dead skin cells clog your pores. This causes pimples, blackheads, and whiteheads, most often on the face, neck, and upper body. Acne usually starts during the teen years and often lasts into adulthood. Many adult women get a few pimples just before their menstrual periods.

Stress and some birth control pills may make acne worse. (However, some birth control pills may help treat acne.)

You can control most mild acne by gently cleansing your skin each day. Nonprescription acne products can also help. If home treatment does not work, or if your acne is severe, your doctor may prescribe stronger creams or lotions, antibiotics that you take by mouth, or other drugs such as isotretinoin (Accutane).

**More**

Treatment for acne often works very well, but you may not see progress for up to 8 weeks. Sometimes acne gets worse before it gets better, even with treatment. Try to be patient.

## Home Treatment

◆ Keep your skin clean. Once or twice a day, gently wash your face, shoulders, chest, and back with warm (not hot) water and a gentle soap, such as Aveeno, Cetaphil, Neutrogena, or Basis. Do not scrub too hard. Do not use soaps that dry out your skin, such as deodorant soaps. Always rinse well.

◆ Wash your hair each day, and keep it off your face and shoulders.

◆ Try not to touch any areas that have acne.

◆ Do not squeeze or pick at pimples. This can cause infection and scars.

◆ Use an acne cream, lotion, or gel that contains benzoyl peroxide. After cleansing your skin, apply a thin layer of the medicine on all the places you get pimples, not just where you have them now. Start with the lowest strength, and increase the strength of the medicine if your skin can tolerate it. Keep in mind that it may take up to 2 months to work. Mild redness and dryness is normal, but if your skin gets too dry and scaly or red and sore, reduce the amount. Do not use more than 5% benzoyl peroxide unless your doctor tells you to.

◆ Use only water-based, oil-free lotions, makeup, and sunscreens that don't clog skin pores. These products may be labeled noncomedogenic. Don't use any product that seems to make your acne worse.

# Alcohol and Drugs

## When to Call a Doctor

### Call 911 if:

◆ A person is unconscious or has trouble breathing after drinking alcohol or taking drugs.

◆ A person who has been drinking alcohol or using drugs threatens to hurt himself or herself or someone else.

◆ A person who suddenly stops using alcohol has trembling, hallucinations, seizures, or other severe withdrawal symptoms.

### Call a counselor or doctor if:

◆ You are worried about an alcohol or drug problem in someone close to you.

◆ You think you have an alcohol or drug problem and are ready to get help. (See Are You a Problem User? on page 74.) Treatment can help you quit.

The overuse or abuse of alcohol or other drugs is called substance abuse. It is common, costly, and can lead to many problems.

## Alcohol Problems

You have an alcohol use problem if you keep drinking even though it's interfering with your health or daily life.

People abuse alcohol in different ways. Some people get drunk every day. Some drink large amounts of alcohol at once. Others may be sober for a long time and then go on drinking binges for weeks or months. All of these are problems.

Long-term heavy drinking causes liver, nerve, heart, and brain damage; high blood pressure; depression; stomach problems; sexual problems; and cancer. Alcohol abuse can also lead to violence, accidents, and trouble at work, at home, or with the law.

### Signs that you are dependent on alcohol:

◆ Not remembering what happened while you were drinking (blackouts).

◆ Drinking more and more for the same high.

◆ Being uncomfortable when you can't drink alcohol.

◆ Gulping or sneaking drinks.

◆ Drinking alone or early in the morning.

◆ Getting "the shakes."

If your body is dependent on alcohol, you may have severe withdrawal symptoms (such as trembling, delusions, hallucinations, sweating, and seizures) if you suddenly stop drinking. It's very hard to stop drinking without help if you are dependent on alcohol. You may need to go through "detox" under medical care.

## Drug Problems

Drug abuse includes the use of marijuana, cocaine, meth, heroin, and other illegal drugs. It also includes the abuse of legal prescription drugs. People most often misuse tranquilizers, sedatives, pain medicines, and amphetamines, but not always on purpose. Some people turn to drugs as a way to get a high or deal with stress.

### Signs of drug use:

◆ Constant red eyes, sore throat, dry cough, and fatigue. This can also just be allergies.

◆ Major changes in sleeping or eating habits.

◆ Being moody, hostile, or abusive.

◆ Work or school problems, especially being absent a lot.

◆ Losing interest in favorite activities.

◆ Withdrawing from friends, or finding a new group of friends.

◆ Stealing, lying, and having poor family relationships.

**More** ▶

Drug dependence or addiction occurs when you develop a physical or psychological need for a drug. You may not know you are dependent on a drug until you try to stop taking it suddenly. Withdrawing from the drug can cause muscle aches, diarrhea, depression, and other symptoms.

The usual treatment for drug dependence is to reduce the dose of the drug slowly until it can be stopped. This often needs to be done under a doctor's care.

## Are You a Problem User?

Answer the questions below honestly. They ask about your use of alcohol and drugs, including prescribed and illegal drugs.

◆ Have you ever felt that you ought to cut down on your drinking or drug use?

◆ Have you ever been annoyed when others criticized your drinking or drug use?

◆ Have you ever felt guilty about your drinking or drug use?

◆ Have you ever taken an early morning drink or used drugs first thing in the morning to steady your nerves or get the day started?

If you answer yes to two or more of these questions, you may have a problem with alcohol or drugs. Talk about it with your doctor or a counselor.

## Home Treatment

◆ Pay attention to early signs that alcohol or drug use is becoming a problem. See Are You a Problem User? on this page.

◆ Go to an Alcoholics Anonymous (AA) or Narcotics Anonymous (NA) meeting. These support groups help members get sober and stay sober.

◆ If you are worried about a friend's or family member's alcohol or drug use:

❖ Don't ignore it. Discuss it as a health problem.

❖ Build up the person's self-esteem. Help the person see that he or she can succeed without alcohol or drugs. Offer your support.

❖ Ask if the person will accept help. If the person agrees, **act that very day** to get help. Call a doctor, AA, or NA for an immediate appointment. Make it easy for the person to get help. If the person says no to help, keep trying.

❖ Go to a few meetings of Al-Anon, a support group for family and friends of alcoholics. Read some 12-step program information. Many programs use the 12-step approach for dealing with addiction.

# Alcohol, Drugs, and Your Children

You can have a strong influence on whether your children will use alcohol or drugs. Here are some ideas to help you deal with this issue.

1. Talk with your children before any substance use has occurred. Help them understand the risks:

   ◆ Remind them that it's against the law.

   ◆ Talk about how alcohol and drug use can lead to poor decisions about school and sex and can hurt their chances of going to college or getting a job.

   ◆ Stay focused on what matters to people their age. Children and teens live in the moment. Lecturing them about long-term health risks may not have much effect.

2. Tell your children what you expect from them and what the punishment will be if they don't follow the rules. If they break the rules, enforce the punishment you agreed on. Be clear, be fair, and be consistent.

3. Talk about what to do if their peers pressure them to drink or use drugs.

4. Be a good role model. If you drink, drink responsibly. If you have a substance abuse problem, get help. Never drink and drive.

5. If you suspect that your child is using alcohol or drugs, check it out now. Do not take a wait-and-see approach.

 For help with what to do if your child may have a drinking or drug problem, go to the Web site on the back cover and enter **k511** in the search box.

# Allergies

## When to Call a Doctor

**Call 911** if you have any signs of a severe allergic reaction soon after you take a drug, eat a certain food, or are stung by an insect. For example:

◆ You faint or feel like you may faint.

◆ You have swelling around the lips, tongue, or face that is causing breathing problems or is getting worse.

◆ You start wheezing or have trouble breathing.

**Call a doctor if:**

◆ Your face, tongue, or lips are swollen, even if you do not have trouble breathing and the swelling is not getting worse.

◆ There is a lot of swelling around the site of an insect sting. (For instance, the entire arm or leg is swollen.)

◆ You get a skin rash, itching, a feeling of warmth, or hives. Also see Hives on page 194.

◆ Allergy symptoms get worse over time, and home treatment does not help. Your doctor may recommend stronger medicine or allergy shots. See page 78.

Most allergies are caused by pollen, dust, and other things in the air. You can often find the cause of an allergy by noting when symptoms occur.

◆ Symptoms that happen at the same time each year are often caused by tree, grass, or weed pollen. You are most likely to have problems during spring, early summer, or early fall.

◆ Allergies that last all year may be caused by dust, dust mites, cockroaches, mold, or animal dander.

◆ An animal allergy is often easy to spot: your symptoms clear up when you stay away from the pet or its bedding.

Allergies to pollen or grass often cause **hay fever**. If you have hay fever, you already know the symptoms: itchy, watery eyes;

sneezing; runny, stuffy, or itchy nose; and fatigue. You may also get dark circles under your eyes.

Allergies seem to run in families. Parents with hay fever often have children with allergies.

## Home Treatment

Decongestants and antihistamines may help with some allergies. Talk to your doctor about the best choice for you, and use caution when you take these drugs.

If you know what you are allergic to, the best treatment is to avoid it whenever you can. Keep a record of your symptoms and the plants, animals, foods, medicines, or chemicals that seem to trigger them.

In general:

◆ Avoid yard work, which stirs up both pollen and mold. If you must do yard work, wear a mask, and take an antihistamine before you start.

◆ If you smoke, quit. See page 316 for help.

◆ Do not use aerosol sprays, perfumes, room deodorizers, or cleaning products that trigger allergy symptoms.

**For seasonal symptoms caused by pollen or grass:**

◆ Keep your house and car windows closed. Do not open your bedroom windows at night.

◆ Limit the time you spend outside when pollen counts are high.

◆ Wash dogs and other pets often, or leave them outside. They can bring lots of pollen into your house.

**For year-round symptoms caused by dust:**

◆ Keep your bedroom and other places where you spend a lot of time as dust-free as you can. Remove "dust collectors," such as stuffed toys, wall hangings, books, knickknacks, and artificial flowers.

◆ Dust and vacuum once or twice a week. This stirs up dust and makes the air worse until the dust settles, so wear a mask if you do the cleaning yourself. Damp-mop tile, wood, or stone floors.

◆ Try not to use carpets, upholstered furniture, and heavy drapes that collect dust. Vacuum cleaners pick up dust but not dust mites. Use leather, vinyl, or plastic furniture that you can wipe clean and small rugs that you can wash.

◆ Cover your mattress and box spring with dustproof cases, and wipe them clean weekly. Do not use wool or down blankets and feather pillows. Wash all bedding in hot water once a week.

◆ Use an air conditioner or air purifier with a special HEPA filter. Rent one before you buy it to see if it helps.

◆ Change or clean heating and cooling system filters often.

## Life-Threatening Allergic Reactions

A few people have severe allergies to insect stings, nuts or other foods, or drugs, especially antibiotics such as penicillin. The reaction is sudden and severe and may cause dangerous swelling in the throat and mouth, trouble breathing, and a drop in blood pressure. This is called anaphylaxis. It needs emergency care.

If you have ever had a severe allergic reaction, your doctor may suggest that you carry an allergy kit (such as EpiPen). These kits include pills and a shot that you can give yourself in case you are exposed to the same thing that caused your severe reaction before. The shot can help prevent a bad reaction and give you time to get help.

If you have ever had an allergic reaction to a drug, wear medical alert jewelry that lists your allergies.

**More**

**For year-round symptoms caused by mold or mildew (worse when weather is damp):**

◆ Keep your home aired out and dry. Keep the humidity below 50 percent. Use a dehumidifier when the weather is humid.

◆ Use an air conditioner, which removes mold from the air.

◆ Change or clean heating and cooling system filters often.

◆ Clean bathroom and kitchen surfaces often with bleach.

◆ Use exhaust fans in the bathrooms and kitchen.

**If you are allergic to a pet:**

◆ Keep the animal outside, or at least out of your bedroom.

◆ If your symptoms are severe and your efforts to reduce dander exposure do not help, the best answer may be to find a new home for the pet.

## What About Allergy Shots?

For many people who have allergies to insect stings, pollen, dust and dust mites, mold, animal dander, or cockroaches, allergy shots can reduce or prevent symptoms.

◆ Shots may take 3 to 5 years to complete.

◆ You may need to get them once a week at first and then once a month.

◆ It may take up to a full year of shots before you see any change in your symptoms.

You will also need skin and blood tests to find out what you are allergic to. The shots treat just one kind of allergy, such as grass pollen. If you are allergic to more than one thing, you may need to get shots for each.

Getting allergy shots takes time and money. But they work for many people and may be worth it for you if:

◆ Your allergies bother you a lot, and medicines do not help well enough.

◆ You can't avoid the things you are allergic to, and your efforts to control them don't solve the problem.

◆ You have had a severe reaction to an insect sting, or your reactions have gotten worse over time.

◆ Allergy shots work for what you are allergic to. For example, they help with allergies to insect stings, but they do not help with many food allergies.

 For help deciding whether to try allergy shots, go to the Web site on the back cover and enter **d751** in the search box.

## Food Allergies in Children

Food allergies are not common. Many parents think their child has a food allergy when the child really has a food intolerance. Unlike a food allergy, a food intolerance does not cause severe symptoms and usually does not come on quickly. A good example is lactose intolerance (see page 139).

By slowly adding simple foods to your child's diet, you may be able to spot an allergy quickly. Eggs, milk, peanuts, wheat, soy, and fish cause most allergic reactions in children.

◆ Most children outgrow allergies to milk, wheat, eggs, and soy between ages 3 and 5.

◆ Allergies to peanuts, fish, or shellfish often last a lifetime.

If your child was allergic to a food when younger, talk to your doctor before you have your child try the food again. A child with a severe food allergy may have a dangerous reaction to even a tiny bit of that food.

**If your child has a severe food allergy:**

◆ Make sure that school or day care knows about it.

◆ Keep an allergy kit nearby at all times.

◆ Have your child wear medical alert jewelry.

# Anger and Hostility

## When to Call a Doctor

**Call 911** if you or someone you know is in immediate danger.

**Call a counselor if:**

◆ Anger has led or could lead to violence or harm to you or someone else.

◆ Anger or hostility upsets your work, family life, or friendships.

Anger tells your body to prepare for a fight. It can be a normal response to daily events. And it is a healthy response to any situation that's a real threat. You can sometimes use anger as a positive, driving force behind your actions.

Hostility is being ready for a fight all the time. Hostile people are often stubborn, impatient, hotheaded, or have an "attitude."

Feeling angry and hostile all or much of the time is not good for you. It keeps your blood pressure high and may make you more likely to have a heart attack, stroke, or other health problem. Constant anger also cuts you off from the people in your life. It may lead to abuse and violence (see page 70).

More ➤

## Home Treatment

◆ Try to understand why you are angry. Is it the current situation that's making you angry or something that happened earlier?

◆ Notice when you start to get angry, and take steps to deal with your anger in a healthy way. Do not ignore your anger until you "blow up."

   ❖ Think before you act. Count to 10 or use some other form of mental relaxation. When you have calmed down, you'll be better able to deal with the problem.

   ❖ Give yourself a "time-out." Go someplace quiet so you can calm down.

   ❖ Go for a short walk or jog.

❖ Talk with a friend about your anger.

❖ Draw or paint to release the anger, or write about it in a journal.

◆ If you are angry with someone, listen to what the other person has to say. Try to understand his or her point of view. Use "I" statements, not "you" statements, to discuss your anger. Say "I feel angry when my needs are not being met" instead of "You make me mad when you are so inconsiderate."

◆ Forgive and forget. Forgiving lowers your blood pressure and eases muscle tension so you can feel more relaxed.

◆ Focus on the things in your life that make you happy.

◆ Read books about anger and how to handle it, or explore other resources through your job or community.

# Anxiety and Panic

### When to Call a Doctor
**Call a counselor or your doctor if:**

◆ Anxiety or fear upsets your daily life.

◆ Sudden, severe attacks of fear or anxiety seem to occur for no reason.

◆ Symptoms of anxiety are still severe after 1 week of home treatment.

◆ You have nightmares or flashbacks to traumatic events.

◆ You cannot feel certain about things (for example, whether you unplugged the iron) no matter how many times you check, especially if it interferes with your daily life.

Feeling worried, anxious, and nervous is a normal part of life. Everyone frets or feels anxious from time to time.

Your body tells you when you are anxious:

◆ You may tremble, twitch, or shake.

◆ You may feel lightheaded or dizzy.

◆ You may feel "butterflies" in your stomach.

◆ Your breathing and heartbeat may speed up.

◆ Your throat or chest may feel full.

◆ You may sweat, and your muscles may get tense.

◆ You may have sleep problems.

Anxiety also affects your emotions:

◆ You may feel hyper, annoyed, or edgy.

◆ You may worry a lot or fear that something bad is going to happen.

◆ You may not be able to concentrate.

◆ You may feel sad all the time.

A specific situation or fear can cause these symptoms for a short time. When the situation passes, the symptoms go away.

When you have an **anxiety disorder**, you get these symptoms for no clear reason or for reasons that don't make sense. This type of anxiety is not normal and can be overwhelming. People with an anxiety disorder may have fears, or phobias, of common places, objects, or situations.

**Panic disorder** is a problem related to anxiety. People with panic disorder have periods of sudden, intense fear and anxiety when there is no clear cause or danger. These panic attacks can cause scary (but not dangerous) symptoms, such as a pounding heart, shortness of breath, and a sense that you are about to lose control or die.

People who have had panic attacks may try hard to avoid anything that might trigger another attack. This often causes an even higher level of anxiety.

On your own or with the help of a counselor, you can learn ways to manage your anxiety and panic. Medicines may also help.

## Home Treatment

Try these tips to relieve anxiety. They can also help if you are getting treatment for anxiety or panic disorder.

◆ Recognize and accept your anxiety. Then, when a situation makes you feel anxious, say to yourself, "This is not an emergency. I feel uncomfortable, but I'm not in danger. I can keep going even if I feel anxious."

◆ Be kind to your body:

❖ Relieve stress and tension with exercise, massage, warm baths, walks, or whatever works for you.

❖ Learn and use a relaxation technique. See page 320.

❖ Get enough rest. If you have trouble sleeping, see Sleep Problems on page 236.

❖ Avoid alcohol, caffeine, and nicotine. They can increase your anxiety, cause sleep problems, or trigger a panic attack.

◆ Use your mind. Do things you enjoy, like going to a funny movie or taking a walk or a hike. Plan your day. Having too much or too little to do can make you more anxious.

◆ Keep a daily record of your symptoms. Discuss your fears with a good friend or family member, or join a support group. Talking to others about the problem sometimes relieves stress.

◆ Get involved in social groups, or volunteer to help others. Being alone may make things seem worse than they are.

# Arthritis

Joint problems that cause pain, swelling, and stiffness are called arthritis. Arthritis can occur at any age but affects older people most often.

There are many types of arthritis. The chart on page 83 describes three common ones.

## Home Treatment

The tips here will help with many types of arthritis and joint pain. The goal is to ease your pain, protect your joints, and help you stay active.

- Take a warm shower or bath to help relieve morning stiffness. Keep moving so your joints don't stiffen up.

- If a joint is stiff or sore but not swollen, put moist heat on it for 20 to 30 minutes, 2 to 3 times a day. You may also try cold packs.

- If the joint is swollen, use cold packs for 10 minutes once an hour. Cold will help reduce pain and swelling.

- When joints are sore, rest them. For a few days, avoid activities that put weight or strain on the joints. Give your joints short rest breaks all through the day.

- Put each of your joints gently through its full range of motion once or twice a day.

- Exercise regularly to help your muscles and joints stay strong and flexible. Swimming, water aerobics, biking, or walking are great ways to be active and do not stress your joints as much as other exercises. Do some stretching every day. To learn how to exercise safely with  arthritis and see examples of good exercises, go to the Web site on the back cover and enter **d288** in the search box.

- Stay at a healthy weight. Being overweight puts extra strain on your joints. If you need to lose weight, see page 300 for help.

- Take nonprescription pain medicines.

  ❖ Try acetaminophen (Tylenol) first.

  ❖ Anti-inflammatory medicines, such as aspirin, ibuprofen (Advil, Motrin), or naproxen (Aleve), also work well but can cause problems in some people. Talk to your doctor about whether these medicines are safe for you and how much to take.

## Common Types of Arthritis

| Type | Symptoms | Comments |
|------|----------|----------|
| Osteoarthritis (breakdown of joint cartilage) | Pain and stiffness; common in knees, fingers, hips, feet, and back | Most common after age 50; most common type of arthritis |
| Rheumatoid arthritis (inflammation of tissue lining the joint) | Pain, stiffness, warmth, and swelling in joints on both sides of the body; common in hands, wrists, elbows, feet, knees, and neck | Often starts around age 40; more common in women |
| Gout (buildup of uric acid crystals in joint fluid) | Sudden burning pain, stiffness, and swelling; usually in the big toe or in the ankle, knee, wrist, or elbow | Most common in men 30 to 50; alcohol and exposure to cold may make gout worse |

◆ Use helpful devices such as special doorknobs, kitchen tools with padded handles, and a higher toilet seat. Braces, splints, canes, or walkers can give your joints a rest while they help you get around.

◆ Join a support group or take a course on how to manage your arthritis. People in these programs often have less pain and fewer limits on what they can do.

**Looking for the Asthma topic? See page 266.**

# Atopic Dermatitis

## When to Call a Doctor

◆ You have new blisters or bruises and do not know why.

◆ The rash spreads and looks like a sunburn.

◆ There are crusting or oozing sores or serious scratch marks.

◆ Fever occurs with the rash.

◆ Joint aches or body aches occur with the rash.

◆ Itching is severe and home treatment does not help.

◆ You cannot control atopic dermatitis with home treatment.

Atopic dermatitis (also called atopic eczema) causes intense itching and a red, raised, scaly, or rough rash. When the rash is severe, it may have fluid-filled blisters. The blisters can get infected, especially if you scratch them too much.

Where the rash is depends partly on age:

◆ In babies, the rash is usually on the face, scalp, arms, thighs, and torso.

**More**

- In older children, it tends to occur in areas that bend, like elbows and knees.

- In adults, it may affect the hands, neck, face, genitals, or legs. The rash is usually smaller than in children.

Atopic dermatitis often occurs in young children who have asthma, hay fever, and other allergies, though it can occur at any age. Most children outgrow it by their early teens.

## Home Treatment

- Take short baths or showers with warm (not hot) water. For areas that need soap (armpits, feet, groin), use a nondrying cleanser, such as Aveeno, Dove, Basis, or Neutrogena.

- Right after bathing, apply a moisturizer while your skin is still damp. Use a cream such as Lubriderm, Moisturel, or Cetaphil that doesn't irritate the skin.

- Keep cool, and stay out of the sun.

- Use a cool-mist humidifier in your bedroom if the air is dry.

- Avoid things that make the rash worse, like cleaning products, chemicals, or certain fabrics. Wear gloves when you have to work with an irritating product.

- When you wash clothes and bedding, use mild detergent and rinse at least twice. Don't use fabric softener if it irritates your skin. Avoid scratchy fabrics.

- Keep fingernails trimmed and filed smooth so you don't hurt your skin if you scratch. Put mittens or cotton socks on your baby's hands.

- Use cold, wet cloths to reduce itching. An oral antihistamine (such as Benadryl) may also help. Do not use antiseptic and antihistamine creams and sprays. Also see Relief From Itching on page 142.

## If Your Child Has Atopic Dermatitis

Atopic dermatitis can be very hard on children. Both the child and the parents may avoid touching, which is a vital part of their bonding. The child avoids it because the skin hurts, and the parents avoid it because the skin feels rough and looks bad.

The child may also feel set apart from other children because of restrictions (on diet or sports, for instance). He or she may feel unattractive because of the rash. And the child may be fussy and hard to deal with because he or she is so itchy.

Here's how you can help:

- Talk to your child, and offer support. Spend time with your child every day.

- Try to be sure your child takes part in activities with other kids.

- Help your child find things to do that keep his or her hands busy and distracted from the itching. (This may take a lot of effort on your part, but it can help.)

- Help your child with proper skin care. Provide soft clothes and bedding. Keep your child cool. Watch for things that make the problem worse, and remove them if you can.

# Back Pain

## When to Call a Doctor

**Call 911** if back pain occurs with chest pain or other symptoms of a heart attack (see page 38).

**Call a doctor if:**

- You suddenly lose bowel or bladder control. This could be a sign of a serious problem.

- You cannot walk or stand at all. If this is because of weakness and not just because it hurts too much, you need medical care right away.

- You have new numbness in the buttocks, genital or rectal area, or legs.

- You have leg weakness that is not solely due to pain. Many people with low back pain say their legs feel weak. If leg weakness is so bad that you cannot bend your foot upward, get up out of a chair, or climb stairs, see your doctor.

- You have new or increased back pain with fever, painful urination, or other signs of a urinary tract infection. See page 251.

- You have a dramatic increase in your chronic back pain, especially if it's not related to physical activity.

- You have a history of cancer or HIV infection and you have new or increased back pain.

- You have severe pain that does not improve after a few days of home treatment.

- Pain wakes you from sleeping.

- You have a new, severe pain in your lower back that does not change when you move and is not related to stress, muscle tension, or a known injury.

- Pain does not improve after 2 weeks of home treatment.

Your back is the whole area from your neck to your tailbone. It includes the bones (vertebrae) and joints of the spine, the spinal discs that separate the bones and absorb shock as you move, and the muscles and ligaments that hold them all together. You can stress or hurt any of these parts of your back.

What causes most back pain?

- Repeating movements or staying too long in positions that strain the back

- Moving suddenly or awkwardly in ways that twist the back

These kinds of movements or postures can strain or sprain the ligaments, muscles, or the joints between the spine and the pelvic bones (sacroiliac joints).

You can hurt a disc in your back the same way, causing it to bulge or tear (rupture). This is called a **herniated disc**. If the tear is large enough, the gel inside the disc may leak out and press against a nerve.

A sprain or strain can cause 2 to 3 days of pain and swelling, followed by slow healing and a gradual decrease in pain. Pain from a herniated disc may last much longer.

**More**

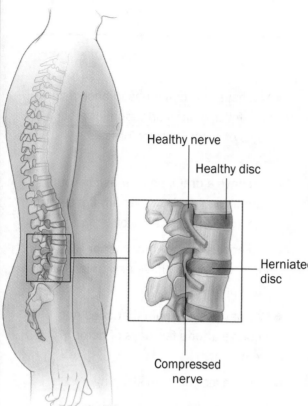

Healthy nerve

Healthy disc

Herniated disc

Compressed nerve

A bulging (herniated) disc can press on a nerve, causing pain.

You may feel the pain in your low back, in your buttocks, or down one or both legs.

With good self-care, most of these back injuries will heal in 6 to 12 weeks. Home treatment can help relieve pain, promote healing, and prevent reinjury.

Back pain can also be caused by problems that affect the bones and joints of the spine.

◆ **Arthritis** pain may be a steady ache, unlike the sharp, sudden pain of back strain and disc injuries. If you think arthritis may be causing your back pain, combine the home treatment for back pain with the treatment for arthritis on page 82.

◆ **Osteoporosis** can weaken the bones of the spine and cause them to break or collapse. See page 214.

## Home Treatment

◆ Follow the First Aid for Back Pain guidelines on page 87. These include rest, ice, pelvic tilts, and short walks.

◆ Sit or lie in positions that feel good and reduce your pain, especially any leg pain.

◆ Do not sit up in bed, and avoid soft couches and twisted positions. Avoid sitting for long periods of time. Follow the tips for good body mechanics on page 89.

◆ Bed rest can help relieve back pain but may not speed healing. Unless you have severe leg pain, 1 to 2 days of bed rest should relieve pain. Do not stay in bed for more than 3 days unless your doctor tells you to.

◆ For bed rest, try one of the following positions (see pictures on page 90):

❖ Lie on your back with your knees bent and supported by large pillows. Or lie on the floor with your legs on the seat of a sofa or chair.

❖ Lie on your side with your knees and hips bent and a pillow between your legs.

❖ Lie on your stomach if it does not make the pain worse.

◆ Take aspirin, ibuprofen (Advil, Motrin), or naproxen (Aleve) for pain and swelling. Do not give aspirin to anyone younger than 20. If your doctor has told you not to take these medicines, try acetaminophen (Tylenol) instead. Read the labels, and do not take more than the highest recommended dose. If you mask the pain completely, you may be tempted to move in ways that could make your back worse.

◆ Relax your muscles. See page 320.

Two to three days after the injury, you can try the following:

◆ Put heat on your sore back for 20 minutes at a time. Moist heat (hot packs, baths, showers) works better than dry heat. Some people like switching between heat and ice packs, or using ice only. Do what works for you.

◆ Keep taking short walks. Increase to 5 to 10 minutes, 3 to 4 times a day.

◆ Try swimming. It may hurt right after a back injury, but lap swimming or kicking with swim fins often helps prevent pain from coming back.

◆ When your pain has improved, try easy exercises that don't increase your pain. One or two of the exercises described on pages 91 to 94 may be a good place to start. Start with 5 repetitions, 3 to 4 times a day, and increase to 10 repetitions if it does not cause pain.

## First Aid for Back Pain

When you first feel a strain in your back, try these steps to avoid or reduce pain. These are the most important home treatments for the first few days of back pain.

**1. Relax:** Lie down in a comfortable position. This will let your back muscles relax.

**2. Ice:** Put ice or a cold pack on your back for 10 to 15 minutes every hour. Cold used for the first 3 days reduces pain and speeds healing.

**3. Pelvic tilts:** This exercise gently moves the spine and stretches the lower back.

   ◆ Lie on your back with knees bent and feet flat on the floor.

   ◆ Slowly tighten your stomach muscles and press your lower back against the floor. Hold for 10 seconds (don't hold your breath). Slowly relax.

**4. Walk:** Take a short walk (3 to 5 minutes) on a flat, level surface every 3 hours. Walk only as far as you can without pain. If your back or legs hurt, stop.

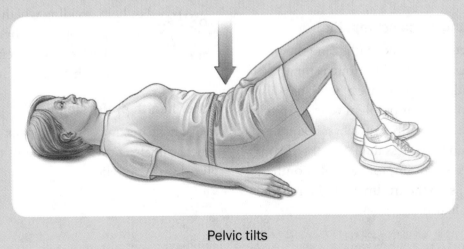

Pelvic tilts

**More**

## Who to See for Back Pain

### Medical doctors

A doctor (MD or DO) can:

◆ Diagnose the cause of back pain and assess injuries.

◆ Help you develop an exercise and home care plan or a modified work plan if you need it.

◆ Prescribe muscle relaxants, anti-inflammatory drugs, and pain medicines. (If you get a strong pain medicine or muscle relaxer, be extra careful to avoid postures and activities that could reinjure your back.)

◆ Suggest physical therapy.

◆ Recommend back surgery.

### Physical therapists

After basic first aid, a physical therapist with training in orthopedic treatment can:

◆ Identify specific muscle or disc problems.

◆ Provide or suggest other therapies, such as massage or acupuncture, if you are not getting better.

◆ Develop an exercise program to help you recover and prevent future problems.

### Chiropractors and osteopaths

Chiropractors and osteopaths can relieve some types of back pain through spinal manipulation. (If you have a herniated disc, this may make your problem worse.) Spinal manipulation usually works best if you have had symptoms for less than 4 weeks. If your symptoms do not improve after 1 month of treatment, stop the treatment and have your pain reevaluated.

## Sciatica

Sciatica is an irritation of the sciatic nerve, which is formed by the nerve roots coming out of the spinal cord into the lower back. The nerve extends down through the buttocks to the feet. Sciatica can occur when a damaged disc presses against a spinal nerve root.

The main symptom is pain, numbness, or weakness that extends from your back down into your leg. The pain is usually worse in the leg.

For relief, see Home Treatment on page 86, and follow these tips:

◆ Do not sit unless you have to (unless it's more comfortable to sit than to stand).

◆ Switch between lying down and taking short walks. You can slowly increase how far you walk as long as it does not cause pain.

◆ Put ice or a cold pack on the middle of your lower back for 10 to 15 minutes once an hour.

 **Go to Web** For help deciding whether to see a chiropractor, go to the Web site on the back cover and enter **i018** in the search box.

### Other health professionals

Acupuncturists, massage therapists, and others can also provide treatments that may give short-term relief.

# How to Have a Healthy Back

The keys to preventing back pain are to:

◆ Use good body mechanics.

◆ Stretch and strengthen your back.

◆ Practice good health habits, such as getting regular exercise, staying at a healthy weight, and not smoking (nicotine weakens the discs in your back).

Some of the tips presented here are things you'll want to do every day, not only because they're good for your back, but because they're good for your overall health. The rest will come in handy if you ever have back pain. They include:

◆ Good body mechanics.

◆ Exercises to make your back stronger and more flexible.

◆ Exercises to avoid.

## Good Body Mechanics

The goal of good body mechanics is to sit, stand, sleep, and move in ways that reduce the stress on your back. Use good body mechanics all the time, not just when you have back pain.

### Sitting

◆ Try not to sit in the same position for more than an hour at a time. Get up or change positions often.

◆ If you must sit a lot, the extension exercises starting on page 91 are particularly important.

◆ If you work at a desk or computer, set up your workstation to reduce stress on your back and neck.

❖ Use a chair that you can adjust and that does not upset the normal curve of your back.

❖ Keep your feet flat on the floor or on a footrest.

❖ Keep your screen at or just below eye level so you do not have to tilt your head or look sideways.

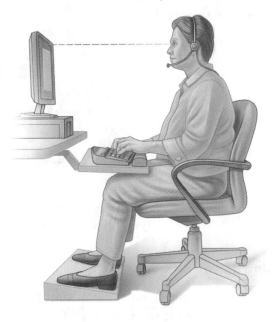

Adjust your chair, keyboard, and screen to reduce back and neck stress.

◆ If your chair does not give enough support, use a small pillow or rolled towel to support your lower back.

◆ When you drive, pull your seat forward so that you can easily reach the pedals and steering wheel. Stop often to stretch and walk around. A small pillow or towel roll behind your lower back might help too.

**More**

## Lifting

◆ Keep your upper back straight. Do not bend forward at the waist.

◆ Bend your knees, and let your arms and legs do the work. Tighten your buttocks and belly to support your back.

◆ Keep the load as close to your body as you can, even if the load is light.

◆ While holding a heavy object, use your feet to turn, not your back. Try not to turn or twist your body.

◆ Do not lift heavy objects above shoulder level.

◆ For very heavy or awkward items, use a hand truck or ask someone to help you.

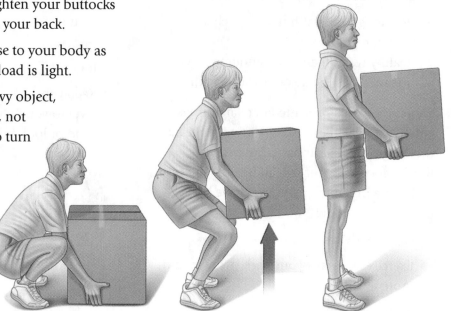

When you lift heavy objects, keep your upper back straight, bend your knees, and keep the load close to your body.

## Lying down

◆ If you have back pain at night, your mattress may be the problem. Try a firmer mattress. Or, if you think your mattress is too firm, try a softer one.

◆ If you sleep on your back, you may want to use a towel roll to support your lower back or put a pillow under your knees.

◆ If you sleep on your side, try placing a pillow between your knees.

◆ Sleeping on your stomach is fine if it does not cause back or neck pain.

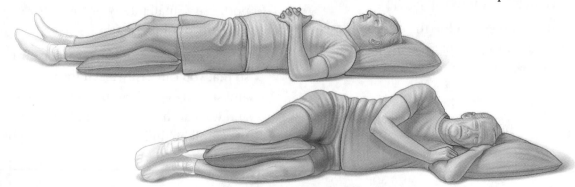

Try placing pillows between or under your knees to relieve back pain while lying in bed.

## Exercise

Regular exercise helps you stay fit and flexible and strengthens the muscles that support your back. It also helps you stay at a healthy weight, which reduces the strain on your lower back.

Although there is no clear evidence that specific exercises can help prevent back pain, the exercises described here are a common, practical approach to helping you stay strong and flexible. You may want to make them a part of your regular fitness routine.

Do not do these exercises if you have just hurt your back. Instead, see First Aid for Back Pain on page 87.

It helps to do both extension exercises and flexion exercises. Extension exercises strengthen your lower back muscles and stretch the stomach muscles. Flexion exercises stretch the lower back muscles and strengthen the stomach muscles—the reverse of extension.

◆ You do not need to do every exercise. Do the ones that help you the most.

◆ If any exercise makes your back pain worse, stop it and try something else. Stop any exercise that makes the pain spread into your buttocks or legs, either during or after the exercise.

◆ Start with 5 repetitions, 3 to 4 times a day, and gradually increase to 10 repetitions. Do all exercises slowly.

### Extension exercises

### Press-ups

This is a good exercise to start and end with.

◆ Lie facedown with your arms bent, palms flat on the floor.

◆ Lift yourself up on your elbows, keeping the lower half of your body relaxed. Press your chest forward.

◆ Keep your hips pressed to the floor. Feel the stretch in your lower back.

◆ Lower your upper body to the floor. Repeat slowly.

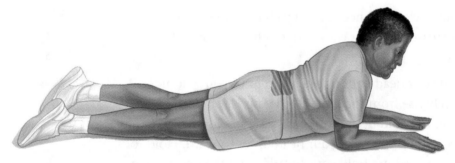

Press-up (shading shows where you should feel the stretch)

**More**

### Shoulder lifts

These strengthen the back muscles.

◆ Lie facedown with your arms beside your body.

◆ Lift your shoulders straight up from the floor as high as you can without pain. Keep your chin down and your eyes facing the floor. Keep your belly and hips pressed to the floor.

Shoulder lift (keep neck straight and chin down)

### Backward bends

These help a lot if you work in a bent-forward position.

◆ Stand with your feet slightly apart. Back up to a countertop if you want extra support.

◆ Place your hands in the small of your back and gently bend backward. Keep your knees straight (not locked), and bend only at the waist. Hold the backward stretch for 1 to 2 seconds.

### Flexion exercises

### Curl-ups

These strengthen your stomach muscles, which help support your spine.

◆ Lie on your back with knees bent, feet flat on the floor, and arms crossed on your chest. Do not hook your feet under anything.

◆ Slowly curl your head and shoulders up until your shoulder blades barely rise from the floor. Keep your lower back pressed to the floor. To avoid neck problems, remember to lift your shoulders, and do not force your head up or forward. Hold for 5 to 10 seconds (don't hold your breath), and then curl down very slowly.

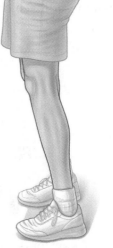

Backward bend
(keep neck straight
and chin down)

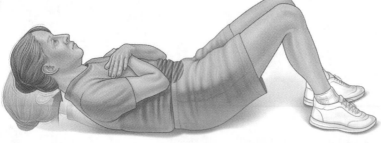

Curl-up (keep neck straight and chin tucked in)

### Knee-to-chest stretch

This stretches the lower back and butt muscles and relieves pressure on the joints in your spine.

◆ Lie on your back with knees bent and feet close to your buttocks.

◆ Bring one knee to your chest, keeping the other foot flat on the floor (or the other leg straight, if that is more comfortable for your lower back). Keep your lower back pressed to the floor. Hold for 5 to 10 seconds.

◆ Relax and lower your knee to the starting position. Repeat with the other leg.

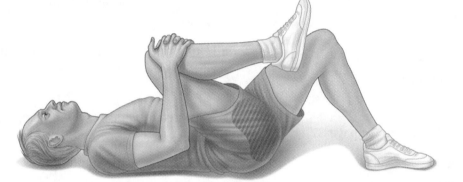

Knee-to-chest stretch (shading shows where you should feel the stretch)

### Hamstring stretch

This stretches the muscles in the back of your thigh, which will let you bend your legs without stressing your back.

◆ Lie on your back in a doorway. Keep one leg resting on the floor of the doorway, and extend the leg you want to stretch straight up, resting the heel on the wall next to the doorway.

◆ Keep the leg straight, and slowly move your heel up the wall until you feel a gentle pull in the back of your thigh. Stretch as far as you can without pain.

◆ Relax in this position for 30 seconds. Then bend the knee to relieve the stretch. Repeat with the other leg.

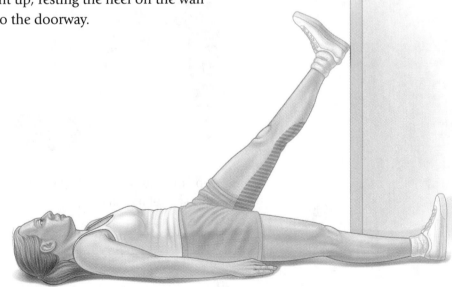

Hamstring stretch (shading shows where you should feel the stretch)

**More** ➤

## Other strengthening and stretching exercises

### Prone buttocks squeeze

This strengthens the butt muscles, which support the back and help you lift with your legs. You may need to place a small pillow under your stomach for comfort.

◆ Lie flat on your stomach with your arms at your sides.

◆ Slowly tighten your buttocks muscles and hold for 5 to 10 seconds. Do not hold your breath. Relax slowly.

### Pelvic tilts

See First Aid for Back Pain on page 87.

### Hip flexor stretch

This stretches the muscles in the front of your hip.

◆ Kneel on one knee with your other leg bent in front of you.

◆ Slowly sink your hips so your weight shifts onto your front foot. The knee of your forward leg should be in a straight line with your ankle. Hold for 10 seconds. You should feel a stretch in the groin of the leg you are kneeling on. Repeat with the other leg.

## Exercises to Avoid

These common exercises actually increase the risk of low back pain.

◆ Sit-ups with your legs straight out in front of you.

◆ Bent-leg sit-ups when you have back pain.

◆ Lifting both legs while lying on your back.

◆ Lifting heavy weights above the waist (military press, biceps curls while standing).

◆ Any stretching done while sitting with the legs in a V.

◆ Toe touches while standing.

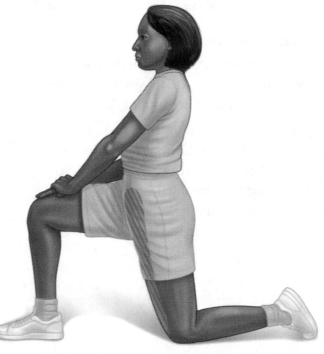

Hip flexor stretch (shading shows where you should feel the stretch)

## Back Surgery

Rest, pain medicines, and exercise can relieve almost all back problems. And back pain usually gets better within 6 to 12 weeks.

Most back surgeries are done to treat problems that have not improved with time. You may need surgery if you have a broken bone in your spine, a spinal infection, or another serious problem. Or you may think about surgery if you have a disc problem that has not improved with time and other treatment.

If you are thinking about having surgery to treat your back pain, get all the facts. Find out:

◆ How much it will cost.

◆ How likely it is to help your problem. For some kinds of surgery, there is no clear evidence about whether it will help.

◆ What risks it has.

 For help deciding whether surgery is right for you, go to the Web site on the back cover and enter **f952** in the search box.

If you do plan to have surgery, using good body mechanics and doing exercises for your back are very important. Having a strong, flexible back will help you recover more quickly after surgery.

# Bed-Wetting

## When to Call a Doctor

Your doctor can rule out or treat any physical causes of bed-wetting and help you and your child manage the problem.

### Call your doctor if:

◆ Bed-wetting occurs with pain or burning during urination or other signs of a urinary infection. See page 251.

◆ Bed-wetting occurs in a child older than 6 years and home treatment has not solved the problem after 4 to 5 weeks.

◆ Your child starts wetting the bed more often, even with home treatment.

◆ Bed-wetting occurs in a child who had been dry for several months.

◆ A child age 4 or older is wetting the bed and leaking stool.

◆ A child over age 3 who has been toilet-trained has bladder control problems during the day.

**More** ➤

Bed-wetting in children who have never been dry is common. Most children will outgrow it by age 5 or 6.

In some cases, a child who has been dry for several months or more may start to wet the bed again. This can happen without a clear cause, or it may be caused by a urinary tract infection or emotional problems.

## Home Treatment

There are a lot of ways to deal with bed-wetting if there is not an infection or other physical cause behind it. Ask your doctor for advice.

◆ Do not punish, embarrass, or blame your child. Praise and reward your child for dry nights.

◆ Have your child empty his or her bladder before bed.

◆ Remind your child to get up during the night to urinate. A night-light may help.

◆ Let your child choose whether to wear diapers, Pull-Ups, or absorbent under-wear at night. Use a thick pad or a vinyl mattress cover to protect the mattress.

◆ If your child is old enough, let him or her help with changing clothes after wetting, putting a dry towel down on the bed, and changing the sheets.

◆ Add ½ cup vinegar to the wash water to get rid of odor in clothing and bedding.

# Birth Control

Birth control helps prevent pregnancy. But no birth control method works every time and is risk-free. The only way to be sure you will not get pregnant is not to have sex.

This topic briefly describes the most common types of birth control. Be sure to think about their pros and cons, including cost, if you are trying to choose a method.

For more help with your options, go to the Web site on the back cover and enter **j225** in the search box. Talk to your doctor about it as well.

Use birth control exactly as your doctor or the package instructions say. Birth control works best when you use it right every time.

## Hormonal Birth Control

This includes birth control pills, Depo-Provera shots, the patch (Ortho Evra), and the vaginal ring (NuvaRing). These types of birth control either stop the release of an egg each month (ovulation) or thicken the mucus at the opening of the uterus so sperm cannot get through to the egg.

These types of birth control work very well if you use them right. All of them require a doctor's prescription. They do not protect you from sexually transmitted diseases (STDs).

## IUD (Intrauterine Device)

The IUD is a piece of plastic or metal that your doctor can place in your uterus. There are two types.

- The copper IUD can stay in place for at least 10 years.

- The levonorgestrel IUD (Mirena) works for at least 5 years, and it reduces menstrual bleeding and cramping.

Both types of IUDs damage or kill sperm. IUDs also change the lining of the uterus so that the egg does not attach there.

IUDs work better than most other types of birth control (IUDs work about as well as surgery). Rarely, an IUD can come out without you noticing it. And some women have problems with IUDs during the first few months of use and decide to have them removed. IUDs don't protect you from STDs.

## Condoms

The male condom is a thin, stretchy tube of latex, polyurethane, or animal skin that is placed over the man's erect penis before sexual intercourse. There are also condoms for women that fit inside the vagina.

Latex condoms are the best protection against STDs, including HIV. If you are allergic to latex, polyurethane condoms are the next best choice. See page 323. Lambskin condoms do not prevent HIV and STDs nearly as well.

Condoms are cheap, and you can get them without a prescription. But many people don't use them properly, and they can break or slip off. For tips on how to use them right, see page 323.

## Emergency Birth Control

Emergency birth control can help prevent pregnancy if you use it soon after you have sex. Sometimes called the morning-after pill, it is usually a high-dose form of birth control pills (Plan B). Inserting a copper IUD (intrauterine device) also works, but a doctor has to do this.

You can take the morning-after pill up to 5 days after having sex. But the sooner you take it, the better your chance of not getting pregnant. The IUD can be used up to 7 days after sex.

Call your doctor or local clinic right away if you want to avoid pregnancy and:

- You just had sex without birth control.

- You just had sex and your birth control failed. (For instance, a condom slipped or broke, or you skipped a pill.)

In some states, you can buy Plan B at your local pharmacy without a prescription.

### For next time

You may want to ask your doctor for a prescription for Plan B in case of a future birth control mistake. That way, you'll have it if you need it. If you have not been using birth control at all, also talk to your doctor about what might work best for you.

**More** ➤

## Diaphragm and Cervical Cap

These are small rubber caps that you fill with spermicide and put in the vagina to cover the opening of the uterus (cervix) before you have sex. You have to leave them in place for 6 hours or longer after sex. And you have to see a doctor to have the diaphragm or cervical cap fitted.

For preventing pregnancy, the diaphragm or cervical cap works better if you use it with another method, such as condoms. The diaphragm offers a little protection from STDs, but condoms are by far the best choice for this.

## Spermicide

Spermicides are foams, jellies, and suppositories that kill sperm. You can buy them without a prescription. Many condoms are lubricated with a spermicide.

Used by itself, spermicide is not a very good birth control method. For better protection, use it with another form of birth control, like a condom, diaphragm, or cervical cap. Spermicide does not protect you from STDs at all and may irritate the vagina.

## Surgery

◆ For men: In a vasectomy, the tubes (vas deferens) that carry sperm from the testicles are clamped or cut off. (See the picture on page 224.) This means there is no sperm in the semen when you ejaculate.

◆ For women: Tubal ligation ties off the tubes that carry eggs from the ovaries to the uterus. (See the picture on page 329.) This keeps eggs from being fertilized or implanting in the uterus.

Surgery is the most effective form of birth control. Both types of surgery are permanent, though you can sometimes reverse them with a second surgery.

Surgery does not protect you from STDs.

## Natural Family Planning

Natural family planning helps a couple know when the woman is most likely to get pregnant (just before or during ovulation). This is sometimes called fertility awareness.

The woman records her temperature, checks her vaginal discharge, and tracks her periods. You can also buy urine test strips that help tell when ovulation occurs.

People may use natural family planning methods to know:

◆ When *not* to have sex if they don't want to get pregnant.

◆ When to have sex if they want to get pregnant.

Like other birth control, these methods work best when you use them correctly. If you don't want to get pregnant, you must agree to use other birth control or not to have sex on fertile days. And it's hard to predict exactly when you are fertile.

Natural family planning does not protect you from STDs.

## How Well Does Birth Control Work?

| Method | Pregnancies per 100 Women* |
|---|---|
| **Surgery:**<br>**Tubal ligation** (women)<br>**Vasectomy** (men) | Fewer than 1 |
| **Birth control pills** | 8 |
| **Patch** (Ortho Evra) | 8 |
| **Shot every 3 months** (Depo-Provera) | 3 |
| **Intrauterine device (IUD):**<br>**Levonorgestrel** (Mirena)<br>**Copper T** (Paragard) | Fewer than 1 |
| **Male condom** (latex or polyurethane) | 15 |
| **Female condom** | 21 |
| **Diaphragm** (with spermicide) | 16 |
| **Cervical cap** (with spermicide) | 16 to 32 |
| **Spermicide by itself** (jelly, cream, foam, suppositories) | 29 |
| **Periodic abstinence** (natural family planning: basal body temperature, mucus, or rhythm/calendar method) | 25 |
| **Withdrawal** (pulling out) | 27 |
| **No birth control** | 85 |

*Typical number of accidental pregnancies per 100 women in 1 year. If you use birth control exactly as directed every time, pregnancy rates are lower.

Adapted from: Trussel J, Kowal D (2004). The essentials of contraception. In RA Hatcher et al., eds., *Contraceptive Technology*, 18th ed. New York: Ardent Media, Inc.

# Bladder Control

## When to Call a Doctor

- Loss of bladder control develops suddenly.

- You have to urinate frequently but cannot pass much urine.

- Your bladder does not feel empty after you urinate.

- You have trouble urinating even when your bladder feels full.

- It burns or hurts when you urinate. See Urinary Tract Infections on page 251.

- Your urine has blood in it.

- Your urine smells strange.

- You want help with your bladder control problem.

If you sometimes cannot control your bladder—a problem called **urinary incontinence**—you are not alone. It happens to many people.

The two most common bladder control problems are stress incontinence and urge incontinence.

If you have **stress incontinence**:

- Small amounts of urine leak out when you exercise, cough, laugh or sneeze. This is more common in women.

- Kegel exercises may help. See page 101.

If you have **urge incontinence**:

- The need to urinate comes on so fast that you don't have time to get to the toilet.

- There may be an illness or disease causing the problem. This can include bladder infection, prostate enlargement, tumors that press on the bladder, and nerve problems such as those caused by Parkinson's disease, multiple sclerosis, and stroke.

Bladder control problems often can be controlled or cured if you can find and correct the cause. Water pills (diuretics) and other common medicines can cause short-term problems. Constipation, urinary tract infections, kidney stones, pregnancy, and being overweight are other causes.

Try not to let a bladder control problem embarrass you. Work with your doctor to treat it.

## Home Treatment

- Avoid caffeine. It can make symptoms worse.

- Do not cut down on fluids. You need them to stay healthy. If having to get up at night bothers you, cut down on fluids before bed.

- If you smoke, quit (see page 316). This may reduce your coughing, which may help with bladder control.

- Lose weight if you need to.

- Practice "double-voiding." Empty your bladder as much as you can, relax for a minute, and then try to empty it again.

- If you have trouble controlling your bladder when you laugh, sneeze, cough, or exercise, try doing Kegel exercises every day. See page 101.

◆ Urinate on a schedule, perhaps every 3 to 4 hours during the day, whether you have the urge or not. This may help you restore control.

◆ Wear clothing that you can take off quickly, such as pants with an elastic waist.

◆ Clear a path from your bed to the bathroom, or place a portable toilet by your bed.

◆ Use absorbent pads or briefs, such as Attends or Depend. No one will know you're wearing an absorbent pad.

◆ Keep skin in the genital area dry to prevent rashes. Use Vaseline or Desitin ointment to help protect the skin from irritation caused by urine.

◆ Ask your doctor or pharmacist whether any medicines you take, including non-prescription drugs, can affect bladder control. Do not stop taking your medicine without first talking to your doctor.

## Kegel Exercises

Kegel exercises strengthen the pelvic muscles that control the flow of urine. This can help cure or improve some bladder control problems.

◆ To locate the muscles, repeatedly stop your urine in midstream and start again.

◆ Practice squeezing these muscles while you are not urinating. If your belly or buttocks move, you are not using the right muscles.

◆ Hold the squeeze for 3 seconds; then relax for 3 seconds.

◆ Repeat the exercise 10 to 15 times a session. Do at least 3 sessions each day.

You can do Kegel exercises anywhere, anytime. No one will know you're doing them but you.

# Blisters

## When to Call a Doctor

◆ You have signs of infection. These may include increased pain, swelling, redness, or warmth; red streaks leading from the blister; pus; and fever.

◆ You get blisters often and do not know why.

◆ You have a band of painful blisters on one side of your body or face. See Shingles on page 122.

◆ You have diabetes or peripheral artery disease and you get blisters on your hands, feet, or legs.

Blisters are usually caused by something rubbing against the skin.

## Home Treatment

◆ If a blister is small and closed, leave it alone. Use a loose bandage to protect it. Avoid the activity or shoes that caused the blister. (Blisters are usually caused by something rubbing against the skin.)

◆ If a small blister is in a weight-bearing area like the bottom of the foot, protect it with a doughnut-shaped moleskin pad. (Moleskin has soft felt on one side and a sticky backing on the other.) Leave the area over the blister open.

**More**

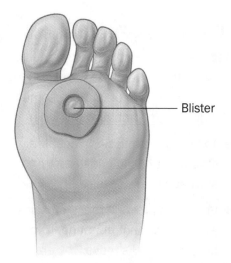

Blister

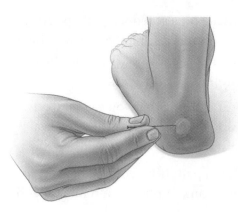

Use a needle to puncture a large blister.

Use a doughnut-shaped pad to protect the blister.

- If a blister is large and painful, it is usually best to drain it. Here is a safe method:
  - ❖ Wipe a needle or straight pin with rubbing alcohol.
  - ❖ Gently puncture the edge of the blister.
  - ❖ Press the fluid in the blister toward the hole so it can drain out.

Once you have opened a blister, or if it has torn open:

- Wash the area with soap and water. Do not use alcohol, iodine, or any other cleanser.
- Do not remove the flap of skin over a blister unless it's very dirty or torn or there is pus under it. Gently smooth the flap flat over the tender skin.
- Apply an antibiotic ointment and a clean bandage.
- Change the bandage once a day or anytime it gets wet or dirty. Remove it at night to let the area dry.

# Boils

## When to Call a Doctor

If needed, your doctor can drain the boil and treat the infection. **Call your doctor if:**

- The boil is on your face, near your spine, or in the anal area.
- You have any other lumps near the boil, especially if they hurt.
- You are in a lot of pain or have a fever.

- The area around the boil is red or has red streaks leading from it.
- You have diabetes and you get a boil.
- The boil is as large as a Ping-Pong ball.
- The boil has not improved after 5 to 7 days of home treatment.
- You get many boils over several months.

A boil is a red, swollen, painful bump under the skin. It may look like an overgrown pimple. Boils are often caused by infected hair follicles. A boil can become large and cause severe pain.

Boils occur most often where there is hair and rubbing. The face, neck, armpits, breasts, groin, and buttocks are common sites.

## Home Treatment

◆ Do not squeeze, scratch, drain, or open the boil. Squeezing can push the infection deeper into the skin. Scratching can spread the infection.

◆ Wash with an antibacterial soap. Dry the area well.

◆ Put hot, wet cloths on the boil for 20 to 30 minutes, 3 or 4 times a day. Do this as soon as you notice a boil. The heat and moisture can help bring the boil to a head, but it may take 5 to 7 days. A hot pack or a waterproof heating pad placed over a damp towel may also help.

◆ Keep using heat for 3 days after the boil opens. Apply a bandage so the draining material does not spread. Change the bandage every day.

◆ Do not wear tight clothing over the area.

# Breast Problems

## When to Call a Doctor

◆ You find a lump in your breast, armpit, or chest area that concerns you, especially if it is hard and not like the rest of your breast tissue.

◆ You find a breast lump after menopause.

◆ You have a bloody or greenish discharge from a nipple, or a watery or milky discharge that occurs without pressing on the nipple or breast.

◆ You have a change in a nipple, such as crusty or scaly skin or a nipple that turns in rather than points out.

◆ One of your breasts changes shape or seems to pucker or pull when you raise your arms.

◆ The skin looks dimpled like an orange peel.

◆ You have a change in the color or feel of the skin of a breast or the darker area around a nipple.

◆ You have new pain in one breast that lasts longer than 1 or 2 weeks and was not caused by an injury.

◆ You have any signs of infection in a breast, such as pain, redness, warmth, or swelling.

◆ You are a man and you find a lump in your chest area.

**More**

# Breast Pain

Many women's breasts get achy, heavy, or sore a week or so before their periods. This is caused by normal hormone changes. The symptoms usually go away at the end of a woman's period.

It may help to:

◆ Avoid salty foods just before your period starts.

◆ Take 400 mg of magnesium each day.

◆ Take 400 to 600 IU of vitamin E each day.

◆ Take evening primrose oil.

◆ Cut down on caffeine.

◆ Take ibuprofen (Advil, Motrin) or naproxen (Aleve) for pain.

◆ Wear a more supportive bra, especially when you exercise.

You will probably stop having this type of breast pain once you complete menopause.

Stress, estrogen therapy, and the use of certain medicines can make breast pain worse. Sore breasts can also be a sign of pregnancy.

Breast pain that is not related to your periods or an injury is usually sharp or burning. This pain tends to be on one side only and may reach up to the armpit. It may come and go. Pain in one spot that does not go away should be checked by a doctor.

# Breast Lumps

Breast lumps are common, especially in women between ages 30 and 50. Many women's breasts feel lumpy right before their periods. Women also may have lumps when they are breast-feeding. Breast lumps usually go away after menopause, but they may occur in women who take hormones after menopause.

**Most breast lumps are not cancer.** Still, you should have a doctor check any lump or thickness that is not like the rest of your breast tissue. (It may be bigger or harder, or feel different.)

How dense or lumpy a woman's breasts are tends to run in the family. If your mother had lumpy breasts, you are likely to as well. It is also common for one breast to be denser than the other. The important thing is to watch for a change in the breast tissue.

# Breast Cancer

Here are a few things you should know:

◆ Breast cancer can often be cured if you find it early.

◆ Regular mammograms and breast exams done by a health professional can help find breast cancer early and save lives.

◆ Self-exams can help you learn what is normal for your breasts and may make you aware of changes sooner. See page 330.

◆ Your risk for breast cancer goes up after age 50. In general, women younger than 50 are at lower risk for breast cancer.

◆ If your mother or a sister had breast cancer before menopause, you are at increased risk for breast cancer. Talk with your doctor about starting mammograms and other tests before age 40.

### What You Can Do to Prevent Breast Cancer

◆ Do not have more than 1 alcoholic drink a day. Moderate to heavy drinking increases your risk for breast cancer.

◆ Eat a low-fat diet (see page 305). Although it has not been proven that a diet low in fat will prevent cancer, women in populations that eat a high-fat diet are more likely to die of breast cancer than those that eat a low-fat diet.

◆ Have a breast exam by a health professional every year starting at age 40.

◆ Have a mammogram every 1 to 2 years starting at age 50. If you are age 40 to 49, discuss the best testing schedule for you with your doctor. See page 330.

◆ If you have a strong family history of breast cancer, you may need to have mammograms before age 40. Also talk with your doctor about tamoxifen or other medicines that may lower your risk of breast cancer.

# Breast-Feeding

## When to Call a Doctor

**Call your doctor if you are nursing and:**

◆ You have signs of a breast infection, such as breast pain, swelling, redness, warmth, or a fever.

◆ You gain or lose more than 1 pound a week for several weeks in a row.

◆ You need to take a medicine and have not talked to your doctor about whether it is safe.

◆ You have trouble breast-feeding and want help.

## Home Treatment for Sore Breasts

◆ Use ice or cold packs on the sore breast for 10 to 15 minutes at a time.

◆ Wear a supportive nursing bra.

◆ Take acetaminophen (Tylenol) or ibuprofen (Advil, Motrin). These will not affect your breast milk.

◆ To soften your breasts before feedings, put a warm, wet cloth on them, massage gently, and use your hands to squeeze a little milk from both breasts.

◆ Although painful for you, breast-feeding from your sore breast is safe for your baby. If starting with the sore breast hurts too much, start feeding on the other side, then switch sides after your milk lets down. If your nipple hurts too much to breast-feed from that breast, use a breast pump to empty the breast of milk each time that you cannot breast-feed.

**More**

105

# Health Tips for Breast-Feeding Mothers

◆ Take in 500 extra calories a day. Although you do not need to drink milk to make milk, extra calcium and protein are important. Your doctor may have you keep taking your prenatal vitamins.

◆ Do not smoke.

◆ Do not drink alcohol.

◆ Limit caffeine to one or two drinks a day.

◆ Talk to your doctor before you take any medicine. Some medicines may pass through the breast milk to your baby.

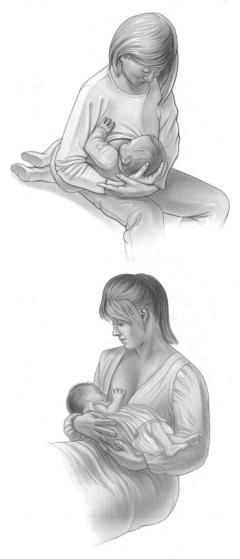

Breast milk is the perfect food for babies.

## Thinking About Breast-Feeding?

Breast milk is the perfect food for babies and the only food they need for the first 6 months.

◆ Breast milk helps your baby resist infections and other diseases. Breast-fed babies have fewer colds and ear infections.

◆ Breast milk is easier for your baby to digest than formula. Breast-fed babies have less diarrhea and vomiting.

◆ Breast-fed babies have a lower risk of problems like obesity and high blood pressure later in life.

For these reasons, the American Academy of Pediatrics recommends that babies be breast-fed for at least the first year.

But whether you breast-feed and for how long also depends on you, your child, and your situation. Babies can get great nutrition from formula too.

If this is your first baby, you may want to take a breast-feeding class before your child is born. Many hospitals offer them. The La Leche League and the Nursing Mothers Counsel are other good sources of breast-feeding advice and support.

**Go to Web** To learn how to breast-feed and how to deal with problems that might come up, go to the Web site on the back cover and enter **g021** in the search box.

# Breathing Problems

## When to Call a Doctor

### Call 911 if:

◆ You cannot breathe, or you have severe trouble breathing. For signs of severe trouble breathing, see page 19.

◆ You have shortness of breath with chest pain or pressure or other symptoms of a heart attack. See page 38.

◆ Your tongue or throat swells quickly and makes it very hard to breathe. This can be caused by an allergic reaction. See page 77.

### Call your doctor if:

◆ You wheeze when you breathe. Wheezing is a high-pitched sound you may make if you have a problem in your airways.

◆ You tire quickly when you talk or eat, or you often have to stop to catch your breath.

◆ You wake up in the night short of breath.

◆ You have trouble breathing or cough a lot when you exercise.

◆ You have any trouble breathing that lasts longer than an hour and is not related to a cold, flu, or other illness.

Be sure to check the Chest, Heart, and Lung Problems chart on page 65 if you do not find your symptoms here.

Breathing problems have many possible causes, from asthma to anxiety to heart problems. A breathing problem can be a sign of something serious, though this is not always the case. Use the When to Call a Doctor list to find out whether you need medical care and how soon.

If you have already been diagnosed with allergies, asthma, COPD (chronic obstructive pulmonary disease), or heart failure, one of these topics may help:

❖ Allergies, page 76

❖ Living Better With Asthma, page 266

❖ Living Better With Heart Failure, page 291

❖ Living Better With COPD, page 271

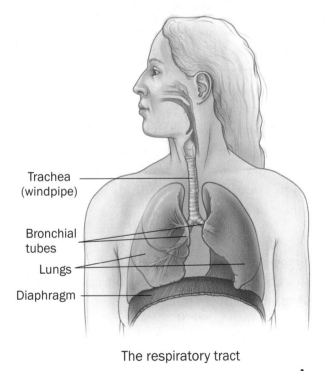

Trachea (windpipe)

Bronchial tubes

Lungs

Diaphragm

The respiratory tract

**More**

# Bronchitis

## When to Call a Doctor

Any of these symptoms may mean that your bronchitis is getting worse or that you have a bacterial infection that needs treatment.

**Call your doctor if:**

◆ A cough occurs with new wheezing or new trouble breathing.

◆ You cough up blood.

◆ You cough up yellow, green, or rust-colored mucus from your lungs (not from your nose or the back of your throat) for more than 2 days and have a fever.

◆ A cough lasts more than 7 to 10 days after other symptoms have gone away, especially if it brings up mucus. (It is normal for a dry, hacking cough to last a few weeks after a cold.)

◆ You have a fever of 104°F or higher.

◆ You have a fever higher than 101°F with shaking chills and a productive cough.

◆ You still have a fever after using home treatment. Bronchitis may cause fevers of 102°F or higher for up to a day. But call a doctor if the fever stays high. See the fever guidelines on page 160.

◆ Your breathing is fast or shallow, and you are short of breath.

◆ You have pain in the muscles of your chest (chest-wall pain) when you cough or breathe.

◆ You are more tired than you would be with a typical cold.

**Also call if:**

◆ You cannot drink enough fluids and are dehydrated, or you cannot eat at all.

◆ The sick person is a baby, an older adult, or someone who has lung problems or another long-term disease.

◆ Any cough lasts longer than 2 weeks.

Bronchitis means that the airways leading to the lungs are irritated. It is usually caused by a virus, such as a cold, and may start 3 to 4 days after a cold goes away. But bronchitis can also be caused by bacteria, cigarette smoke, or air pollution.

You may have a dry cough, mild fever, fatigue, pain or tightness in the chest, and wheezing. As your cough gets worse, it may bring up mucus (sputum).

If you get bronchitis often—especially if you smoke—you may reach a point where your airways are inflamed and irritated all the time. This is called chronic bronchitis. If you smoke, you are also at high risk for emphysema. Chronic bronchitis, emphysema, and other lung diseases are known as **COPD (chronic obstructive pulmonary disease)**. If you have COPD, see page 271.

## Home Treatment

◆ If your doctor prescribes medicine, take it as directed. But don't be surprised if your doctor does not prescribe medicine. Bronchitis often goes away without it.

◆ Drink plenty of water. Extra fluids help thin the mucus in your lungs so you can cough it out.

◆ Get some extra rest.

◆ Take aspirin, ibuprofen (Advil, Motrin), or acetaminophen (Tylenol) for fever and body aches. But do not take aspirin if you have asthma, and do not give aspirin to anyone younger than 20.

◆ Use a nonprescription cough suppressant with dextromethorphan. This will help quiet a dry, hacking cough so you can sleep. Read the label on the bottle, and don't take cough medicines that have more than one active ingredient.

◆ Breathe moist air from a humidifier, a hot shower, or a sink filled with hot water. The heat and moisture will thin mucus so you can cough it out.

◆ Do not smoke.

◆ If you have classic flu symptoms, try home treatment for flu, and see how you're doing after another day or two. See Flu on page 165.

# Bunions and Hammer Toes

### When to Call a Doctor

◆ You have sudden, severe pain in your big toe and you have not been diagnosed with gout.

◆ Your big toe starts to partly cover your second toe.

◆ You have diabetes, poor blood flow, peripheral artery disease, or a weakened immune system and you develop any kind of foot problem. Irritated skin over a bunion or hammer toe can easily get infected.

◆ You have a sore over a bunion or hammer toe.

◆ Pain does not get better after 2 to 3 weeks of home treatment.

A **bunion** is a bump on the outside of the joint at the bottom of your big toe. You get a bunion when the big toe bends toward and sometimes partly covers the second toe.

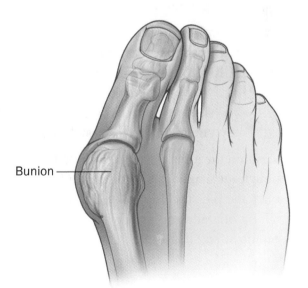

Bunion

**More**

A **hammer toe** is a toe that bends up at the middle joint.

These foot problems sometimes run in families. Tight or high-heeled shoes increase the risk of both. If you already have a foot problem, wearing tight shoes or high heels may make it worse.

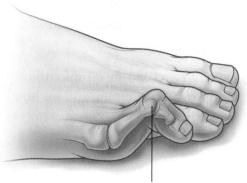

Hammer toe

## Home Treatment

Once you have a bunion or a hammer toe, there is usually no way to get rid of it. Home treatment will help relieve pain and keep the problem from getting worse.

◆ Wear roomy, low-heeled shoes that have wide, deep toe areas and good arch support. To find the best footwear for  your problem, go to the Web site on the back cover and enter **v561** in the search box.

◆ Cushion the joint with moleskin or a doughnut-shaped pad to prevent rubbing and pressure. (Moleskin has soft felt on one side and a sticky backing on the other.)

## What About Foot Surgery?

If you have tried home treatment but you have severe pain or an oddly shaped joint that affects your walking, you may want to think about surgery.

◆ Surgery can help reduce pain and help you walk better, but it may not cure the problem.

◆ If you want surgery to improve how your foot looks rather than to relieve pain, you may not be happy with the result.

◆ Surgery can sometimes cause other problems.

◆ Surgery costs a lot.

 For help deciding whether surgery is worth the cost and risks, go to the Web site on the back cover and enter **b064** in the search box.

◆ Take an old pair of shoes, and cut out the area over the toe. Wear these shoes around the house. Or wear comfortable sandals that do not press on the area.

◆ Try ibuprofen (Advil, Motrin) or acetaminophen (Tylenol) to relieve pain. Ice or cold packs may also help.

◆ Ask your doctor about bunion pads, arch supports, or custom-made supports called orthotics. These can hold your foot in a healthy position and take pressure off your big toe.

# Bursitis and Tendinosis

## When to Call a Doctor

- You have fever with sudden joint swelling or redness.

- You cannot use a joint at all.

- You have severe pain when the joint is at rest, and ice does not help.

- Pain lasts longer than 2 weeks even with home treatment. Your doctor or a physical therapist can help you create a plan for exercise and home treatment.

If you have had a sudden injury, see Strains, Sprains, and Broken Bones on page 50 or Sports Injuries on page 242.

Bursitis and tendinosis are common reasons for pain and swelling in the legs, knees, hips, wrists, elbows, and shoulders.

A bursa is a small sac of fluid that helps the tissues around a joint slide over one another easily. Injury, overuse, or constant direct pressure on a joint can cause pain, redness, heat, and swelling of the bursa. This is called **bursitis**. Bursitis often develops quickly, over just a few days.

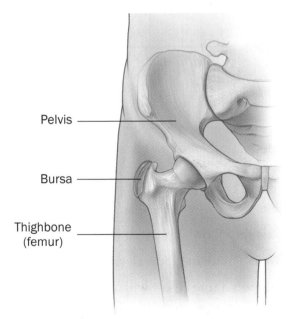

The fluid-filled bursa helps cushion a joint like the hip.

Pelvis

Bursa

Thighbone (femur)

Tendons are tough, ropelike fibers that connect muscles to bones. **Tendinosis** develops when wear and tear or overuse of a tendon causes tiny tears in the tissue. This leads to pain, inflammation, and breakdown in the tendons or the tissues surrounding them.

Both bursitis and tendinosis can be caused by jobs, sports, or things you do around the house that require a lot of twisting or fast moving of the joints or constant pressure on a joint (kneeling, for example).

The same home treatment is good for both problems.

## Home Treatment

Bursitis or tendinosis will usually get better in a few days or weeks if you avoid the activity that caused it. But the mistake many people make is thinking that the problem is gone when the pain is gone.

To keep the problem from coming back, you will need to strengthen and stretch the muscles around the joint and change the way you do some activities.

More

◆ Rest the area. Change the way you do the activity that causes pain so that you can do it without pain. See the joint-specific guidelines later in this topic. To stay fit, try activities that do not stress the area.

◆ As soon as you notice pain, use ice or cold packs for 10 minutes at a time, once an hour or as often as you can for the next 2 days. Keep using ice (10 minutes, 3 times a day) as long as it relieves pain. See Ice and Cold Packs on page 243. Heating pads or hot baths may feel good, but they don't help you heal.

◆ Take aspirin, ibuprofen (Advil, Motrin), or naproxen (Aleve) to ease pain and swelling. But do not use the medicine to control the pain while you keep over-using the joint. Do not give aspirin to anyone younger than 20.

◆ To prevent stiffness, gently move the joint through as full a range of motion as you can without pain. As the pain gets better, keep doing range-of-motion exercises, and add exercises that strengthen the muscles around the joint.

◆ When you are ready to try the activity that caused the pain, start slowly and do it for short periods only or at a slower speed. Increase the intensity slowly and only if the pain does not come back.

◆ Warm up before and stretch after the activity. Use ice after exercise to prevent pain and swelling.

Along with the home treatment information for bursitis and tendinosis above, the following tips will help for problems with a specific joint.

## Wrists

Wrist pain may be caused by tendinosis. Although this is not the same as carpal tunnel syndrome, the same home care may help. See page 116.

## Elbows

Elbow pain is often caused by tendinosis in the forearm or bursitis in the elbow.

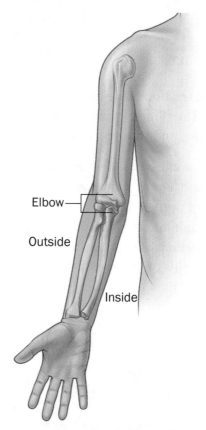

Tennis elbow causes pain on the outside of the elbow. Golfer's elbow hurts on the inside.

To relieve elbow pain and prevent further injury:

◆ Rest the elbow and give it time to heal.

◆ Wear a brace or elbow sleeve.

◆ Support a sore elbow with a sling for 1 to 2 days (see page 52). Do range-of-motion exercises daily.

◆ Strengthen the wrist, arm, shoulder, and back muscles.

◆ Avoid activities that make you repeat a wrist motion many times.

◆ Make changes in your activities so you don't irritate the tendon:

❖ Use tools with larger handles.

❖ Use a two-handed tennis back-hand stroke and a more flexible, midsize racket.

❖ Try not to hit divots when you play golf.

❖ Do not throw sidearm pitches or curveballs.

## Shoulders

Shoulder pain that occurs on the outside of the upper arm is often caused by bursitis or tendinosis around the shoulder joint. Pain on the top of the shoulder or in the neck may be caused by tension in the trapezius muscles, which run from the back of the head across the back of the shoulders. See Neck Pain on page 211.

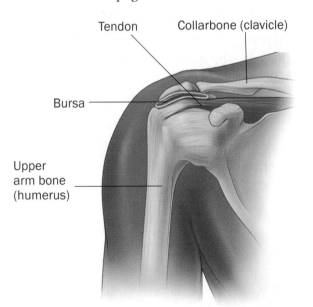

Bursitis, tendinosis, and muscle tension are common causes of shoulder pain.

Common symptoms of shoulder bursitis or tendinosis are pain, pinching, and stiffness when you raise your arm. The symptoms are often brought on by doing repeated overhead movements. Pain and swelling can occur when you keep using your shoulder without giving it time to rest.

To relieve shoulder pain and stiffness:

◆ Avoid activities that involve overhead reaching, but keep using your shoulder.

◆ Try the "pendulum" exercise: Bend forward and hold the back of a chair with the hand of your healthy arm. Let the other arm hang straight down from the shoulder. Move the hanging arm in circles; start with small circles and slowly make them bigger. Then switch directions. Again, go from small circles to large ones. Next, swing the arm forward and backward, then from side to side. Do this exercise 10 times a day.

◆ Use proper throwing techniques for baseball and football.

◆ Use a different swim stroke. Try breaststroke or sidestroke instead of the crawl or butterfly.

◆ Put your shoulder through its full range of motion every day.

## Hips

Hip pain may be caused by tendinosis or bursitis. You may feel it at the side of your hip when you rise from a chair and take the first few steps, while you climb stairs, or while you drive. If pain is severe, sleeping on your side may also hurt.

Pain in the front of the hip may also be caused by arthritis (see page 82).

Hip pain can also cause knee or thigh pain. This is called referred pain.

To relieve hip pain and avoid further problems:

◆ Wear well-cushioned shoes. Do not wear high heels.

◆ Avoid activities that force one side of your pelvis higher than the other, such as running in only one direction on a track or working sideways on a slope.

◆ Sleep on your "good" side with a pillow between your knees, or on your back with pillows under your knees.

◆ See the hip stretches on page 94. Stretch after activity, when your muscles are warm.

### Knees

Knee pain may be caused by bursitis or tendinosis. Also see Knee Problems on page 201.

### Legs and Feet

Heel or foot pain may be caused by plantar fasciitis or Achilles tendinosis. See page 185. Pain in the front of the lower leg may be due to shin splints. See page 205.

# Calluses and Corns

## When to Call a Doctor

Call your doctor if a callus or corn breaks open and starts to hurt.

Calluses and corns are areas of skin that have gotten thick and hard in response to friction and pressure. Calluses are common on the soles of the feet, the heels, and the hands. Corns are often on the toes.

## Home Treatment

◆ If you have diabetes or peripheral artery disease, talk to your doctor before you try to remove a callus or corn on your own.

◆ If a callus or corn hurts, soak your foot in warm water for 5 to 10 minutes. Then rub the callus or corn with a towel or pumice stone. You may need to repeat this a few times over several days until the thickened skin is gone.

◆ You can also use a nonprescription product for removing calluses and corns.

◆ To prevent pain and rubbing, cushion the area with a doughnut-shaped pad or moleskin patch. (Moleskin has soft felt on one side and a sticky backing on the other.)

◆ Do not try to cut or burn off a callus or corn.

# Canker Sores

## When to Call a Doctor

◆ You have mouth sores and a fever.

◆ You get mouth sores after you start a new medicine.

◆ A mouth sore does not heal in 2 weeks, or you get several sores.

◆ A sore hurts a lot or goes away and then comes back.

◆ You have white spots in your mouth that are not canker sores and that have not gone away after 1 to 2 weeks.

Canker sores are painful, open sores on the inside of the mouth. The sores usually heal in 7 to 10 days. You can get them because of mouth injury, infection, certain foods, hormone changes, and other reasons.

## Home Treatment

◆ Avoid coffee, spicy and salty foods, nuts, chocolate, and citrus fruits when you have open sores in your mouth.

◆ Use a nonprescription canker sore medicine to protect the sore, ease pain, and speed healing. Or put a thin paste of baking soda and water on the sore to relieve pain.

◆ Rinse your mouth with an antacid (such as Maalox or Mylanta) or with a mixture of 1 tablespoon of hydrogen peroxide in 8 ounces of water.

◆ Do not smoke or chew tobacco.

◆ Use a soft-bristled toothbrush to brush your teeth and gums.

# Carpal Tunnel Syndrome

## When to Call a Doctor

◆ You have tingling, numbness, weakness, or pain in your fingers and hand even after 2 weeks of home treatment.

◆ You often have little or no feeling in your fingers or hand.

◆ You cannot do simple hand movements, or you drop things a lot because you can't hold on to them.

◆ You cannot pinch your thumb and first finger together, or you have no thumb strength.

◆ You have problems at work because of pain in your fingers or hand.

More

The carpal tunnel is a narrow space in your wrist. The nerve that controls feeling in some of your fingers and controls some of the hand muscles passes through this space.

Carpal tunnel syndrome develops when there is pressure on the nerve where it goes through the carpal tunnel.

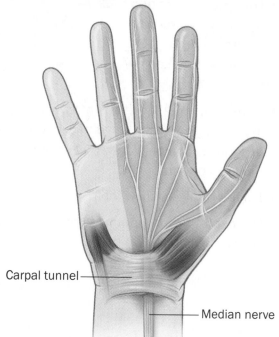

Carpal tunnel syndrome causes pain and tingling in the shaded area.

You may have:

◆ Numbness or pain in your hand or wrist that wakes you up at night.

◆ Numbness or tingling in your fingers, except for the little finger and half of the ring finger.

◆ Numbness or pain that gets worse when you use your hand or wrist, especially when you grip an object or flex your wrist.

◆ Aching pain in your arm between your hand and your elbow. The pain may come and go.

◆ A weak grip.

Activities that make you use the same finger or hand movements over and over can cause carpal tunnel syndrome or make it worse. You may do things at work, at home, or during sports or hobbies that cause this problem.

## Home Treatment

◆ Stop any activity that you think may be causing numbness or pain. If the problem improves when you stop, return to that activity slowly. Try to keep your wrist straight or only slightly bent.

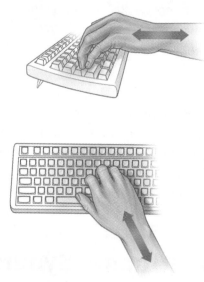

When you type, keep your fingers lower than your wrists. Try to keep your wrist straight or only slightly bent.

◆ Watch your posture. When you type, keep your fingers lower than your wrists. A keyboard wrist support and arm supports on your chair may help. When your arms are at your sides, relax your shoulders.

◆ Use your whole hand (not just your fingers and thumb) to hold objects.

◆ Reduce the speed and force of repeated hand movements. For instance, type a little slower, and don't hit the keys too hard.

- Switch hands and change positions often when you have to repeat the same motions a lot.

- Rest your hands frequently.

- Use ibuprofen (Advil, Motrin) or naproxen (Aleve) to relieve pain and reduce swelling.

- Use ice or a cold pack on the palm side of your wrist. See Ice and Cold Packs on page 243.

- Don't sleep on your hands.

- Ask your doctor about a wrist splint. This can relieve pressure and keep your wrist in a good position when you sleep.

- Do simple range-of-motion exercises with your fingers and wrist to prevent stiffening and keep your muscles strong. Stop if it hurts.

Losing weight, quitting smoking, reducing alcohol and salt, and controlling diabetes may help reduce swelling in your wrist. Use the index in the back of the book to find information that can help.

## What About Surgery?

Most cases of carpal tunnel syndrome can get better without surgery. If you are thinking about surgery, learn as much as you can about its pros and cons, including the cost of the surgery.

 To help you decide whether surgery is right for you, go to the Web site on the back cover and enter **b941** in the search box.

## Preventing Carpal Tunnel Syndrome

You are more likely to get carpal tunnel syndrome if:

- You spend a lot of time doing activities that make you repeat the same finger and hand movements.

- You work with tools or machines that vibrate in your hand, like sanders or drills.

But there are ways you can reduce your risk, as well as any pain or weakness you already have. To learn how to keep your  wrist healthy, go to the Web site on the back cover and enter **v714** in the search box.

# Cataracts

A cataract is a painless, cloudy area in the lens of the eye (see the picture on page 172). By blocking some of the light that comes into the eye, a cataract may cause cloudy, foggy, filmy, or double vision. Glare is also a common problem.

Cataracts can be caused by:

- Normal changes in your eyes as you get older.

- Eye injury.

- Certain medicines.

- Eye disease and other health problems, especially diabetes.

Some children are born with cataracts.

## Home Treatment

Home treatment may help you avoid or delay cataract surgery. There are many things you can do to make the changes in your vision easier to live with.

- Move room lights and use window shades to prevent glare.

- Use more lighting or higher-watt bulbs in your home.

## Do You Need Surgery?

For most adults, the need for cataract surgery depends on how much the cataract affects their quality of life. Most cataracts grow slowly. At first, you may just need stronger glasses. Many people get along very well with the help of glasses, contact lenses, and other vision aids.

Later, if the cataract grows and starts to seriously affect your vision, you can have surgery to remove it. Some cataracts, such as those caused by injury, need to be removed right away.

For most people with cataracts, whether and when to have surgery is up to them. For help with your decision, go to the Web site on the back cover and enter **p502** in the search box.

◆ Use contrasts in color and brightness to make things easier to find. For example, use dark switch plates on light-colored walls. Use bright labels to "color code" medicines, spices, and stove dials.

◆ Use a magnifying glass to help you read. Look for large-print books and other reading material. You sometimes can get bank checks, medicine labels, and other items in large print.

◆ Have your eyes checked regularly. Update your glasses when needed.

◆ Wear sunglasses to reduce glare and block out harmful sunlight. Buy sunglasses that screen out UVA and UVB rays.

◆ If you smoke, quit. Smoking can make cataracts worse.

# Chest Pain

## Are You Having a Heart Attack?

You may be having a heart attack if:

❏ You have chest pain that feels like pressure, tightness, squeezing, crushing, intense burning, or aching in your chest.

❏ The pain or pressure lasts longer than 5 minutes and does not go away with rest or nitroglycerin.

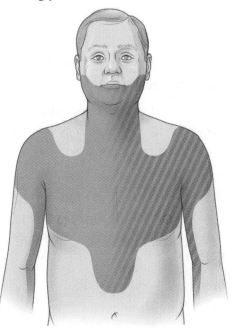

A heart attack may cause discomfort in any of the shaded areas as well as the upper back.

Other signs include:

❏ Pain spreading to your back, shoulders, neck, jaw or teeth, or arms.

❏ Sweating.

❏ Shortness of breath.

❏ Dizziness and fainting.

❏ Nausea or vomiting.

❏ Sudden, unusual weakness.

❏ Fast or uneven heartbeat.

❏ Sense of doom.

The more boxes you check, the more likely it is that you are having a heart attack. Women and people with diabetes may not have chest pain but may have some of the other symptoms.

**More**

119

## When to Call a Doctor

### Call 911 if:

◆ You think you may be having a heart attack. Do not wait to see if you feel better.

◆ You have been diagnosed with angina and you have chest pain that does not go away with rest or is not getting better within 5 minutes after taking a dose of nitroglycerin.

After calling 911, chew one adult aspirin (unless you are allergic to it). If an ambulance is not an option, have someone drive you to the hospital. Do not drive yourself unless you have no choice.

### Call a doctor if:

◆ You think you have angina and have not seen a doctor about it.

◆ You have been diagnosed with angina and are having chest pain more often than usual.

◆ You have any chest pain and have a history of heart disease or blood clots in the lungs.

◆ You have mild but constant chest pain that does not go away with rest.

◆ You have chest pain with other symptoms of pneumonia. See page 216.

◆ Mild chest pain lasts longer than 2 days without getting better.

## Angina

Angina is pain, pressure, heaviness, or numbness behind the breastbone or across the chest. It occurs when your heart does not get enough oxygen. This can happen during moments of stress, exercise, or anything that works your heart too hard. The pain goes away when you stop and rest or take a medicine called nitroglycerin.

A heart attack is caused by blocked blood flow to the heart muscle, not just lack of oxygen. The pain of a heart attack is usually more severe than angina, lasts longer, and does not go away with rest or nitroglycerin.

Angina is a sign of coronary artery disease. Having coronary artery disease means you are at high risk for a heart attack. To learn how to reduce your risk, see page 276.

## Other Causes of Chest Pain

Chest pain is not always caused by a heart problem.

◆ Heartburn (see page 183) or gas can cause chest pain.

◆ Hyperventilation (see page 23) can also cause chest pain.

◆ Chest pain that gets worse when you take a deep breath or cough may be a sign of pneumonia (see page 216) or an illness called pleurisy.

◆ An ulcer (see page 249) can cause chest pain, usually below the breastbone. The pain may be worse when your stomach is empty.

◆ Gallstones (see page 170) may cause pain in the right side of the chest or around the shoulder blade. The pain may get worse after a meal or in the middle of the night.

◆ Shingles (page 122) may cause a sharp, burning, or tingling pain that feels like a tight band around one side of the chest.

A shooting pain that lasts a few seconds, or a quick pain at the end of a deep breath, is usually not a cause for concern.

## Chest-Wall Pain

If you can point to the exact spot in your chest that hurts and it hurts more when you press on it, you probably have chest-wall pain.

If you have chest-wall pain, you may have strained a muscle in your chest or hurt a rib. Or the cartilage in your chest wall could be inflamed for no obvious reason. This is called **costochondritis**. It usually goes away in a few days.

## Home Treatment

If you have angina caused by coronary artery disease, there are many things you can do to control it. See page 275.

### For chest-wall pain caused by injury

◆ Take aspirin, ibuprofen (Advil, Motrin), or acetaminophen (Tylenol) for pain. Do not give aspirin to anyone younger than 20.

◆ Use an ice pack to help relieve pain the first 2 to 3 days after an injury.

◆ After the first 2 to 3 days (or once the swelling has gone down), you can use heat for the pain. Use a heating pad set on low or heat that is no warmer than bath water. Don't go to sleep while using a heating pad.

◆ Use products such as Bengay or Icy-Hot to help soothe sore muscles.

◆ Avoid any activity that strains the chest. As your pain gets better, slowly return to your normal activities.

# Chickenpox

## When to Call a Doctor

◆ A child who takes steroid medicines, is being treated for cancer, or has a weakened immune system gets chickenpox or is exposed to it.

◆ You are pregnant, you have never had chickenpox, and someone in your household gets chickenpox.

◆ A child age 3 months to 3 years has a fever of 103°F or higher for 24 hours. See page 158.

◆ Bruising appears for no clear reason.

◆ Your child has sores in his or her eyes.

◆ Your child has signs of a serious illness called **encephalitis** (see page 161). These include:

❖ Fever, severe headache, and stiff neck.

❖ Unusual sleepiness or lack of awareness.

❖ Vomiting.

◆ A teenager or adult gets chickenpox.

◆ You cannot control severe itching.

**More**

Chickenpox is a common viral infection. In most children, it is a minor illness.

◆ For the first couple of days, your child will feel ill with a fever and headache. He or she may not want to eat and will feel very tired.

◆ Red spots will appear. There may be as few as 30 spots, or the rash may cover the whole body, including the throat, mouth, ears, groin, and scalp. The rash itches a lot.

◆ The spots turn into blisters that break open and crust over.

◆ More spots will appear for 1 to 5 days and then go away over 1 to 2 weeks.

Chickenpox spreads easily. Symptoms usually start 14 to 16 days after you come in contact with the virus. You can spread chickenpox 2 to 3 days before the rash appears (when there is a fever) and until all the spots have crusted over.

Children can usually go back to school or day care after the sixth day of the rash, as long as clothing covers any blisters that have not crusted over. The same rule applies to adults going back to work.

### Preventing Chickenpox

◆ **Children 12 months and older:** Make sure they get the chickenpox vaccine. See page 325.

◆ **Teens and adults who have not had the vaccine or the illness:** Get the vaccine. Until then, avoid anyone who has chickenpox or shingles (see this page). Chickenpox can be serious if you get it as an adult.

◆ **Pregnant women who have not had the vaccine or the illness:** Avoid anyone who has chickenpox or shingles. The virus can harm your unborn baby, and the vaccine is not safe for pregnant women.

## Shingles

If you have ever had chickenpox, you still have the virus in your body. If the virus becomes active again, years after the original illness, it is called **shingles**.

Shingles usually affects one or two of the large nerves that spread outward from the spine. This causes pain and a rash in a band around one side of the chest, belly, or face. The rash will blister and scab, then clear up over the course of a few weeks.

If you think you have shingles, call your doctor right away. There is medicine that can limit the pain and rash. It works best if you start it as soon as symptoms appear.

Avoid close contact with people until your blisters have healed. A person who has not had chickenpox can get shingles from exposure to your rash. Be extra careful to avoid contact with pregnant women, babies, and anyone who has a hard time fighting infection (such as someone with HIV, diabetes, or cancer).

## Home Treatment

◆ Use acetaminophen (Tylenol) to relieve fever if your child feels bad or has a high or fast-rising temperature. Do not give aspirin to anyone younger than 20. It can put your child at risk for a rare but very serious illness called Reye's syndrome.

◆ Reduce itching with an oral antihista-mine (such as Benadryl) and warm baths with baking soda or Aveeno colloidal oatmeal added to the water. Do not use antihistamine creams, because they make it hard to control how much medicine you are using.

◆ Cut your child's nails short to prevent scratching. If he or she scratches off the scabs too early, the sores may get infected.

**Looking for the Chronic Obstructive Pulmonary Disease (COPD) topic? See page 271.**

# Cold Sores

## When to Call a Doctor

◆ You have cold sores and a fever.

◆ A sore lasts longer than 2 weeks.

◆ You often have outbreaks of cold sores. Your doctor can prescribe a medicine that may help.

Cold sores (fever blisters) are small, red blis-ters on the lips and outer edge of the mouth. They often weep a clear fluid and scab over after a few days.

Sometimes people confuse cold sores with impetigo (see page 195), which is usually between the nose and upper lip. The fluid from impetigo is cloudy and honey-colored, not clear like the fluid from a cold sore.

The herpes simplex virus causes cold sores. Herpes viruses (chickenpox is another kind) stay in the body after the first infec-tion. Later, something triggers the virus to become active again. You can get a cold sore after a cold, a fever, or stress. A woman's menstrual period can be another trigger. Sometimes you get cold sores for no clear reason.

Sunlight triggers cold sores in some people. Wear lip balm with sunscreen in it when you are going to be outdoors.

## Home Treatment

◆ Do not kiss or have oral sex with anyone while you have a cold sore. This can spread the virus.

◆ Put ice or a cool, wet cloth on the area 3 times a day. This may help reduce red-ness and swelling.

◆ Use petroleum jelly to ease cracking and dryness.

◆ Use a lip protector such as Blistex or Campho-Phenique to ease the pain. Do not share the product with anyone else.

◆ Apply vitamin E gel or a product that has aloe vera, goldenseal, or bee propolis.

◆ Be patient. Cold sores usually go away in 7 to 10 days.

# Colds

## When to Call a Doctor

- You have trouble breathing.
- You have a high fever. See page 160.
- You have new shortness of breath, or it gets worse.
- You cough up yellow, green, or bloody mucus (sputum) from your lungs and have a fever.
- Mucus from your nose is thick (like pus) or bloody.

- You have redness in your face or around your eyes, or you have pain in your face, eyes, or teeth that does not get better with home treatment.
- Your symptoms are worse than what you would expect with a cold, and you don't think you have the flu. See Flu on page 165.

Everyone gets a cold from time to time. The average child has six colds a year; adults have fewer.

Lots of different viruses cause colds, but the symptoms are usually the same:

- Runny nose and sneezing
- Red eyes
- Sore throat and dry cough
- Headaches and body aches

You will probably feel a cold come on over the course of a couple of days. As the cold gets worse, your nose may get stuffy with thicker mucus. Most colds last a week or two.

There is no cure for the common cold. Antibiotics will not help. If you catch a cold, treat the symptoms.

If you feel like you have a cold all the time, or if cold symptoms last more than 2 weeks, you may have allergies (see page 76) or sinusitis (see page 232).

## Home Treatment

Sometimes a cold will lead to a worse infection like bronchitis or pneumonia. Good home treatment of a cold can help prevent this and will help you feel better.

- Get extra rest. Slow down just a little from your usual routine. You don't need to stay home in bed, but try not to expose others to your cold.
- Drink plenty of fluids. Hot water, herbal tea, or chicken soup will help relieve a stuffy nose and head.
- Take aspirin, ibuprofen (Advil, Motrin), or acetaminophen (Tylenol) to relieve aches. Do not give aspirin to anyone younger than 20.
- Use a humidifier in your bedroom and take hot showers to relieve a stuffy nose and head.
- If you have streaks of mucus in the back of your throat (postnasal drip), gargle with warm water.

- Use throw-away tissues, not handkerchiefs. This will reduce the chance of spreading the cold to others.

- If your nose is red and raw from rubbing it with tissues, put a dab of petroleum jelly on the sore area.

- Do not take cold remedies that use several drugs to treat different symptoms. Treat each symptom on its own. Take a decongestant for a stuffy nose and a cough medicine for a cough. See Home Treatment for coughs on page 132.

- Do not use nasal decongestant sprays for more than 3 days in a row. Doing so may lead to a "rebound" effect, which makes the mucous membranes in your nose swell up even more.

- Do not take antihistamines for a cold. They don't help.

## How to Avoid Colds

- Wash your hands often! Be extra careful during the winter and when you are around people with colds.

- Keep your hands away from your nose, eyes, and mouth. These are the most likely places for a cold virus to enter your body.

- Eat well, and get plenty of sleep and exercise. This keeps your body's immune system strong.

- Do not smoke.

# Colic

## When to Call a Doctor

Colic does not need medical care unless it occurs with vomiting, diarrhea, or other signs of a more serious illness. If your baby looks healthy and acts normally when he or she is not crying, and if your emotions can stand the noise for the first 3 to 4 months, you do not need to worry.

But if colic lasts more than 4 hours a day, or if you feel like you need help, call your doctor for advice.

In rare cases, colic may be so severe that you and your doctor may consider a medicine for the baby. Ask about side effects.

## Does Your Baby Have Colic?

All babies cry, but colic usually follows the "rule of three": Crying starts in the first 3 to 6 weeks after birth and goes on for more than 3 hours a day, on more than 3 days a week, for more than 3 weeks. The crying tends to be worse at night.

There is no way to prevent colic. It is equally common among boys and girls and among breast-fed and bottle-fed babies.

The good news is that colic goes away as the baby gets older, almost always by the end of the fourth month. It ends sooner for many babies.

**More**

## Home Treatment

A colicky baby may cry no matter what you do, but there are several things you can try. What works one time may not work the next. Be creative, and don't give up.

◆ Most important: Stay calm. If you start to lose control, take a minute to calm down. Never shake a baby. It can cause brain damage and even death. If you have the option, let family members or friends take a turn trying to comfort the baby.

◆ Make sure your baby is getting enough to eat, but not too much. The problem may be hunger, not colic.

◆ Make sure your baby does not swallow too much air while eating.

  ❖ Feed the baby slowly, holding him or her almost upright. Burp your baby regularly. Prop your baby up for 15 minutes after feeding.

  ❖ If your baby is bottle-fed, use nipples with holes large enough to drip cold formula at least 1 drop per second. Babies will swallow more air from around the nipple if the hole is too small.

◆ Heat formula to body temperature. Don't make it too hot.

◆ Babies may need to suck on something for up to 2 hours a day to be satisfied. If feedings are not enough, use a pacifier.

◆ Set a schedule for meals, naps, and play. Keep feedings calm and quiet.

◆ Make sure that your baby does not have a dirty diaper, is not too hot, and is not bored.

◆ Try to keep the environment around your baby calm. Some babies cry because there is too much light, noise, or activity, or too many people around them.

◆ Try rocking or walking your baby. Putting him or her stomach-down over your knee or arm may help.

◆ Calm your baby with a car ride or a walk outside. The hum of a clothes dryer, dishwasher, or bubbling fish tank may soothe your baby.

◆ Don't worry about spoiling a baby during the first few months of life. Comforting a baby makes both of you feel better.

◆ Do not leave your baby alone for more than 5 to 10 minutes while he or she is crying. After 10 minutes, try the suggestions here again.

# Colorectal Cancer

When to Call a Doctor

## When to Call a Doctor

◆ Your bowel habits have changed for no clear reason.

◆ You have bleeding from your rectum or blood in your stools.

◆ You have constant or frequent diarrhea, constipation, or a feeling that your bowel does not empty completely.

◆ Your stools have become very thin (they may be as thin as a pencil).

◆ You have frequent belly pain or new problems with gas or bloating.

◆ You are losing weight and don't know why.

◆ You have a family member with colon cancer and want to know how to prevent it in yourself.

◆ You want to talk about your test options.

Cancer of the colon and rectum is a leading cause of cancer deaths in the United States. Treatment works very well early in the disease and can cure the cancer. But because the cancer usually does not cause symptoms early on, it is often not found until later.

This is why screening tests are important. These tests can help find cancer early, when treatment can work the best. They can also find growths and changes in the colon before they lead to cancer.

## Screening Tests

Your doctor may suggest one or more of these tests:

**Colonoscopy.** For this test, doctors use a flexible lighted tube to view the rectum, the colon, and part of the small intestine. They can remove any growths or polyps at the same time. Colonoscopy is the most thorough screening test. It also costs the most and is probably the least convenient (you have to do some preparation at home). But if the first result is normal and you are not at high risk, you would only need to have the test every 10 years.

**Flexible sigmoidoscopy.** As in a colonoscopy, the doctor uses a lighted tube to look for growths and cancers. But the doctor can only view the rectum and part of the colon. If the test finds any growths, you may need a colonoscopy. If the first result is normal and you are not at high risk, you would need to have a sigmoidoscopy every 5 years.

**Fecal occult blood test.** This test can find hidden blood in your stool. It does not cost much and is easy to do at home, but it's only a first step. If the test finds blood in your stool, you will need more tests. If this is your only screening test (not recommended), you need it every year.

**Barium enema.** This is an X-ray exam of the colon and rectum. The colon is filled with a white liquid called barium so that it shows more clearly on the X-ray. Barium enema is not used very often to screen for colorectal cancer. If you are not at high risk, you would need to have the test every 5 years.

More

## Who Should Get Tested?

◆ All adults starting at age 50.

◆ Adults older than 40 who are at high risk. You are at high risk if you have a family history of this cancer or if you have had colon polyps, ulcerative colitis, or Crohn's disease.

Which test should you have? Some tests may cost less, but you need to have them more often. And in some cases, you may wind up having to have a more expensive test anyway.

*Go to Web* For help deciding which tests are right for you and how often you need them, go to the Web site on the back cover and enter **i924** in the search box. Then talk with your doctor.

# Confusion and Memory Loss

## When to Call a Doctor

### Call 911 if:

◆ Confusion occurs with other signs of a stroke, such as sudden, severe headache; new trouble seeing or speaking; new weakness or numbness; and loss of balance.

◆ Confusion and memory loss develops quickly, over a few hours or days. This can be a sign of many serious problems, such as a medicine problem, an infection, an alcohol or drug problem, or a worsening of a long-term illness like heart disease or diabetes.

### Call a doctor if:

◆ You are worried that confusion or memory loss is caused by medicine or a health problem.

◆ Confusion or memory loss occurs with changes in behavior or personality.

◆ You have new trouble with familiar things, like how to read or how to tell time, or you get lost in places you know well.

◆ Confusion or memory loss starts to upset your daily life.

It's normal to forget a person's name or lose a set of keys from time to time. But more serious confusion or memory loss needs to be checked out by a doctor. If it comes on quickly, it may be caused by something that needs urgent care.

We all forget things as we get older. It also may take a little longer to remember things as you age. This is normal. But if your memory keeps getting worse—especially if you start to have other problems too—see your doctor.

## Home Treatment

The best way to keep your mind sharp and avoid the problems that can cause confusion is to stay healthy and fit.

◆ Eat a healthy diet, and drink plenty of water (unless your doctor has told you to limit fluids).

◆ Get enough sleep. If you have trouble sleeping, see Sleep Problems on page 236.

◆ Try to reduce stress. Slow down and focus on what you're doing. People often forget things because they have too much on their minds. See Dealing With Stress on page 318.

◆ Keep your body active. Try to get some exercise most days of the week.

◆ Keep your brain active. This is the "use it or lose it" approach.

❖ Learn new things. Read. Take a class.

❖ Play "brain" games like cards and Scrabble. Do crossword puzzles or other word or number games.

❖ Spend time with other people.

◆ Do not drink alcohol.

◆ Do not use illegal drugs.

◆ Some people take an herb called ginkgo biloba to help with memory. Talk to your doctor before using this or any other treatment to make sure that it's safe for you. Ginkgo seems to have few side effects, but it can cause bleeding problems and may not react well with other medicines.

◆ If you feel depressed (see Are You Depressed? on page 156), tell your doctor. Treatment can help.

## Alzheimer's Disease

Alzheimer's disease damages the part of the brain involved in memory, problem solving, judgment, language, and behavior. It is the most common type of **dementia** in older adults.

Alzheimer's usually starts with mild memory loss and gets worse over a few years. Medicines may for a short time improve some of the thinking and memory problems, but they do not cure the disease. Over time, Alzheimer's robs people of the ability to take care of themselves. They may become confused and frightened and may strike out at others.

You may wonder how to tell whether memory loss is normal or related to Alzheimer's. Early on, it's not always clear.

But there are some warning signs you can look for. Here are a few:

◆ Trouble learning or remembering new information

◆ Trouble with familiar tasks like cooking a meal or driving a car

◆ Problems with language and finding the right words to say

◆ Poor or decreased judgment, such as dressing improperly for the weather or giving away large sums of money to strangers

◆ Losing things in strange places, like putting an iron in the freezer or a wristwatch in the sugar bowl

◆ Confusion about time and place

**More** ➤

## Be Careful With Medicines

Misuse of medicines is a common cause of confusion. This is especially true in older adults, but it can happen at any age. You can help prevent problems by using medicines safely.

◆ Take as few medicines as possible. Do not take medicines that you don't need. If you have a medicine and are not sure what it's for, take it to your pharmacist or doctor and ask.

◆ Keep a list of the medicines, vitamins, and herbal products you use. Review the list with your doctor, and bring a copy to anyone who treats you or any pharmacist who fills a prescription for you. Some medicines do not work well together and can cause a bad reaction.

◆ Always take your medicines exactly as your doctor says. Take them at the right time and in the right amount. If you are supposed to take a medicine with food, then do so.

◆ For people who have to take several medicines, it can be hard to keep track of them all. Use a calendar or notepad to list each medicine and what time of day you should take it. Post it on your refrigerator or bathroom cabinet—any place where you will see it several times a day. Your pharmacist may be able to suggest products, such as medicine organizers, to help you stay on schedule.

◆ Never take someone else's prescription medicine.

# Constipation

## When to Call a Doctor

◆ Constipation gets worse or does not improve with home treatment.

◆ Rectal bleeding is heavy (more than a few bright red streaks), the blood is reddish brown or black, or your stools look like black tar.

◆ Rectal bleeding lasts longer than 2 to 3 days after constipation has improved, or any bleeding occurs more than once.

◆ You have sharp or severe belly pain.

◆ You still have rectal pain after you pass a stool, or pain keeps you from passing stools at all.

◆ You have any leaking of stool.

◆ Stools have become consistently thinner (they may be no wider than a pencil).

◆ You cannot pass stools unless you take laxatives.

Constipation means you have trouble passing stools. Some people pass stools 3 times a day; others do it 3 times a week. No matter what your normal schedule is, if your stools are soft and pass easily, you are not constipated.

Constipation causes cramping and pain in the rectum that gets worse when you try to pass hard, dry stools. If a stool gets stuck in the rectum, mucus and fluid may leak out around it. This may cause you to go back and forth between constipation and diarrhea.

Lack of fiber and too little water in the diet are common reasons for constipation. Other causes include not getting enough exercise, delaying bowel movements, taking certain medicines, and using laxatives too often. Irritable bowel syndrome (see page 197) may also cause constipation.

Toilet training may lead to constipation in young children. Kids who are playing or busy and ignore the urge to pass stools may get constipated. Children and adults who do not like to use toilets away from home may get constipated.

## Home Treatment

◆ Eat more fiber (see page 308).

❖ Eat plenty of fruits, vegetables, and whole grains.

❖ Eat bran cereal that has at least 10 grams of bran in a serving.

❖ Add 2 tablespoons of wheat bran to cereal or soup.

❖ Try a product that contains a bulk-forming agent, such as Citrucel, FiberCon, or Metamucil. Start with 1 tablespoon or less, and drink extra water to avoid bloating.

◆ Avoid foods that are high in fat and sugar.

◆ Drink plenty of water and other fluids.

◆ Get some exercise every day. A walking program is a good start.

◆ Set aside a relaxed time for each bowel movement. Urges usually occur sometime after meals. A daily routine (after breakfast, for example) may help.

◆ Go when you feel the urge, and teach your children to do the same. The bowel sends signals when a stool needs to pass. If you ignore it, the urge will go away and the stool will become dry and hard.

◆ If you need more help, use a stool softener or a very mild laxative such as Milk of Magnesia. Do not give laxatives or enemas to a child without talking to your child's doctor first. And don't use mineral oil or any other laxative for more than 2 weeks unless your doctor tells you to.

If your child is constipated and has pain, try this:

◆ Put the child in a warm bath, and add about ½ teaspoon of baking soda to the tub. This may help relax the muscles that keep stool inside the rectum.

◆ If your child is 6 months old or older and the warm bath doesn't work, use 1 or 2 glycerin suppositories to make the stool easier to pass. Use these suppositories only once or twice. If they don't help, talk to your doctor.

**Looking for the Coronary Artery Disease topic? See page 275.**

# Cough

## When to Call a Doctor

◆ You have a fever and a cough that brings up yellow, green, or bloody mucus from the lungs.

◆ A cough lasts more than 7 to 10 days after other symptoms have cleared, especially if the cough brings up mucus from the lungs. (It is normal to have a dry, hacking cough for several weeks after a cold.)

◆ Any cough lasts longer than 2 weeks.

Coughing is the body's way of keeping the lungs clear.

◆ **Productive coughs** bring up mucus (sputum) from the lungs. If you have this kind of cough, you should not try to stop it with cough medicine.

◆ **Nonproductive coughs** are dry coughs that do not bring up mucus. You may get a dry, hacking cough after a cold or after being exposed to dust or smoke. A dry cough that follows a viral illness like a cold may last several weeks and get worse at night.

Longtime smokers often have a frequent dry cough. If you have a "smoker's cough," it means your lungs are always irritated.

A common type of blood pressure medicine can cause a dry cough. If your cough began after you started taking an ACE inhibitor for high blood pressure, tell your doctor. You may need to switch to another medicine.

Chronic coughs are often caused by the backflow (reflux) of stomach acid into the lungs and throat. If you think problems with stomach acid reflux may be causing your cough, see Heartburn on page 183.

## Home Treatment

◆ Drink plenty of water. Water helps loosen mucus and soothe the throat. Or try hot tea or hot water with honey or lemon juice in it. Do not give honey to a child younger than 1 year.

◆ Suck on cough drops or hard candy if your throat hurts. Expensive, medicine-flavored cough drops do not work any better than cheap, candy-flavored ones or hard candy.

◆ To ease a dry cough at night, use extra pillows to raise your head.

◆ Do not take cold remedies that use several drugs to treat different symptoms. Treat each symptom on its own.

◆ Use cough medicines wisely. Coughing can be good, because it brings up mucus from the lungs and helps prevent infection. People with asthma and other lung diseases need to cough. But if you have a dry, hacking cough that doesn't bring anything up, ask your doctor to suggest a good cough suppressant.

◆ Do not take anyone else's prescription cough medicine.

◆ Avoid dust and smoke, or wear a mask to protect yourself.

◆ If you smoke, quit. See page 316 for help.

| Type of Cough | Possible Causes and Treatment |
|---|---|
| Baby's loud cough like a seal's bark | Croup (see below) |
| Dry cough in the morning that gets better as the day goes on | Dry air; smoking. Drink more fluids. Humidify the bedroom. Stop smoking. Also see Cough, p. 132. |
| Hacking, dry cough; may be worse at night. Common for several weeks after a cold. | Postnasal drip, smoking, or mild asthma. Drink more fluids. Try a decongestant. Stop smoking. Also see Cough, p. 132, and Asthma, p. 266. |
| Productive cough after a cold or flu | Bronchitis, p. 108; pneumonia, p. 216; sinusitis, p. 232 |
| Dry cough that starts suddenly after a choking episode, most often in a baby or young child | Object in the throat. See Choking, p. 28. |

# Croup

## When to Call a Doctor

### Call 911 if:

◆ Your child stops breathing or starts to turn blue. Give rescue breaths (see page 19) until help arrives.

◆ Your child has serious trouble breathing. It can be hard to know for sure, but a child who is having trouble breathing may:

❖ Breathe very fast.

❖ Drool or grunt with each breath.

❖ Not be able to speak, cry, or make sounds.

❖ Use the neck, chest, and belly muscles to breathe. The skin may "suck in" between the ribs with each breath, and the child may need to sit up and lean forward to tilt the nose up.

❖ Flare the nostrils with each breath.

❖ Have a gray, blotchy, or blue color to the skin. Look for color changes in the nail beds, lips, and earlobes.

### Call a doctor if:

◆ Your child has a bad cough and some trouble breathing and does not get any better after 30 minutes of home treatment.

◆ Your child's cough has not started getting better after 2 days.

More

Croup can be scary but is not usually serious. The main symptom of croup is a harsh cough that sounds like a seal's bark. A fever up to 101°F is also common.

Croup may last 2 to 5 days. It usually gets worse at night, but it tends to get better with each passing night.

Croup occurs most often in children from 6 months to 4 years of age. It usually happens when a child has a viral infection, like a cold.

## Home Treatment

◆ Do whatever you can to calm your child. Crying can make it harder to breathe.

◆ Get moisture into the air to make it easier for your child to breathe. Use water in a cool humidifier. Set your child in your lap, and let the cool vapor blow into your child's face. Do not use a hot vaporizer.

◆ If your child does not improve after several minutes, take him or her into the bathroom and turn on all the hot-water faucets to create steam. Close the door, and sit with your child while he or she breathes the moist air for several minutes.

◆ If your child's breathing still does not improve, bundle him or her up and go outside into the cool night air for a few minutes.

# Dandruff

## When to Call a Doctor

Call if daily shampooing or shampooing with a dandruff shampoo does not control dandruff.

You get dandruff when the skin cells of the scalp flake off. This flaking is natural and occurs all over your body. On the scalp, though, flakes can mix with oil and dust to form dandruff. Some people are more likely to get it than others.

## Cradle Cap

Cradle cap is an oily, yellow scaling or crusting on a baby's scalp. It is caused by a buildup of normal oils on the skin.

### If your baby has cradle cap:

◆ Wash your baby's head with baby shampoo once a day. Wet your baby's head, then gently scrub the scalp with a soft-bristled brush for a few minutes to remove the scales. A soft toothbrush works well. Shampoo and rinse well.

◆ It may help to rub mineral oil on your baby's scalp an hour before you shampoo it. This will loosen the scales.

◆ If baby shampoo doesn't work, try a dandruff shampoo, such as Selsun Blue, Head & Shoulders, or Sebulex. Be careful to keep these shampoos out of your baby's eyes.

◆ If the rash looks irritated and red, a mild hydrocortisone cream (such as Cortaid) may help.

## Home Treatment

◆ Wash your hair every day with any shampoo you choose. This is often enough to control dandruff.

◆ If you have a lot of dandruff or itching, try a dandruff shampoo such as Head & Shoulders, Sebulex, T/Gel, or Tegrin. Work the shampoo into your scalp, and leave it on for several minutes. Then rinse well.

◆ You can treat eyebrows, ears, and beards with a gentle shampoo.

**Looking for the Depression topic? See page 280.**

**Looking for the Diabetes topic? See page 284.**

# Diaper Rash

### When to Call a Doctor

◆ The diaper rash is very red or raw, looks very sore, or has blisters, pus, peeling areas, or crusty patches.

◆ The rash is mainly in the skin creases. This may mean your baby has a yeast infection.

◆ A rash does not get better after 3 days.

Diaper rash is a skin reaction, usually to the moisture and bacteria in a baby's urine and stools, to the soap used to wash diapers, or to the diapers. The rash is uncomfortable but usually not serious.

Symptoms of the rash are a red bottom and thighs. It will be easy to recognize diaper rash after you have seen it the first time.

## Home Treatment

If your baby gets diaper rash often, these are good tips to follow all the time.

◆ Change wet or dirty diapers as soon as you can. Check the diaper at least every 2 hours. Use a washcloth and water to rinse the skin in the diaper area at every diaper change. Let the diaper area air-dry for 5 to 10 minutes when you can. Wash the area with a mild soap once a day.

◆ Do not use plastic pants. They trap moisture against the skin.

◆ Protect healthy skin near the rash with Desitin, Diaparene, A & D Ointment, or zinc oxide cream. Put the cream only on dry, unbroken skin. Stop using the cream if a rash develops or if it seems to slow down the healing.

◆ Try another brand of diapers. Some babies handle one kind better than another. Unscented, white diapers may not irritate the skin as much as scented or colored ones.

◆ Do not use bulky diapers or ones with lots of layers.

◆ If you use cloth diapers, wash them with mild detergent, and rinse twice. Do not use bleach or fabric softeners.

◆ Try changing laundry soaps if a rash does not clear.

# Diarrhea, Age 11 and Younger

## When to Call a Doctor

### Call 911 if:

◆ Your child faints or you cannot wake him or her.

◆ Your child has signs of severe dehydration. These include sunken eyes, no tears, and a dry mouth and tongue; a sunken soft spot on your baby's head; little or no urine for 8 hours; skin that sags when you pinch it; and fast breathing and a fast heartbeat.

### Call a doctor if:

◆ The diarrhea is bloody or dark red, or looks like tar.

◆ The urine is bloody or cola-colored.

◆ Your child refuses to drink or cannot take in enough liquid to replace lost fluids.

◆ Severe diarrhea (large loose stools every 1 to 2 hours) lasts longer than:

  ❖ 4 hours in a baby younger than 3 months.

  ❖ 8 hours in a baby 3 to 6 months old.

  ❖ 24 hours in a child 7 months to 11 years old.

◆ Mild to moderate diarrhea continues without obvious cause or other symptoms for longer than:

  ❖ 24 hours in a baby younger than 3 months.

  ❖ 1 to 2 days in a baby 3 to 6 months old.

  ❖ 4 days in a child 7 months to 11 years old.

◆ Your child has a fever of 103°F or higher. Also see the fever guidelines on page 160.

◆ Your child has a low fever with diarrhea for more than 12 hours.

◆ Your child has severe belly pain.

◆ Your child has pain in just one part of the belly, especially the lower right belly. See the picture on page 69. It may be hard to tell where the pain is in a small child.

Diarrhea in children is often caused by:

◆ Eating unusual kinds or amounts of food. A baby's digestive system sometimes cannot handle large amounts of juice, fruit, or even milk. Breast-fed babies are less likely to get diarrhea.

◆ Viral stomach flu or another illness. Stomach flu often starts with vomiting that is followed in a few hours (sometimes 8 to 12 hours or longer) by diarrhea. Sometimes there is no diarrhea.

Babies and young children need special care when they have diarrhea because they can quickly get dehydrated. This means the body has lost too much fluid. If your child has bad diarrhea, watch for signs that he or she is looking sicker, and make sure your child gets enough fluids.

## Home Treatment

### Diarrhea in babies up to 1 year

◆ If your baby is breast-fed, breast-feed more often than usual to replace lost fluids.

◆ If your baby is formula-fed, feed him or her more often than usual with small amounts at each feeding to make up for lost fluids.

◆ If there are signs of dehydration (see When to Call a Doctor), give your child a children's oral electrolyte solution (such as Pedialyte, Infalyte, or a store brand) along with the feedings. The amount your baby needs depends on his or her weight and how dehydrated he or she is. You can give the electrolyte solution a little at a time in a dropper, spoon, or bottle. For children over 6 months, add a pinch of NutraSweet, sugar-free Kool-Aid, or gelatin powder to make it taste better.

◆ Do not use oral electrolyte solutions as the only source of fluid for more than 12 to 24 hours.

◆ Do not use sports drinks, fruit juice, or soda to treat dehydration. These drinks have too much sugar and not enough of the minerals your baby needs.

◆ Do not give your baby plain water.

◆ Offer your baby solid foods that are easy to digest (cereal, strained bananas, mashed potatoes) if he or she was eating them before.

◆ Protect the diaper area with Desitin, Diaparene, A & D Ointment, or zinc oxide cream. Babies often get diaper rash after diarrhea.

### Diarrhea in children 1 through 11 years

◆ Give ½ cup to 1 cup of a children's oral electrolyte solution, fruit juice mixed to half strength with water, or plain water (if the child is eating food) each hour. Add NutraSweet flavoring if needed. Let your child drink as much as he or she wants.

◆ Do not use an electrolyte solution as the only source of fluids and nutrients for more than 24 hours.

◆ Do not give your child full-strength juice, chicken broth, sports drinks, soft drinks, or ginger ale. These drinks do not have the right mix of minerals and sugar to restore lost fluids and may make the diarrhea worse.

◆ Give your child frequent small meals with foods that are easy to digest. Cooked cereal, crackers, mashed potatoes, applesauce, and bananas are good choices. Avoid foods that have a lot of sugar.

As the child gets better, the stools will be smaller and less frequent. Some types of diarrhea may cause watery stools for 4 to 6 days. You can treat the illness at home as long as the child gets enough fluids and nutrients, is urinating normal amounts, and seems to be getting better.

# Diarrhea, Age 12 and Older

## When to Call a Doctor

**Call 911** if you have signs of severe dehydration. These include little or no urine for 8 hours, sunken eyes, no tears, and a dry mouth and tongue; skin that sags when you pinch it; feeling very dizzy or lightheaded; fast breathing and heartbeat; and not feeling or acting alert.

**Call a doctor if**:

◆ Symptoms of mild dehydration (dry mouth, dark urine, not much urine) get worse even with home treatment.

◆ Belly pain gets worse or focuses in one area, especially the lower right or lower left part of the belly. This could be serious.

◆ You have large, loose bowel movements every 1 to 2 hours for more than 24 hours.

◆ Your stools are bloody or black.

◆ You have diarrhea and a fever.

◆ Diarrhea gets worse or more frequent.

◆ You get diarrhea after drinking untreated water.

◆ Diarrhea lasts longer than 2 weeks.

For diarrhea in a child 11 years or younger, see page 136.

Diarrhea has many causes—stomach flu, food poisoning, antibiotics and other medicines, certain foods, and food additives such as sorbitol and olestra. For some people, stress or anxiety can be a cause. Irritable bowel syndrome (see page 197) may cause frequent or long-term diarrhea.

Drinking untreated water that contains parasites, viruses, or bacteria is another cause. Just because water looks clean does not mean it is. You may get diarrhea a few days to a few weeks later.

## Home Treatment

◆ Do not eat any food for several hours or until you feel better. Keep taking small sips of water or a rehydration drink (see page 33).

◆ Do not take diarrhea medicines like Pepto-Bismol or Imodium during the first 6 hours. After that, use them only if you do not have a fever, cramping, bloody stools, or other symptoms.

 ❖ Do not take more than the label tells you to.

 ❖ Stop the medicine as soon as stools thicken.

After the first 24 hours (or sooner, if you feel better), try some mild foods. Bananas, rice, applesauce, dry toast, and crackers are all good choices. Avoid spicy foods, fruits other than bananas, alcohol, and caffeine until 48 hours after all symptoms have gone away. Avoid milk and dairy products for at least 3 days.

Be careful not to get dehydrated. This can happen when your body loses a lot of fluids. See page 31.

## Lactose Intolerance

People whose bodies produce too little of the enzyme lactase have trouble digesting the lactose (sugar) in milk. If you are lactose-intolerant, you may get gas, bloating, cramps, and diarrhea after you drink milk or eat milk products.

**To reduce your symptoms:**

◆ Do not eat or drink large amounts of milk products at once.

◆ Try cheese instead of milk. It may be easier on your stomach because most of the lactose is removed during processing.

◆ Eat yogurt made with active cultures. These have enzymes that digest the lactose in milk.

◆ Drink pretreated milk (such as Lactaid), or try enzyme tablets (such as Lactaid or Dairy Ease).

◆ You may be able to tolerate milk if you drink it with snacks or meals.

**If you have severe lactose intolerance:**

◆ Read food labels to avoid all forms of lactose.

◆ Be sure to include nondairy sources of calcium in your diet. You can get good calcium from tofu, broccoli, certain greens, and calcium-fortified orange juice. Ask your doctor or dietitian if you need to take a calcium supplement.

◆ Plan your diet so it gives you the nutrients that milk products would normally provide.

# Dizziness and Vertigo

## When to Call a Doctor

### Call 911 if:

◆ Vertigo occurs with severe headache, confusion, loss of speech or sight, weakness in the arms or legs, or numbness in any part of the body.

◆ Lightheadedness occurs with chest pain or pressure or any other symptoms of a heart attack. See page 38.

◆ Someone who is feeling dizzy faints and you cannot wake the person.

◆ Vertigo or loss of balance occurs with severe headache, stiff neck, fever, seizure, or feeling grouchy or confused.

◆ Severe lightheadedness lasts a long time and occurs with a sudden change in heart rate.

### Call a doctor if:

◆ You are lightheaded or have vertigo after an injury.

◆ You have severe vertigo, or vertigo with hearing loss.

◆ You think a medicine may be making you dizzy.

◆ You have vertigo often and have not seen your doctor about it.

◆ Vertigo lasts longer than 5 days.

◆ Your vertigo is a lot different than past attacks.

◆ You feel lightheaded several times during just a few days.

◆ You feel lightheaded and your pulse is less than 50 or more than 150 beats per minute. See page 48 to learn how to take your pulse.

Dizziness is a word people use for two different feelings: lightheadedness and vertigo. Knowing what these mean may help you and your doctor narrow down the list of possible problems.

**Lightheadedness** is a feeling that you are about to faint.

◆ You may feel unsteady but do not feel like you are moving.

◆ You may feel sick to your stomach, vomit, or faint.

◆ It usually improves when you lie down.

Feeling lightheaded now and then is common. There are many reasons why you might feel lightheaded. Some of the most common ones are in the chart on page 141.

Lightheadedness is usually not a cause for concern unless it is severe, happens often, or occurs with symptoms like heartbeat changes or fainting.

| Problem | Possible Causes |
|---|---|
| **Lightheadedness** | Drop in blood pressure from getting up too fast |
| | Flu, cold, or allergies |
| | Dehydration, see p. 31 |
| | Medicines |
| | Stress or anxiety, see p. 80 |
| | Blood loss (could either be visible or hidden inside the body; see Bleeding Emergencies on p. 17) |
| | Heart rhythm problem, see p. 181 |
| | Heart attack, see p. 38 |
| **Vertigo** | Inner ear problem (benign positional vertigo, labyrinthitis, Meniere's disease) |
| | Migraine headache, see p. 177 |
| | Multiple sclerosis or other nerve problems |
| | Stroke, see p. 53 |
| | Brain tumor (rare) |

**Vertigo** is the feeling that you or your surroundings are spinning, whirling, or tilting when there is no actual movement. It may make you sick to your stomach. You may have trouble standing or walking and may lose your balance.

Vertigo is often related to an inner ear problem. The most common form is triggered by moving your head. This is called **benign positional vertigo**.

## Home Treatment

◆ If you feel lightheaded, lie down for a minute or two. This lets more blood flow to your brain. Then sit up slowly. Stay seated for a minute or two before you slowly stand up.

◆ If you are having vertigo, do not lie flat on your back. Propping yourself up slightly may help. Keep your eyes open.

◆ If you have a cold or the flu, rest and drink extra fluids.

◆ Do not drive, operate machinery, or do anything else that might be dangerous if you have vertigo or feel lightheaded. You might hurt yourself if you fall or faint.

 There are balance exercises that can help if you have problems with vertigo. To learn how to do them, go to the Web site on the back cover and enter **t822** in the search box.

More

141

# Dry Skin

## When to Call a Doctor

◆ You itch all over your body, but there is no obvious cause or rash.

◆ Itching is so bad that you cannot sleep, and home treatment does not help.

◆ You have open sores from scratching, or your skin is red and swollen.

Dry, itchy, flaky skin is the most common skin problem, especially in winter. Dry indoor air is a common cause. Taking a lot of hot showers or baths can also dry your skin.

## Home Treatment

◆ Take baths instead of showers. Showers strip the natural oil that helps hold moisture in the skin. Baths are much kinder to the skin. If you take showers, keep them short and not too hot.

◆ Use bath oils when you bathe. Be careful not to slip.

◆ Use mild soaps, such as Dove or Cetaphil. You may only need to use soap under your arms and in the groin area.

◆ Use a moisturizing lotion right after you bathe.

◆ For very dry hands or feet, try this for a night: Apply a thin layer of petroleum jelly, and wear thin cotton gloves or socks to bed.

◆ Try not to scratch. It can damage the skin.

## Relief From Itching

◆ Keep the itchy area well moisturized. Dry skin may make itching worse.

◆ Take an oatmeal bath: Wrap 1 cup of oatmeal in a cotton cloth, and boil as you would to cook it. Use this as a sponge, and bathe in cool-to-warm water without soap. Or try an Aveeno colloidal oatmeal bath.

◆ Use calamine lotion on itchy insect bites or plant rashes.

◆ Try a nonprescription 1% hydrocortisone cream for small itchy areas. Do not use it on the face or genitals. If itching is severe, your doctor may prescribe a stronger steroid cream or ointment.

◆ Try a nonprescription oral antihistamine such as Benadryl or Chlor-Trimeton.

◆ Cut nails short or wear gloves at night to prevent scratching.

◆ Wear cotton or silk clothing. Do not wear wool and acrylic fabrics next to the skin.

◆ Do not use soap on the dry skin.

# Ear Infections

This topic covers the two most common kinds of ear infections:

◆ **Swimmer's ear,** which affects the ear canal.

◆ **Middle ear infections.** These are very common in children. Middle ear infections are worse than ear canal infections because they are deeper in the ear and can cause more problems.

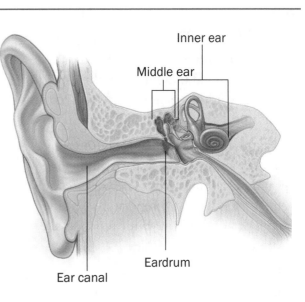

Infections can occur in the ear canal, middle ear, or inner ear.

## Swimmer's Ear

### When to Call a Doctor

◆ There is pus or blood draining from the ear.

◆ Both the ear canal and the outer ear are red.

◆ There is redness or swelling around or behind the ear.

◆ The ear canal is swollen, red, and very painful.

◆ Ear pain follows a cold.

◆ You feel dizzy or unsteady.

◆ Symptoms do not get better after 3 days of home treatment.

Swimmer's ear is an irritation or infection of the ear canal. It often develops after water, sand, or dirt gets in the ear canal.

Other causes include a cut inside the ear or an injury from a cotton swab or other object; too much earplug use; soap or shampoo buildup; and skin problems such as eczema and psoriasis.

If you have swimmer's ear, your ear will probably hurt, itch, and feel full. The ear canal may be swollen. A bad infection can cause discharge from the ear and possibly some hearing loss.

Unlike in a middle ear infection (see page 145), the pain of swimmer's ear is worse when you press on the "tag" in front of the ear, touch your earlobe, or chew.

**More**

## Home Treatment

◆ Make sure there is not an object or insect in the ear. See page 33.

◆ If the eardrum may have ruptured or there is pus or blood draining from the ear, do not put eardrops or anything else into the ear unless a doctor has told you to.

◆ Gently rinse the ear using a bulb syringe and a mixture of equal parts white vinegar and rubbing alcohol. Make sure the mixture is at body temperature. Putting cool or hot fluids in your ear may make you dizzy.

◆ Keep water out of the ear until the irritation clears up. You can use cotton lightly coated with petroleum jelly as an earplug. Do not use plastic earplugs.

◆ If the ear itches, try nonprescription swimmer's eardrops before and after your ears get wet.

◆ To insert eardrops, have the person lie down, ear facing up. Warm the drops by rolling the container between your hands. Place drops on the outer ear near the opening of the ear canal, and gently wiggle the ear until the drops flow in. Pulling the ear up and back will help.

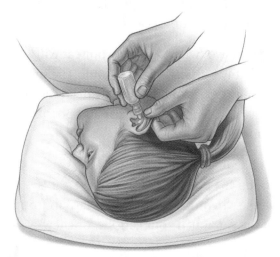

Never stick a dropper into the ear canal.

### Preventing Swimmer's Ear

◆ Keep ears dry. After you swim or shower, shake your head to get water out of the ear canals. (Never shake a baby's head.) Gently dry the ears with the corner of a tissue or towel. You can also use a hairdryer set on low.

◆ After you swim or shower, put a few drops of rubbing alcohol, or alcohol mixed with an equal amount of white vinegar, in the ear. Pull the ear up and back to let the liquid go deep into the ear canal. Then tilt your head and let it drain out. You can also use nonprescription drops (Star-Otic, Swim-Ear).

◆ Never use cotton swabs, hairpins, or other objects to clean wax out of the ears. This can damage the ear. See page 148 for tips on removing earwax safely.

◆ Avoid wearing earplugs for long periods of time.

◆ Try to keep soap and shampoo out of the ear canal. To remove dirt or sand that gets into the ear, spray a gentle stream of warm water from the shower or a bulb syringe into the ear; then tip your head to let the water drain out.

◆ Put a warm, moist cloth on the ear to ease ear pain, or use a heating pad set on low. Do not use a heating pad on a baby or a child who cannot tell you if it's too hot. Do not send your child to bed with a heating pad.

◆ Take acetaminophen (Tylenol) or ibuprofen (Advil, Motrin) for pain. Do not give aspirin to anyone younger than 20.

# Middle Ear Infections

## When to Call a Doctor

◆ Ear pain is severe or gets worse even with home treatment.

◆ Ear pain occurs with other signs of serious illness, such as headache with severe stiff neck, fever, or feeling grouchy or confused. See page 161.

◆ Your baby keeps pulling or rubbing an ear and seems to be in pain (crying, screaming).

◆ Your child has a fever over 102°F with other signs of an ear infection.

◆ A baby younger than 3 months has a fever of 100.4°F or higher.

◆ There is pus or blood draining from the ear.

◆ Your child is not getting better after 48 hours of treatment with an antibiotic.

◆ Your child has ear tubes and has an earache or ear drainage.

◆ There is redness or swelling around or behind the ear.

◆ Your child cannot move the muscles in his or her face normally.

◆ Mild ear pain lasts longer than 3 to 4 days.

A middle ear infection (otitis media) often develops during a cold. Colds can cause the eustachian tube, which connects the middle ear to the throat, to swell and close. Fluid then builds up in the middle ear. Bacteria or viruses can grow in the fluid, causing an infection.

Symptoms of a middle ear infection include:

◆ Ear pain. Children who can't talk yet may tug on their painful ears.

◆ Dizziness.

◆ Ringing or a feeling of fullness in the ear.

◆ Hearing loss.

◆ Fever, headache, and runny nose.

The trapped, infected fluid puts pressure on the eardrum. If there is pus or blood draining from the ear, the eardrum may have ruptured. Ear pain caused by an infection usually improves once an eardrum ruptures.

A single eardrum rupture usually is not serious. Repeated eardrum ruptures can lead to hearing loss.

Fluid buildup (effusion) in the middle ear may also occur after an infection has cleared. There may be no symptoms, or there may be minor hearing loss and mild discomfort. Fluid buildup that occurs after an infection usually does not need treatment unless it lasts longer than 3 or 4 months and causes hearing loss. See What About Ear Tubes? on page 147.

**More**

## Home Treatment

◆ Put a warm washcloth on the ear to relieve pain, or use a heating pad set on low. Do not use a heating pad on a baby or a child who cannot tell you if it's too hot. Do not send your child to bed with a heating pad.

◆ Give your child acetaminophen (Tylenol) or ibuprofen (Advil, Motrin) for pain. Do not give aspirin to anyone younger than 20.

◆ Have your child drink plenty of clear liquids.

◆ If the eardrum ruptures, avoid getting water in the ear for 3 to 4 weeks. Showers or baths are fine, but do not let your child soak his or her head in the tub. Swimming in pools is fine also, as long as the child uses earplugs.

## Does Your Child Need Antibiotics?

Antibiotics can treat ear infections, but most children with ear infections get better without them. If the care you give at home relieves pain, and your child is feeling better after a few days, your child may not need antibiotics.

There are exceptions to this. Your child may need antibiotics right away if:

◆ He or she is younger than 2. The risk of other problems is higher for very young children. Also, a loss of hearing for even a short time may affect how your child learns to talk.

◆ Your child is very ill, has a high fever, or is in severe pain.

◆ Your child has a serious long-term health problem (like heart disease or cystic fibrosis).

In most other cases, your doctor may suggest that you wait 48 hours before you give your child antibiotics. If after 48 hours your child has not improved and needs antibiotics, you will have to wait at least another 48 hours for the antibiotics to take effect.

There are good reasons not to use antibiotics unless you really need them:

◆ Antibiotics can cost a lot.

◆ You will probably have to see the doctor to get a prescription. This costs you time and money.

◆ Antibiotics can have harmful side effects, such as diarrhea, vomiting, and skin rashes.

◆ The most important reason of all: If you take antibiotics when you don't need them, they may not work when you do need them. Each time you take antibiotics you are more likely to carry some bacteria that were not killed by the medicine. Over time, these bacteria get tougher and can cause worse infections. To treat them, you may need different, stronger, and more costly antibiotics.

If you are not sure what's best for your child and need help deciding, go to the Web site on the back cover and enter **i279** in the search box.

## Preventing Childhood Ear Infections

◆ Breast-feed your baby. Breast-fed babies have fewer ear infections. If you bottle-feed your baby, hold the baby upright to drink. Never let a baby or young child lie down with or go to sleep with a bottle.

◆ Do not smoke in your home or around your children.

◆ Take your child to a smaller day care center. Fewer children means less contact with germs and illness.

◆ Wean your child from his or her pacifier by about 6 months of age. Babies who use their pacifiers after 12 months of age are more likely to get ear infections.

◆ Wash your hands and your child's hands often.

◆ Make sure your child's immunizations are up to date. See page 324.

### What About Ear Tubes?

Some children seem to get ear infections all the time. These children often develop fluid behind the eardrum and hearing loss. The hearing loss is usually temporary, but it is more of a concern in children age 2 and younger. Normal hearing is important when young children are learning to talk.

If your baby or young child often has ear infections and fluid in the ear, you may want to talk to your child's doctor about ear tubes. Ear tubes are put in the eardrums to drain fluid and help restore good hearing.

The doctor may want to test your child's hearing first. If there is no hearing loss, you may choose to take a "wait and see" approach for a few months.

 To help you decide whether ear tubes are right for your child, go to the Web site on the back cover and enter **e339** in the search box.

# Earwax

### When to Call a Doctor

◆ Earwax is still hard, dry, and packed after 1 week of home treatment.

◆ Earwax causes ringing in your ears, a full feeling in your ears, or hearing loss.

◆ You have nausea or balance problems along with earwax.

◆ An earwax problem develops in a person who has a ruptured eardrum or ear tubes or who has had previous ear surgery.

Earwax helps keep the ears clean and keeps out dust and water. Normally, earwax drains freely from the ears and does not cause problems.

As a rule, it is best to leave earwax alone. You can avoid most earwax problems by not using cotton swabs in your ears.

**More**

Once in a while, earwax will build up, get hard, and cause some hearing loss or discomfort. Poking at the wax with cotton swabs, fingers, or other objects will only push the wax deeper into the ear canal and pack it against the eardrum.

You should be able to take care of most earwax problems with home treatment. But when wax is tightly packed, you may need professional help to remove it.

## Home Treatment

Do not use home treatment if you think the eardrum is ruptured, if there is pus or blood draining from the ear, or if the person has ear tubes.

To remove earwax safely, try one of these methods:

◆ Place 2 drops of warm (body temperature) mineral oil in the ear twice a day for 1 or 2 days to soften and loosen the wax. Then use the spray from a warm, gentle shower or a bulb syringe to remove the wax. Spray the water into the ear, and then tip the head to let the wax drain out.

◆ Each night for 1 to 2 weeks, use a nonprescription wax softener (such as Debrox or Murine), then gently flush the ear with warm water from a bulb syringe. Make sure the water is warm but not hot. Putting cool or hot fluids in the ear may make you dizzy.

# Eating Disorders

## When to Call a Doctor

**Call a counselor or your doctor** if you notice any of these warning signs:

◆ Unrealistic body image or an intense fear of gaining weight

◆ Extreme weight loss in a short period of time

◆ Frequent vomiting

◆ Frequent use of laxatives or diuretics (water pills)

◆ Constant dieting or a constant focus on food

◆ Excessive, rigid exercise routines

◆ Loss of menstrual periods in a young woman

◆ Withdrawal from family and friends

In a culture where "thin is in," many of us have skipped meals or dieted to try to lose weight. But unlike typical dieters, people who have eating disorders are affected by strong psychological issues that cause abnormal eating. The problem tends to run in families.

Anorexia, bulimia, and binge eating are the most common eating disorders.

### Anorexia

People with anorexia force themselves to follow strict, severe diets even when they do not need to lose weight. The problem occurs most often in teenage girls and young women.

Signs of anorexia include:

◆ Refusing to eat but being focused on food.

◆ Exercising all the time.

◆ Extreme weight loss and loss of menstrual periods.

◆ Thinking you are fat when in fact you are very thin.

◆ Low self-esteem.

◆ Denying the problem.

## Bulimia

People with bulimia eat large amounts of food at once and then vomit or use laxatives or diuretics to get rid of the food. This pattern is called binge eating and purging. Emotional stress, not hunger, usually triggers binges.

Signs of bulimia include:

◆ Dry skin and brittle hair.

◆ Swollen lymph nodes under the jaw (from vomiting).

◆ Depression and mood swings.

◆ Thinking you are fat when you are a normal weight. Most people with bulimia look healthy.

◆ Secrecy. People with bulimia usually know they have a problem but will try to hide it.

## Binge Eating

Binge eaters eat huge amounts of food at once. They will take in thousands of calories at a time, quickly and without pleasure. Because they do not purge the food (vomit), people with this problem often become obese.

## What to Do

If you know or suspect that you or someone in your family has an eating disorder, get help. Eating disorders need professional treatment. Without it, they can lead to major health problems or even death.

Treatment usually involves nutrition counseling, therapy for the person and the family, and medicine. In extreme cases, the person may need to stay in a hospital.

## Teach Healthy Attitudes

You can help your children build healthy relationships with food and their bodies.

◆ Teach and model healthy eating and exercise habits at home and at school.

◆ Help young people build confidence and self-esteem. Accept them for who they are, not how they look.

◆ Be careful about urging a young person to lose weight. Let people know that you love them no matter how much they weigh.

◆ Set realistic expectations for your child. Trying to live up to unrealistic ones may lead to an eating disorder.

◆ Be alert to the stress in your child's life. Let your child know you are there to listen and help.

# Erection Problems

## When to Call a Doctor

- An erection lasts longer than 4 hours after you use an erection-producing medicine, such as Viagra, Cialis, or Levitra.

- You took an erection-producing medicine in the past 24 hours and you are having chest pain. **Do not take nitroglycerin!** See Chest Pain on page 119.

- You cannot have an erection at all, or you think the cause may be physical.

- You have erection problems along with urinary problems, pain in your lower belly or lower back, or fever.

- Your erection problems started after a recent injury.

- You think your erection problems may be caused by a medicine.

Erection problems are common. At some time in their lives, most men have trouble getting an erection or having one that lasts long enough to have sex.

Having an erection problem from time to time is normal and is usually nothing to worry about. But if you often cannot get or maintain an erection, you may want to work with your doctor to find the cause.

Erection problems can be caused by:

- Problems with blood vessels, nerves, or hormones. These can be related to diabetes, heart disease, injuries, and other health problems.

- Medicines. Blood pressure medicines, water pills (diuretics), and mood-altering drugs can all have sexual side effects.

- Alcohol.

- Smoking.

- Depression, stress, grief, or relationship problems.

As you get older, it may take longer to get erections, and they may be less firm. But with the right approach, healthy men can have erections at any age.

## Home Treatment

- Rule out medicines as a cause. Ask your doctor or pharmacist whether any that you take can have sexual side effects.

- Limit alcohol. Have no more than 2 drinks a day.

- If you smoke, quit. Smoking makes it harder for the blood vessels in the penis to relax and let blood flow in. If you need help quitting, see page 316.

- Try to reduce stress. See page 319. Regular exercise may help too.

- Take time for more foreplay.

◆ Talk to your partner about your concerns. If you and your partner have trouble talking about sex, see a therapist who can help you talk about it together. Reading books with your partner about sex may also help.

◆ Find out if you can have erections at other times. If you get erections when you masturbate or have them when you first wake up, the cause is more likely emotional than physical.

◆ Talk to your doctor about medicines that can help, such as Viagra, Levitra, or Cialis. These drugs can make heart problems worse in some people, so check with your doctor first. For help deciding whether these medicines  are right for you, go to the Web site on the back cover and enter **j763** in the search box.

◆ There are also devices that can help with erections. Talk to your doctor if you want to learn more about them.

# Eye Problems

This topic covers three common problems:

◆ Pinkeye

◆ Dry eyes

◆ Blood in the eye

If you have other symptoms, be sure to check the Eye and Vision Problems chart on page 63.

## Pinkeye

### When to Call a Doctor

◆ There is a new difference between the sizes of the pupils.

◆ The skin around the eye or eyelid is red.

◆ You have blurring or loss of vision that does not clear at all when you blink.

◆ You have pain in the eye, rather than irritation.

◆ Light is very painful for your eye.

◆ You think you may have an object in the eye. See page 35.

◆ The eye is red and there is a yellow, green, or bloody discharge that does not begin to go away in 24 hours. You may need antibiotics.

◆ Pinkeye lasts longer than 7 days.

◆ Your eye has not improved within 48 hours after you start using antibiotics.

◆ You wear contact lenses and you have had pinkeye more than once.

**More**

Pinkeye is inflammation of the conjunctiva, which lines the eyelid and covers the surface of the eye. Pinkeye is also called conjunctivitis.

Pinkeye may be caused by:

◆ Infection with a virus or bacteria. This kind of pinkeye spreads very easily.

◆ Dry air, allergies, smoke, and chemicals. This kind of pinkeye does not spread from person to person.

If you have pinkeye, you may have redness in the whites of your eyes; red and swollen eyelids; lots of tears; itching or burning; and a sandy feeling in your eyes. Light may hurt your eyes more than usual. And there may be fluid or pus in your eyes that crusts over and makes your eyelids stick together when you sleep.

Although pinkeye will often clear on its own in 7 to 10 days, pinkeye that is caused by a virus can last many weeks. Antibiotics will help if you have pinkeye that is caused by bacteria. If you have pinkeye because of allergies or chemicals, it will not go away unless you can avoid the cause.

## Home Treatment

Good home care will speed healing and help you avoid spreading pinkeye to others.

◆ Wash your hands often. Always wash them well before and after you treat pinkeye or touch your eyes or face.

◆ Put cold or warm wet cloths on your eye several times a day if your eye hurts.

◆ Use moist cotton or a clean, wet cloth to remove any crust. Wipe from the inside corner (next to the nose) to the outside. Use a clean part of the cloth for each wipe.

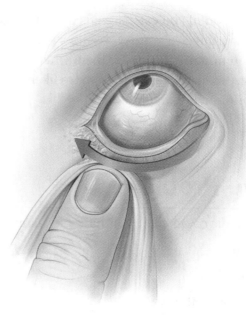

Wipe from the inside corner to the outside to remove crusts.

◆ Do not wear contact lenses or eye makeup until the pinkeye is gone. Throw away any eye makeup you were using when you got pinkeye. Clean your contacts and storage case. If you wear disposable contacts, use a new pair once it is safe to wear contacts again.

◆ If the doctor prescribes eyedrops, use them as directed.

❖ For older children and adults: Pull the lower lid down with two fingers to create a small pouch. Put the drops there. Close the eye for 30 to 60 seconds to let the drops move around.

❖ For younger children: Ask the child to lie down with eyes closed. Put a drop in the inner corner of the eye. When the child opens the eye, the drop will run in.

❖ Be sure the bottle tip is clean and does not touch the eye, eyelid, or eyelashes. If the tip does touch the eye area, throw the bottle away and replace it.

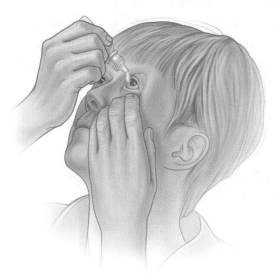

Do not let the bottle tip touch the eye, eyelid, or eyelashes.

◆ Putting antibiotic ointment in the eye can be tricky, especially with children. If you can get it on the eyelashes, it will melt and get into the eye.

◆ Make sure any medicine you buy without a prescription is ophthalmic (for eyes), not otic (for ears).

◆ Do not share towels, pillows, eye makeup, or contact lens equipment while you have pinkeye.

# Dry Eyes

## When to Call a Doctor

Call a doctor if dry eyes are a problem and artificial tears do not help.

Eyes that do not have enough moisture in them may feel dry, hot, sandy, or gritty. Dry air, smoke, aging, and certain diseases can cause dry eyes. Some common medicines also can make your eyes dry. These include antihistamines, decongestants, drugs for depression, and birth control pills.

## Home Treatment

◆ Rest your eyes. When you read, watch TV, or use a computer, take breaks often and close your eyes. As you work, try to blink your eyes more often.

◆ Try "artificial tears" eyedrops. Preservative-free tears are the gentlest on your eye.

◆ Do not use eyedrops that reduce redness (such as Visine) to treat dry eyes. Your eyes may get even worse when you stop using the drops.

◆ Avoid smoke and fumes from chemicals.

## Avoiding Problems With Your Contacts

If you wear contact lenses, these tips will help you avoid problems.

◆ Keep your lenses and anything that touches them (hands, storage cases, makeup) very clean. Wash your hands before you touch your contacts.

◆ Follow the cleaning instructions for your lenses, and use a store-bought contact lens solution. Generic brands are just as good as name brands, and they cost less. Do not make your own solution. It can get contaminated too easily.

◆ Never wet your lenses with saliva. It has bacteria that may infect the eye. Don't use tap water either.

◆ Put in your contacts before you put on eye makeup. Do not put makeup on the inner rim of the eyelid. Replace eye makeup every 3 to 6 months.

◆ If you use extended-wear contacts, follow the wearing and cleaning schedule your eye care professional recommends. When worn for long periods of time, these lenses are more likely to cause severe eye infections.

Symptoms of a possible problem with your contacts include redness, pain, or burning in the eye; discharge from the eye; blurred vision; or extreme sensitivity to light. Take out your lenses, clean them, and don't put them back in until your symptoms are gone. If symptoms last longer than 2 to 3 hours after you take out your contacts, call your eye doctor or optometrist.

Visit your eye doctor or optometrist as directed or at least once a year.

## Blood in the Eye

### When to Call a Doctor

◆ Bleeding starts after a blow to the head or injury to the eye.

◆ There is blood in the colored part of the eye.

◆ Your eye is bloody and painful.

◆ You often get blood spots in your eyes.

◆ Bleeding occurs while you are taking blood thinners (anticoagulants).

Sometimes blood vessels in the whites of the eyes break and cause a red spot or speck. This is called a subconjunctival hemorrhage. The blood may look alarming, especially if the spot is large. But it is usually not a cause for concern, and the red spot will go away in 2 to 3 weeks.

If you have a black eye, see Bruises on page 24.

# Fatigue and Weakness

## When to Call a Doctor

- You have sudden muscle weakness and you don't know why.

- You are so tired that you have to limit your usual activities for longer than 2 weeks.

- You have lost or gained weight for no clear reason.

- You do not feel better after 4 weeks of home treatment.

- Fatigue gets worse even with home treatment.

**Fatigue** is a feeling of being very tired or exhausted or not having any energy. Most fatigue is caused by lack of exercise, stress or overwork, lack of sleep, depression, worry, or boredom. You can usually treat fatigue with self-care.

**Weakness** is a lack of physical or muscle strength and the feeling that moving an arm, a leg, or any other part of your body takes a lot of extra effort. Unexplained muscle weakness is usually more serious than fatigue. It may be caused by diabetes (see page 284), thyroid problems, stroke (see page 53), or other problems related to the brain and spinal cord.

Colds, flu, and other short-term illnesses often cause fatigue and weakness while you are sick.

### Low Thyroid

Not having enough thyroid hormone (hypothyroidism) is a common cause of fatigue, especially in middle-aged and older women. When your thyroid gland does not make enough thyroid hormone, your body slows down. This may make you feel tired and sluggish, have trouble concentrating or remembering things, and slowly gain weight.

A blood test can tell if your thyroid hormone is too low.

Low thyroid is an easy problem to treat with medicine. Most people with this problem need to take thyroid medicine for the rest of their lives.

### Anemia

Anemia means that you do not have enough red blood cells, which carry oxygen to your body's tissues. This can make you pale, weak, and tired.

Lack of iron is the most common cause of anemia. You may not be getting enough iron in your diet, or your body may have trouble absorbing it. To boost your iron:

- Eat foods rich in iron, such as beef, shellfish, chicken, eggs, beans, raisins, whole-grain breads, and leafy green vegetables.

- Use iron pots for cooking.

- Steam vegetables instead of boiling them (they lose iron if you boil them).

**More**

155

You can also get anemia from a gradual loss of blood, such as from heavy menstrual periods or from bleeding in your stomach or colon. If a health problem is causing your anemia, treating that problem may correct your anemia and help you feel better.

## Home Treatment

These self-care tips help with most cases of fatigue. If you have low thyroid, anemia, or another health problem, talk to your doctor about what other home treatment you should do.

◆ Get some exercise every day. Daily exercise balanced with plenty of rest is often the best treatment for fatigue. If you feel too tired to exercise hard, try a short walk.

◆ Eat a healthy diet. This can help you stay at your best.

◆ Make sure you get enough sleep. See page 236.

◆ Do not ignore emotional problems like depression or anxiety. There are treatments that can help. See Living Better With Depression on page 280 and Anxiety on page 80.

◆ Take steps to control your stress and workload. See page 318.

◆ Ask your doctor or pharmacist whether any of your medicines can make you tired. Cold and allergy medicines are common causes of fatigue.

◆ Drink less caffeine and alcohol.

◆ If you smoke or chew tobacco, think about quitting.

◆ Watch less TV. Spend time with friends instead, or try new activities.

◆ Be patient. It may take a while before you feel energetic again.

## Are You Depressed?

If you have been feeling very tired for no clear reason, you may want to think about whether you are depressed.

Depression is more than just the normal sadness and moodiness that come and go with the ups and downs of life. It's an illness. You may be depressed if:

◆ You feel sad, anxious, or hopeless much of the time, and these feelings do not go away.

◆ You have lost interest in many of the things you once enjoyed—hobbies, work, time with friends and family.

You may also have changes in your sleep or eating patterns, weight gain or loss, and trouble concentrating and making decisions. You may feel worthless or guilty for no reason and think about death a lot.

If you think you might be depressed and have felt this way for more than 2 weeks, talk to your doctor or a counselor. If you want to take a self-test for depression, go to the Web site on the back cover and enter **x453** in the search box. If you have already been diagnosed with depression, see Living Better With Depression on page 280.

Treatment can almost always help. If you are just mildly depressed, home treatment may be all you need. Or you may need to try counseling and antidepressant medicines. Without any treatment, your depression is likely to get worse.

# Chronic Fatigue Syndrome

Chronic fatigue syndrome can make you so tired and weak that you can't do your normal activities. Even after you rest, you still may not have your usual energy. You may also have memory problems, headaches, a sore throat, painful lymph glands, muscle and joint pain, and sleep problems.

Chronic fatigue syndrome is hard to diagnose. Depression, thyroid problems, mono, and many other illnesses can cause the same symptoms. You may need tests to rule out some of these other causes. If fatigue and other symptoms go on for at least 6 months and there is no other explanation for them, your doctor may diagnose chronic fatigue syndrome.

Feeling tired and weak may make it hard to get through the day sometimes. But many people do get better over time. Your doctor may be able to help with specific symptoms.

To feel better overall:

◆ Look for ways to adjust your schedule so that it's easier on you. Schedule rest breaks. Resist the urge to do too much when you have energy. If you overdo it, you may get too tired. Then you may be even more tired the next day.

◆ If you have problems sleeping, try to improve your sleep habits. See page 236.

◆ Get light exercise every day. Gentle stretching, light aerobics, swimming, walking, and cycling can help relieve your symptoms.

◆ Eat a healthy diet. You may feel better if you avoid heavy meals and eat more fruits and vegetables.

◆ Join a support group with other people who have chronic fatigue syndrome. These groups can be a good source of information and tips for what to do to feel better.

# Fever, Age 3 and Younger

## When to Call a Doctor

All temperatures listed in this section are rectal temperatures.

- Fever occurs with vomiting, severe headache, sleepiness, not acting alert, stiff neck, or a bulging soft spot on a baby's head. See page 161.

- Fever occurs with a seizure. See page 161.

- Fever occurs with:

  - Fast, difficult breathing. See page 19.

  - Drooling or inability to swallow. See page 19.

  - A purple rash that does not lighten when you press on it. See page 161.

  - Vomiting, diarrhea, and belly pain.

  - Signs of dehydration (see page 31).

  - Unexplained skin rash. See page 227 for common childhood illnesses that cause rashes.

  - Ear pain. Babies often pull at painful ears. See Middle Ear Infections on page 145.

  - Pain or crying when urinating (not caused by painful diaper rash).

- New swelling, pain, redness, or warmth in one or more joints.

  - Any unusual or severe pain.

- A baby younger than 3 months of age has a fever of 100.4°F or higher.

- A child 3 months to 3 years old has a fever of:

  - 105°F or higher.

  - 104°F or higher that does not come down after 4 to 6 hours of home treatment.

  - 102°F to 104°F for more than 12 hours.

  - 100.4°F to 102°F for more than 24 to 48 hours.

- Your child has a fever and seems sicker than you would expect from a viral illness like a cold or the flu.

- Your child acts strangely, seems confused, or hallucinates.

- Your child's fever began after he or she took a new medicine.

For fever in people age 4 and older, see page 160.

---

Fever is usually defined as a rectal temperature above 100.4°F. Rectal temperatures are the most accurate for checking for fever in a child. To learn how to take an accurate rectal temperature, see page 159.

In most but not all cases, fever means your child has an illness. (Sometimes it may mean your baby is dressed too warmly or the room is too warm.)

Common causes of fevers in children are:

◆ Colds, flu, chickenpox, and other infections caused by a virus. Flu can cause a high fever for 5 days or longer.

◆ Ear infections, strep throat, and other infections caused by bacteria.

Teething does not cause a fever. If a baby is teething and has a fever, look for other signs that your child is sick.

By itself, fever is not harmful. It may even help the body fight infection. Children tend to get higher fevers than adults do. Although high fevers are uncomfortable, they do not often cause medical problems. A very fast-rising temperature can cause a fever seizure, but this is not very common. See page 161.

The body limits a fever caused by infection from going above 106°F. But if there is heat from an outside source like sun on a parked car, the body temperature can go above 107°F. This can cause brain damage.

## Home Treatment

It can be hard to know when to call your doctor when your child has a fever, especially during the cold and flu season. How high a fever is may not be a good measure of how sick your child is. The way your child looks and acts is a much better guide.

Most children will be less active when they have a fever. If your child is comfortable and alert, eating well, drinking enough fluids, urinating normal amounts, and seems to be improving, home treatment is all that is needed.

◆ Give your child extra fluids, or let him or her suck on frozen juice pops.

◆ Dress the child lightly. Do not wrap your child in blankets.

## Taking a Rectal Temperature

Taking a rectal temperature gives you the most accurate reading in a child. Rectal temperature is about 0.5° to 1°F higher than an oral temperature.

To take a rectal temperature in a baby or small child:

◆ Clean the thermometer. Use only a rectal thermometer to take a rectal temperature.

◆ Put Vaseline or another lubricant on the bulb.

◆ Hold the child bottom-up across your lap.

◆ Hold the thermometer about an inch from the bulb, and gently insert it into the child's rectum no more than 1 inch. Hold the thermometer right at the anus so it can't slip in any farther. Do not let go.

◆ Wait until the thermometer beeps, and then remove it. (Glass thermometers containing mercury are no longer advised. If you have one, call your local health department to find how to get rid of it safely.)

If the fever is higher than 102°F and your child feels bad:

◆ Give acetaminophen (Tylenol) or ibuprofen (Advil, Motrin). Never give aspirin to your child unless your doctor has told you to.

◆ Urge your child to drink extra fluids, and watch for signs of dehydration. See page 31.

# Fever, Age 4 and Older

## When to Call a Doctor

◆ You have a fever of 104°F or higher.

◆ You have a fever of 103°F to 104°F that does not come down after 12 hours of home treatment.

◆ You have a long-lasting fever. Many viral illnesses cause fevers of 102°F or higher for short periods of time (up to 12 to 24 hours). Call a doctor if the fever stays high:

  ❖ 102°F to 103°F for 1 full day

  ❖ 101°F to 102°F for 3 full days

  ❖ 100.4°F to 101°F for 4 full days

◆ Body temperature rises to 102.3°F or higher, all sweating stops, and the skin is hot, dry, and red. These are signs of heat stroke. See page 39.

◆ You have fever with signs of a wound infection (such as red streaks, pus, or increased pain, swelling, warmth, or redness).

◆ You have fever with a very stiff neck, headache, vomiting, and confusion. These may be signs of a serious illness. See page 161.

◆ You have fever with shortness of breath and cough. See Pneumonia on page 216.

◆ You have fever with pain above the eyes or the cheekbones. See Sinusitis on page 232.

◆ You have fever with pain or burning when you urinate. See Urinary Tract Infections on page 251.

◆ You have fever with belly pain, nausea, and vomiting. See Appendicitis on page 69 and Food Poisoning on page 167.

◆ Fever occurs with confusion, decreased alertness, strange behavior, or other troubling symptoms.

◆ You get a fever after you start a new medicine.

For fever in children under age 4, see page 158.

A fever is a high body temperature. By itself, a fever is not dangerous unless it gets too high. In fact, it can help your body fight illness and infection. Most healthy adults can handle a fever as high as 103°F to 104°F for a short time without problems.

## Home Treatment

◆ Drink plenty of water and other fluids.

◆ Take acetaminophen (Tylenol), aspirin, or ibuprofen (Advil, Motrin) to lower a fever. Do not give aspirin to anyone younger than 20.

◆ Take and record your temperature every 2 hours and whenever symptoms change.

◆ Take a sponge bath with warm (not hot) water if you feel uncomfortable.

◆ Watch for dehydration. See page 31.

◆ Dress lightly.

◆ Eat light foods that are easy to digest, such as soup.

◆ If you have classic flu symptoms, try home treatment for flu and see how you are doing in another day or two. See Flu on page 165.

## Encephalitis and Meningitis

Encephalitis is an inflammation of the brain. It may happen after a virus like chickenpox, flu, measles, mumps, mono, cold sores, or genital herpes. You can also get it from ticks or mosquitoes (see page 16).

Meningitis is an inflammation of the brain and spinal cord. It may follow an ear or sinus infection or other illness, though it may also occur even if you have not been sick.

Either illness can be quite serious. The symptoms are:

◆ Fever with a bad headache, stiff neck, and vomiting.

◆ Trouble staying awake, confusion, or seizures.

◆ A rash that develops quickly and looks like bruises or tiny purple or red blood spots under the skin.

Call your doctor right away if you get these symptoms, especially if you have recently been ill or been bitten by mosquitoes.

# Fever Seizures

## When to Call a Doctor

### Call 911 if:

◆ The child stops breathing for longer than 15 to 20 seconds or has severe trouble breathing. Start rescue breathing (see page 19) while you wait for help to arrive.

◆ A seizure lasts longer than 3 minutes, or the child has a second seizure.

◆ Seizure occurs with fever, vomiting, severe headache, sleepiness, not being alert or active, stiff neck, or a bulging soft spot on a baby's head.

### Call a doctor if:

◆ It is the child's first seizure, or you have not discussed with your doctor what to do if there is another one.

◆ A child younger than 6 months or a child 5 years or older has a seizure.

◆ The seizure affects only one side of the body.

◆ A seizure occurs without fever.

See pages 158 and 160 for when to call a doctor because of fever.

**More**

Fever seizures are uncontrolled muscle spasms that can happen while a child's temperature rises quickly. Sometimes the seizure occurs before you even know the child has a fever.

A child having a fever seizure may faint. The child's muscles will get stiff, and his or her teeth will clench. Then the arms and legs will start to jerk. The child's eyes may roll back, and he or she may stop breathing for a few seconds and turn slightly blue. The child might also vomit, urinate, or pass stools. Seizures usually last 1 to 5 minutes.

Fever seizures are scary, but in children age 6 months to 5 years they usually are not serious and do not cause harm. Some children in this age group just seem to get fever seizures, though there is no clear reason why. About a third of children who have a fever seizure will have another one in the future.

## Home Treatment

### During a seizure

◆ Try to stay calm. This will help calm the child.

◆ Protect the child from injury. Ease the child to the floor, or hold a very small child facedown on your lap. Do not restrain the child.

◆ Turn the child onto his or her side. This will help clear the mouth of any vomit or spit and will keep the airway open so the child can breathe.

◆ Do not put anything in the child's mouth to prevent tongue biting, because it may injure the child.

◆ Time how long the seizure lasts, if you can.

### After a seizure

◆ If the child is having trouble breathing, turn his or her head to the side. Use your finger to gently clear the mouth of any vomit or spit so the child can breathe.

◆ Check for injuries.

◆ Give acetaminophen (Tylenol) or ibuprofen (Advil, Motrin) and lukewarm sponge baths if the fever is higher than 102°F and your child feels bad. Do not give your child aspirin unless your doctor tells you to.

◆ Put the child in a cool room to sleep. Feeling drowsy is common after a seizure. Check the child often. The child should return to his or her normal behavior and activity level within 1 hour after the seizure.

# Fibromyalgia

## When to Call a Doctor

◆ You have severe joint or muscle pain.

◆ You feel sad, helpless, or hopeless; lose interest in things you used to enjoy; or have other symptoms of depression. See Are You Depressed? on page 156.

◆ You think you have injured a muscle or joint, and the pain does not go away in a few days.

Fibromyalgia is a painful condition that can make you ache all over and feel tired and weak. It also causes tender spots at specific points of the body that hurt only when you press on them. You may have trouble sleeping. These problems can upset your work and home life.

Symptoms tend to come and go, though they may never go away completely. Fibromyalgia does not harm your muscles, joints, or organs.

Fibromyalgia is not very well understood by anyone. Its cause is unknown. Your doctor may suggest prescription medicines to help with some of your symptoms.

## Home Treatment

◆ Get regular exercise, such as walking, biking, or swimming. This is the best thing you can do for fibromyalgia. It may help with pain and sleep problems and help you feel better.

◆ Try to get a good night's sleep every night. Go to bed and get up at the same time each day, whether you feel rested or not. Make sure you have a good mattress and pillow. See page 236 for more tips.

◆ Reduce stress. Avoid things that cause you stress, if you can. If not, work at making them less stressful. Learn to use biofeedback, meditation, or other methods to relax. See page 320.

◆ Use a heating pad set on low or take warm baths or showers for pain. Using cold packs for up to 15 minutes at a time can also relieve pain. Put a thin cloth between the cold pack and your skin. A gentle massage might help too.

◆ Take acetaminophen (Tylenol), ibuprofen (Advil, Motrin), or naproxen (Aleve) for pain.

◆ Think about joining a support group with others who have fibromyalgia to learn more and get support.

# Fifth Disease

## When to Call a Doctor

- Your child seems very sick.

- Your child feels weak and tired, and his or her skin is pale.

- Your child has a rash with high fever. See the fever guidelines on pages 158 and 160.

- You are pregnant and think you may have been exposed to a child with fifth disease. Although fifth disease is harmless in children, there is a small chance that it could harm your unborn baby.

- You are pregnant and get a rash that looks like fifth disease ("slapped cheeks" rash on the face, or a lacy, pink rash on the arms, legs, torso, and buttocks).

Fifth disease causes a rash and, in some cases, mild flu-like symptoms. It mostly affects children, though adults can get it too.

A child with fifth disease may have:

- A red rash on the face that looks like slapped cheeks.

- A lacy, pink rash on the backs of the arms and legs, torso, and buttocks.

Most children will have only the rash. But some may get a low fever, runny nose, sore throat, headache, and achy joints 7 to 10 days before the rash appears.

The rash may come and go for several weeks in response to changes in temperature and sunlight.

Sneezing and coughing spreads the illness. A child with fifth disease is most likely to give it to others the week before the rash appears, when there is a fever. By the time the rash appears, the child can no longer spread the illness.

## Home Treatment

Rest and fluids are the main treatment for fifth disease. Keep your child comfortable, and watch for signs that he or she is getting worse and needs a doctor's care.

If the rash itches, try the tips in Relief From Itching on page 142.

# Flu

## When to Call a Doctor

It is common for adults with flu to have high fevers (up to 104°F) for 3 to 4 days. When trying to decide if you need to see a doctor, think about how likely it is that you have the flu rather than some other illness. If it is flu season and lots of people have been getting the flu, chances are good that you have it too.

**Call your doctor if:**

◆ You have fever with a stiff neck or severe headache. You may have a serious illness. See page 161.

◆ A baby, an older adult, or a person with a long-term health problem may have the flu. Antiviral medicine can help prevent problems.

◆ You have the flu and want to take antiviral medicine to make it less severe.

◆ You start to get signs of a worse infection, such as fast or shallow breathing; a cough that brings up colored mucus from the lungs; or pain, fever, and fatigue that are getting a lot worse.

◆ You seem to get better and then get worse again.

Flu (influenza) is a viral illness that tends to occur in the winter and often affects many people at once. If you have the flu, you may feel very tired and have fever and shaking chills, lots of aches and pains, headache, and a runny nose.

The flu is not the same as the common cold.

◆ The symptoms are worse and come on faster.

◆ It lasts for up to 10 days, and you feel pretty bad the whole time.

For most people, the flu does not usually lead to more serious problems. But flu can be dangerous, especially for babies, older adults, pregnant women, and people with health problems like diabetes, asthma, or heart disease.

Antiviral medicine is advised for some of these high-risk people. The medicine can make the illness shorter and less severe if you take it before you have symptoms or within 48 hours after they appear. Even those who are not at high risk may want to take these medicines so that they feel better faster.

Antibiotics will not help you get over the flu. Home treatment will help you feel a little better until the illness ends.

### Should You Get a Flu Shot?

Flu shots help prevent the flu. They are not foolproof, because there is more than one flu virus and it can change from year to year. But flu shots give you the best chance of avoiding the illness.

**More**

Get a flu shot every fall if:

◆ You are over 50.

◆ You are at high risk for other problems from flu for reasons other than your age. See page 326.

◆ Someone you live or work with closely is at high risk for problems from flu. Think about whether you would expose a baby, older adult, or other high-risk person to the flu if you got it.

Flu shots are also recommended for:

◆ Pregnant women.

◆ Babies age 6 to 23 months.

◆ Anyone who takes care of a child 0 to 23 months old.

Even if you are not at high risk, yearly flu shots are a good idea for most people. No one wants to get the flu.

## Stay Well During Flu Season

◆ Wash your hands often!

◆ Keep your hands away from your nose, eyes, and mouth.

◆ Keep up your resistance to infection by eating a healthy diet, getting plenty of rest, and getting regular exercise.

◆ Consider getting a flu shot before flu season starts.

## Home Treatment

◆ Stay home from work, school, and public places for several days after you get sick so you don't give the flu to anyone else.

◆ Rest.

◆ Drink plenty of water to replace fluids lost from fever, to ease a scratchy throat, and to keep nasal mucus thin. Other good choices are hot tea with lemon, plain water, fruit juice, and soup.

◆ Take acetaminophen (Tylenol), aspirin, or ibuprofen (Advil, Motrin) to relieve fever, headache, and muscle aches. Do not give aspirin to anyone younger than 20.

◆ Do not smoke or let others smoke around you.

# Food Poisoning

## When to Call a Doctor
### Call 911 if:

◆ You have signs of severe dehydration. These include little or no urine; sunken eyes, no tears, and a dry mouth and tongue; skin that sags when you pinch it; feeling very dizzy or lightheaded; fast breathing and heartbeat; and not feeling or acting alert.

◆ You think you may have food poisoning from a canned food and you have symptoms of botulism (blurred or double vision, trouble swallowing or breathing, muscle weakness).

### Call a doctor if:

◆ Severe diarrhea (large, loose stools every 1 to 2 hours) lasts longer than 2 days in an adult.

◆ Vomiting lasts longer than 1 day in an adult.

◆ Symptoms of mild dehydration (dry mouth, dark urine, not much urine) get worse even with home treatment.

Food poisoning may occur when you eat food that has been contaminated with bacteria. Meats, dairy foods, sauces, and spreads like mayonnaise are often the source of the problem. Bacteria can grow in these foods if they are not handled right, cooked well, or stored at a temperature below 40°F.

You may start to feel sick as soon as 1 or 2 hours or as late as 2 days after you eat the food. Nausea, diarrhea, and vomiting are the usual symptoms.

Suspect food poisoning when:

◆ Others who ate the same food now have the same symptoms.

◆ Symptoms start after you eat foods that were left out (at a party, picnic, or buffet).

Botulism is a rare but often deadly type of food poisoning. It is most often caused by improper home canning methods for low-acid foods like beans and corn. Bacteria that survive the canning process may grow and produce poisons in the jar. Symptoms include blurred or double vision and trouble swallowing or breathing.

## Home Treatment

◆ Symptoms of food poisoning will usually go away in a day or two. Good home care can help you get well faster. For adults and older children, see Diarrhea on page 138 and Vomiting and Nausea on page 261. For babies and young children, see pages 137 and 259.

◆ Watch for and treat early signs of dehydration. See page 31. Older adults and young children can quickly get dehydrated from diarrhea and vomiting.

## Food Safety

◆ If food looks or smells spoiled, throw it out.

◆ Keep hot foods hot and cold foods cold.

◆ Follow the 2-40-140 rule. Do not eat meat, dressings, salads, or other foods that have been kept between 40°F and 140°F for more than 2 hours.

More

- Use a thermometer to check your refrigerator. It should be between 34°F and 40°F.

- Defrost meats in the refrigerator or microwave, not on the kitchen counter.

- Keep your hands and your kitchen clean. Wash your hands, cutting boards, and counters with hot, soapy water. After you touch raw meat, especially chicken, wash your hands and utensils very well before you prepare other foods.

- Cook meat until it's well done. Use a meat thermometer to make sure you have cooked meat, chicken, and fish to a safe temperature. This temperature varies depending on the food.

- Never eat undercooked hamburger. It's the main source of *E. coli* infection. All of the pink should be gone, and all of the meat (not just the surface) should have reached a temperature of at least 160°F.

- Do not eat raw eggs or uncooked dough or sauces made with raw eggs.

- Throw away cans or jars with bulging lids or leaks.

- Follow home canning and freezing instructions carefully. Contact your county agricultural extension office for advice.

## Hepatitis A

Hepatitis A is a virus that affects the liver. It is spread mainly by oral contact with stool that contains the virus. If the stool gets into the water or food supply, the virus may infect anyone who drinks the water or eats the food.

The United States does not tend to have this problem with its water and food supply. But sometimes a large group of people who eat at the same restaurant gets infected. This usually happens when an employee with hepatitis A does not wash his or her hands well after using the bathroom and then prepares food.

- Symptoms of hepatitis A may not appear for 2 to 7 weeks after you are exposed.

- You may have fatigue, nausea, fever, sore muscles, headaches, and pain in your upper right belly. Your skin and the white part of your eyes may turn yellow. Symptoms usually last less than 2 months.

- Hepatitis A usually goes away on its own and does not cause long-term liver problems.

If you or someone in your home has hepatitis A, take care not to spread it to others. Always wash your hands well after using the bathroom, after changing a baby's diapers, and before preparing or eating food.

If you live in an area where hepatitis A is common or you are at high risk, you may want to get the hepatitis A vaccine. See page 326.

# Fungal Infections

## When to Call a Doctor

◆ You have signs of a worse infection, such as increased pain, redness, swelling, or warmth; pus; and fever.

◆ You have diabetes and get athlete's foot.

◆ You have sudden hair loss, along with flaking, broken hairs, and redness of the scalp, or others in your household start losing hair.

◆ Ringworm is severe and spreading or is on the scalp. You may need prescription medicine.

◆ A fungal infection does not improve after 2 weeks or clear up after 1 month even with home treatment. You may want to ask your doctor about prescription medicine.

Fungal skin infections most often affect the feet, groin, scalp, or nails. Fungi grow best in warm, moist areas, such as between the toes, in the groin, and in the area just beneath the breasts.

| Common Fungal Infections | Symptoms | Comments |
|---|---|---|
| Athlete's foot | Itching and cracked, blistered, peeling areas between the toes and on the soles of the feet | Often comes back; needs to be treated each time |
| Jock itch | Severe itching and moistness in groin and on upper thighs; red, scaly raised areas that may ooze pus or fluid | Similar to athlete's foot |
| Ringworm of the skin | Patches that are clear in the center and red, peeling, or bumpy on the edges; itching | Can spread quickly to other areas |
| Ringworm of the scalp and beard | Bald patches that are scaly, red, crusty, or swollen with small bumps | Hair or beard may have flakes that look like dandruff |
| Nail infections | Discolored (often yellow), cracking, thickened, or softened nails | Hard to treat |
| Thrush of the mouth (yeast infection) | White coating inside the mouth that looks like milk but is hard to remove | Common in babies; may occur after taking antibiotics |

More

## Home Treatment

◆ For athlete's foot and jock itch, use a nonprescription antifungal powder or lotion, such as Micatin, Lamisil, or Lotrimin AF. Always wash and dry the area well before you apply the powder or lotion. Use the medicine for 1 to 2 weeks after the symptoms clear up so the infection doesn't come back. Do not use hydrocortisone cream on a fungal infection.

◆ For ringworm on the body, use one of the antifungals listed above.

◆ Keep your feet clean, cool, and dry. Dry well between your toes after you swim or shower. Use antifungal powder such as Desitin or Zeasorb in your shoes and socks and on your feet to prevent reinfection.

◆ Wear leather shoes or sandals that let your feet "breathe," and wear cotton socks to absorb sweat. Give shoes 24 hours to dry before you wear them again.

◆ Wear flip-flops or shower sandals in public pools and showers.

◆ Keep your groin area clean and dry. Shower or bathe soon after you exercise, or at least change out of sweaty clothes. Wear cotton underwear, and avoid tight pants and panty hose.

◆ Do not share hats, combs, brushes, or towels.

# Gallstones

## When to Call a Doctor

If you have not been diagnosed with gallstones, see When to Call a Doctor on page 68 in Abdominal Pain.

If you know you have gallstones, **call your doctor if**:

◆ You have sudden, severe belly pain. Severe belly pain can be a sign of a serious or even life-threatening problem.

◆ You develop a yellow tint to your skin and the white part of your eyes, dark yellow-brown urine, or light-colored stools.

◆ You have another attack of gallstone symptoms.

Gallstones are stones (usually made of cholesterol) that form in the gallbladder or bile duct, which carries bile from the gallbladder to your intestines. Bile helps you digest fats. Gallstones may be as small as a grain of sand or as large as a golf ball.

Most people who have gallstones do not have any symptoms, but sometimes stones can irritate the gallbladder. When this happens, you may have:

◆ A dull aching or cramping pain that starts in your upper right belly (see the picture on page 69) and may spread to the center of your upper belly or to your right upper back or shoulder blade.

◆ Sudden, severe pain that lasts several hours and then quickly fades.

◆ Fever and vomiting.

Symptoms often occur at night, usually at about the same time every night. Pain may or may not be related to a meal.

# Home Treatment

There is no home treatment for gallstones. You may be able to avoid more gallstones if you:

◆ Stay at a healthy weight.

◆ Eat a healthy, low-fat diet. Avoid foods that cause symptoms, especially fatty foods.

◆ Get regular exercise.

Esophagus

Liver

Gallbladder

Large intestine (colon)

Appendix

Stomach

Small intestine

Rectum

The digestive tract
(the gallbladder is in the upper right part of the belly)

## Do You Need Gallbladder Surgery?

◆ People who have frequent or severe pain from gallstones often have surgery to remove the gallbladder.

◆ If your first attack of gallstone pain is mild, it is often safe to wait and see if you have another attack before you get treatment. You may not need surgery if gallstones do not cause problems for you.

◆ Besides the pain of gallstones, there may be other medical reasons why you need the surgery.

◆ Surgery costs a lot and has some risks. If you don't need it, don't have it.

For help deciding whether surgery is right for you, go to the Web site on the back cover and enter **g126** in the search box. Then talk to your doctor.

# Glaucoma

## When to Call a Doctor

**Call 911 if:**

◆ You have sudden vision loss or blurring that does not clear.

◆ You have sudden, severe eye pain.

**Call your doctor if:**

◆ You have blind spots in your side vision.

◆ Your vision has gotten worse.

◆ You have a family history of open-angle glaucoma, you are age 40 or older, and you have not had an eye exam in the past year.

Glaucoma is an eye disease that damages the optic nerve at the back of the eye. (The optic nerve carries signals from the eye to the brain, which turns them into images that you see.) The damage is often related to increased pressure in the eye.

Open-angle glaucoma is the most common form. It tends to affect side (peripheral) vision. It's usually painless and can develop slowly over several years without you knowing. You may not notice any vision changes until a lot of damage has occurred.

**Closed-angle glaucoma** is not common but can be very serious. It occurs when the flow of fluid in the eye gets blocked. This can cause a quick rise in eye pressure that causes sudden vision changes and severe pain. You can lose vision within just a few hours.

## Home Treatment

◆ Use eyedrops and medicines for glaucoma as directed.

◆ Make sure your other doctors know you have glaucoma. You may need to avoid certain medicines, such as antihistamines. Check with your doctor before you take any medicines, including ones you buy without a prescription.

### Finding Glaucoma Early

Untreated glaucoma is a leading cause of blindness in adults. But the disease is easy to find in an eye exam. It responds well to treatment if you find it early.

Talk with your doctor about how often to have a glaucoma test. This may be based on your age and risk factors.

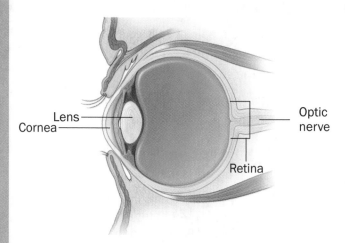

Lens — Cornea — Optic nerve — Retina

Glaucoma damages the optic nerve at the back of the eye.

# Grief

## When to Call a Doctor

Normal grieving can last for days, weeks, months, or years. Only you know how much grieving is reasonable for you. But if your grief continues and you have any of the following problems, you may need to get some help.

**Call a counselor or doctor if:**

◆ You feel hopeless and cannot stop yourself from thinking about death or suicide. **Call 911 or the national suicide hotline at 1-800-784-2433.**

◆ You are starting to do things that hurt you physically or financially or hurt others.

◆ You cannot control your anger toward people you blame for the loss.

◆ You are overwhelmed by guilt.

◆ You feel more and more isolated from other people.

◆ You have been grieving longer than you think is good for you.

Grieving is a natural healing process that lets you adjust to a major change or loss. Grief hurts, but it also helps you heal.

Grief can affect your body as well as your emotions. You may feel tired or restless, have trouble sleeping, get headaches, and not feel like eating. You may feel sad, angry, guilty, or depressed.

No person or book can tell you what your grief should be like. We each have our own ways of grieving. And grief doesn't stick to a schedule.

Although you may not get over a major loss, you can find ways to get through it. Your life may never be the same as it was before. But a time will come when you feel better and more at ease.

## Home Treatment

There is no formula for getting over grief. Some of these ideas may help:

◆ Take as much time as you need to grieve.

◆ Let yourself cry. Don't fight the emotions you feel. Look at photos, and read old letters.

◆ Try to cut back on some of your usual responsibilities for a little while. Do not make major decisions while you're grieving unless you have no choice.

◆ Talk to friends who will listen and who will encourage you to reconnect with the world. Join a support group, or talk to a counselor or clergy member.

◆ Find ways to express your grief. Keep a journal. Paint or draw.

◆ Take care of yourself. Get enough rest and eat nourishing foods.

◆ Exercise. Move around. Take a walk. It's a good way to relieve stress.

◆ As you start to move past your grief, renew old interests and pursue new ones. Do things that give you a sense of control and hope.

# Hair Loss

## When to Call a Doctor

◆ Hair loss is sudden or severe.

◆ You have patchy hair loss, or hair falls out in clumps.

◆ You have hair loss after starting a new medicine.

◆ Hair loss occurs with a scalp rash or any other skin change on your scalp.

◆ You are losing your hair bit by bit and want to talk about treatment.

Many people lose hair as they age. While men tend to lose hair from the hairline and crown of the head, women's hair gets thinner all over. This hair loss is natural and tends to run in families. It increases your risk of sunburn and skin cancer of the scalp, but you can avoid both of these by wearing sunscreen and a hat.

If you are thinking about medicine (such as minoxidil) or surgery for hair loss, make sure you understand the risks of treatment, how many treatments you will need, what it costs, and how long the results will last.

**Bald spots** are not the same as baldness.

◆ Wearing tight braids or having a habit of tugging or twisting your hair may cause bald spots.

◆ Ringworm is a fungal infection that causes scaly bald spots. See page 169.

◆ Alopecia areata causes patchy hair loss that may need treatment with medicines. Alopecia totalis can cause total hair loss, even the eyelashes and eyebrows.

**Thinning hair** can be a sign of problems such as thyroid disease or lupus. Mental or physical stress can cause short-term hair loss all over the head. So can hormone changes during pregnancy or menopause.

# Hand-Foot-and-Mouth Disease

## When to Call a Doctor

◆ Your child has a high fever. See the fever guidelines for children under age 4 on page 158 and for older children on page 160.

◆ Your child is dehydrated and has a fever with blisters in the mouth or a blistering rash on the hands and feet. See page 31.

Hand-foot-and-mouth disease is a viral illness that most often affects children under age 10. It usually occurs during the summer and fall.

Fever, a sore throat or mouth, and loss of appetite are early symptoms. Within 2 days, mouth and tongue blisters appear. Children often get a blistering rash on the fingers, tops of the hands, and tops and sides of the feet. There may be blisters on the buttocks.

The virus that causes hand-foot-and-mouth disease spreads easily through saliva, mucus from the nose, and stools. Children should not go to school or day care while they have symptoms. They are most contagious in the first 7 to 10 days, but they may be able to spread the disease for a few weeks. Good hand-washing can help prevent this.

## Home Treatment

◆ Give your child acetaminophen (Tylenol) to reduce fever and mouth pain. Do not give aspirin to anyone younger than 20.

◆ Have your child drink plenty of fluids.

◆ Give your child soft, bland foods and cool or warm (not hot) drinks if the mouth is sore. Frozen juice pops may also help.

◆ If the rash hurts or itches, put calamine lotion on it.

◆ Wash hands well after blowing a runny nose or changing a diaper. This will help prevent spreading the illness to others.

# Headaches

## When to Call a Doctor

### Call 911 if:

◆ You have a sudden, severe headache unlike any you have had before. The headache may seem to "explode" out of nowhere.

◆ You have a headache with signs of a stroke. These may include sudden weakness, numbness, inability to move, loss of vision, slurred speech, confusion, behavior changes, or seizure. See page 53.

### Call a doctor if:

◆ You have a headache with stiff neck, fever, vomiting, drowsiness, or confusion. You may have a serious illness. See page 161.

◆ You have had a recent head injury and your headaches are getting a lot worse.

◆ You have a headache with severe eye pain. See page 172.

◆ You have a headache with dizziness and vomiting, and others in your household have the same symptoms. These may be signs of **carbon monoxide poisoning**.

◆ You often have severe headaches with no clear cause.

◆ You think your headaches are migraines but have not talked to your doctor about it. There may be medicine that can help prevent them.

◆ You have a lot more headaches than you used to, or they are worse than they used to be.

◆ You often get headaches during or after exercise, sex, coughing, or sneezing.

◆ Headaches wake you from a sound sleep or are worse first thing in the morning.

◆ You are using pain medicine to control headaches more than once a week, or you need help dealing with your headaches.

If your headache seems unusual or occurs with other symptoms, you may want to check the chart on page 62.

Most headaches are **tension headaches**, which get worse when you are under stress. You may have tightness or pain in the muscles of your neck, back, and shoulders with the headache. A past neck injury or arthritis in the neck can also cause tension headaches.

A tension headache may cause pain all over your head, pressure inside your head, or a feeling that you have a tight band around your head. Some people feel a dull, pressing, burning sensation above the eyes. With a tension headache, you can rarely point to an exact spot where it hurts.

## Are your headaches migraines?

They may be if:

◆ The pain is severe, throbbing, or piercing.

- Headaches occur with nausea and vomiting, or sound seems too loud or light too bright when you get a headache.

- The pain is on one side of the head.

- You have an "aura"—flashing lights, blind spots, numbness or tingling, strange smells or sounds—about an hour before you get the headache. (Some people may have less noticeable symptoms like hunger or mood changes a day or two before the headache.)

- Headaches seem to be related to your menstrual period.

## Preventing Headaches

- Reduce emotional stress. Take time to relax before and after you do something that has caused a headache in the past. Try relaxation techniques such as meditation or progressive muscle relaxation. See page 320.

- Reduce physical stress. When you sit at a desk, change positions often, and stretch for 30 seconds each hour. Try to relax your jaw, neck, shoulder, and upper back muscles.

- Check your neck and shoulder posture at work. See page 213.

- Exercise every day. It can help reduce stress and muscle tension.

- Get regular massages. Some people find this very helpful in relieving tension.

- Limit caffeine to 1 to 2 drinks a day. People who drink a lot of caffeine often get a headache several hours after they have their last caffeine drink. Or they may wake with a headache that does not go away until they drink caffeine. Cut down slowly to avoid caffeine-withdrawal headaches.

### If you get migraines

You may find that certain foods, events, medicines, or activities tend to "trigger" your headaches. Learning what your triggers are and finding ways to limit or avoid them can help you prevent headaches. Tracking your headaches is one thing that can help.

For help figuring out what triggers your migraines, go to the Web site on the back cover and enter **u300** in the search box.

## Tracking Your Headaches

If you have headaches often, keep a record of your symptoms. This record will help your doctor if you need to be checked or treated. It may also help you take control of your headaches, especially if they are migraines.

Write down:

1. The date and time each headache starts and stops.

2. Anything that could have triggered the headache. This might be food, smoke, bright light, stress, or activity.

3. Where the pain is. Is it in one spot or all over your head?

4. What kind of pain you have. Is it throbbing, aching, stabbing, or dull?

5. How bad the pain is. Rate it from 1 to 10 (10 is the worst).

6. Any other symptoms you have, such as nausea, vomiting, vision changes, or sensitivity to light or noise.

7. (Women only) Any link between your headaches and your menstrual cycle, birth control pills, or hormone therapy.

**More** ▶

## Home Treatment

◆ If you get migraines and your doctor has prescribed medicine for them, take it at the first sign that you're getting a migraine.

◆ Stop what you're doing, and sit quietly for a moment. Close your eyes, and breathe slowly. If you can, go to a quiet, dark place and relax. If you have a migraine, sleeping may help.

◆ Some people find that taking a pain medicine such as acetaminophen (Tylenol) or ibuprofen (Advil, Motrin) at the first sign of a headache helps. But using these medicines too often may make headaches worse or more frequent when the medicine wears off. This is called rebound headache.

◆ Put a cold pack on the painful area or on your forehead.

◆ Gently massage your neck and shoulder muscles. Try the neck exercises on page 212.

◆ Put a heating pad on painful or tight muscles, or take a hot shower. But do not use heat if you have a migraine.

◆ Try a relaxation exercise such as progressive muscle relaxation. See page 320.

## Headaches in Children

People often start getting migraine headaches during childhood or the teen years. Migraines are the most common headaches in children. Home treatment for migraines in children is the same as for adults, although some of the medicines may be different.

### Cluster Headaches

Cluster headaches occur in "clusters" over a period of days or months and then disappear for months or even years. During a cluster period, you may have several headaches each day.

These headaches cause sudden, very severe, sharp, stabbing pain on one side, usually in the temple or behind the eye. The eye and nostril on that side may be runny, and the eye may be red. The headaches often start at night and may last from a few minutes to about an hour.

To prevent headaches during a cluster period:

◆ Avoid alcohol and tobacco.

◆ Get plenty of sleep.

◆ Reduce stress.

If you think you are having cluster headaches, talk to your doctor.

Children's headaches can also be caused by:

◆ Stress about school, sports, relationships, or peer pressure. Even fun activities can be overdone. Many times, just talking about a problem with your child may help.

◆ Hunger. A healthy breakfast and after-school snack may prevent headaches.

◆ Eyestrain. Have your child's eyes checked.

◆ Lack of sleep. Set bedtimes and enforce them. Make sure your child gets enough rest.

◆ Colds, sinus problems, and other illnesses.

### When Your Child Has a Headache

◆ Check the When to Call a Doctor list on page 176.

◆ If your doctor has prescribed a specific treatment for your child's headaches, start treatment as soon as your child says he or she has a headache.

◆ For mild headaches that occur only once in a while, let your child rest quietly in a dark room with a cool, wet cloth on his or her forehead. If rest does not help, try acetaminophen (Tylenol) or ibuprofen (Advil, Motrin). Never give aspirin to your child unless your doctor has told you to.

◆ If your child often gets mild headaches, encourage him or her to go on with normal activities. Do not let your child avoid chores, homework, or other things unless the pain is bad. It helps to practice what you preach in this area. When you have a headache, deal with it in a calm, matter-of-fact way, and try to keep up your own usual activities. Your child may follow your example.

◆ Talk to your child. Let him or her know you care. Extra attention and quiet time may be enough to relieve the headache.

# Hearing Problems

This topic covers two common hearing problems:

◆ Hearing loss

◆ Ringing in the ears (tinnitus)

## Protect Your Hearing

◆ Avoid harmful noise. The noise from machines, guns, snowmobiles, motor-cycles, lawn mowers, power tools, household appliances, high-volume music, and other sources can damage your hearing.

◆ Use hearing protectors such as earplugs or earmuffs when you have to be around harmful noise. These can greatly reduce the noise that reaches the ear. Cotton balls or tissues stuffed in the ears do not help much.

◆ Control the volume when you can. Don't buy noisy toys, appliances, or tools when there are quieter choices. Turn down the stereo, the TV, the car radio, and personal music players with earphones.

◆ Never use cotton swabs, hairpins, or other objects to remove earwax or to scratch your ears. They can damage the ear. See page 148 to learn how to remove earwax safely.

◆ Ask your pharmacist if any medicines you take can affect your hearing. For example, antibiotics, blood pressure medicines, ibuprofen (Advil, Motrin), and large doses of aspirin can cause hearing loss.

◆ During air travel, swallow and yawn a lot when the plane is coming down. If you have a cold, the flu, or a sinus infection, take a decongestant a few hours before the plane lands.

◆ If you scuba dive, learn how to dive safely.

**More**

# Hearing Loss

## When to Call a Doctor

◆ Hearing loss develops suddenly (within a matter of days or weeks).

◆ You have hearing loss in one ear only.

◆ You develop a hearing problem while taking medicine, including aspirin or ibuprofen (Advil, Motrin).

◆ Hearing loss occurs with vertigo (you feel like the room is spinning) or loss of movement in your face.

◆ You think your hearing is slowly getting worse.

◆ You wonder if you need a hearing aid.

◆ You think your baby or child may not be hearing well.

Millions of people cope with reduced hearing. In adults, the most common causes are:

◆ **Noise.** Over time, the noise you are exposed to at work, at play (such as listening to very loud music), or even during common chores (like mowing the lawn) can lead to hearing loss. Your hearing usually gets worse over many years.

◆ **Age.** Changes in the inner ear that occur as you grow older cause a gradual but steady hearing loss. This is called **presbycusis**.

Other causes of hearing loss include earwax buildup, an object in the ear, injury to the ear or head, ear infection, and other ear problems. Some common medicines—aspirin, ibuprofen (Advil, Motrin), antibiotics—can affect your hearing. Check with your pharmacist. Sometimes hearing loss can be a sign of a serious health problem.

## Home Treatment

Hearing loss can affect your work and home life. It can make you feel lonely, depressed, or helpless. But there are things you can do to hear better and feel connected to others.

◆ Protect the hearing you have. Always wear hearing protection around loud noises. Avoid loud noise when you can.

◆ Learn to pay close attention to a speaker's face, posture, gestures, and tone of voice. These clues can help you understand what a person is saying. Face the person you're talking to and have him or her face you. Make sure the lighting is good so that you can see the other person's face clearly.

◆ Consider a hearing aid. See an expert who can help you pick one that fits. Be sure to have your hearing tested and the hearing aid adjusted over time.

◆ Use other helpful devices, such as:

❖ Telephone amplifiers.

❖ Hearing aids that can connect to a TV, stereo, radio, or microphone.

❖ Devices that use lights or vibrations to alert you to the doorbell, a ringing phone, or a baby monitor.

❖ TV closed-captioning that shows the words at the bottom of the screen. Most new TVs have this option.

❖ TTY (text telephone), which lets you type messages back and forth on the phone instead of talking or listening. These devices are also called TDD.

# Ringing in the Ears

## When to Call a Doctor

◆ Tinnitus starts suddenly and affects only one ear.

◆ You have new tinnitus with hearing loss, vertigo (you feel like the room is spinning), loss of balance, nausea, or vomiting.

◆ Ringing in your ears does not stop or change.

◆ You get tinnitus after an injury to your head or ear.

◆ Tinnitus lasts longer than 2 weeks, even with home treatment. There may be no cure, but your doctor can help you learn how to live with the problem.

Most people have ringing, roaring, hissing, or buzzing in their ears from time to time. The sound usually lasts only a few minutes. If it does not go away or it happens often, you may have a problem called tinnitus.

Tinnitus is most often caused by being around too much loud noise. But it can have other causes like ear infections, dental problems, and medicines (especially antibiotics and large amounts of aspirin). Be sure to discuss it with your doctor. Drinking alcohol or lots of caffeine can add to the problem.

## Home Treatment

◆ Cut back on alcohol and caffeine.

◆ Limit your use of aspirin, ibuprofen (Advil, Motrin), and naproxen (Aleve).

◆ If you have an earwax problem, remove the wax safely. See page 148.

Looking for the **Heart Failure** topic? See page 291.

# Heart Palpitations

## When to Call a Doctor

**Call 911** if you have chest pain or pressure, especially if it occurs with other symptoms of a heart attack (sweating, shortness of breath, nausea or vomiting, feeling dizzy or lightheaded). See page 38.

**Call your doctor if:**

◆ Heart palpitations occur with:

❖ Weakness or fatigue.

❖ Confusion.

❖ Feeling lightheaded.

❖ Feeling as if something bad is going to happen.

◆ It feels like your heart skips beats or beats unevenly all the time.

◆ Heart palpitations are new or different than before and do not go away with home treatment.

**More** ➤

Heart palpitations are an uncomfortable feeling that your heart is beating very fast or in an odd rhythm. You may feel like:

- Your heart is pounding, or there is a fluttering in your chest.

- Your heart is doing a "flip-flop" or is skipping a beat.

- Your heart is racing, or there is an extra heartbeat.

- Your heart is beating in your neck.

Palpitations may be caused by a heart problem. But they also occur because of:

- Stress or fatigue.

- Too much alcohol, caffeine, or nicotine.

- Illegal drugs like meth and cocaine.

- A high thyroid level.

- Medicines, including diet pills, antihistamines, decongestants, and some herbal products.

Nearly everyone has heart palpitations from time to time. There is usually no reason to worry.

But if you are at higher risk for heart disease (for example, if you smoke or are not very active, or you have high blood pressure, high cholesterol, or a lot of stress), see your doctor for a checkup. Finding and treating heart problems early is the best way to prevent serious illness.

## Home Treatment

- Take deep breaths and try to relax.

- If you start to feel like you may faint, lie down so that you don't fall.

- Write down the date and time; your pulse rate; what you were doing when the problem started; how long it went on; and any other symptoms. Having a record can help you and your doctor figure out the cause of the problem.

To prevent further problems:

- Do not smoke. If you need help quitting, see page 316.

- Cut down on caffeine and alcohol.

- Check with your pharmacist or doctor to see whether any of your medicines can cause heart palpitations.

- Reduce stress. See page 319. If you have problems with anxiety, see page 80.

- Get regular exercise. If you often have heart palpitations, talk to your doctor before you start an exercise program.

# Heartburn

Heartburn occurs when stomach juices flow backward into the esophagus, the tube that leads from the mouth to the stomach. The backflow, called **reflux**, causes a feeling of burning, warmth, or heat beneath the breastbone. You may feel it spread in waves up into your neck and get a sour taste in your mouth.

Heartburn can last up to 2 hours or longer. It gets worse when you lie down or bend over and improves when you sit or stand up.

Don't worry if you have heartburn now and then. Nearly everyone does. Use the home treatment tips to get relief.

But if you have heartburn often, you may have **gastroesophageal reflux disease (GERD)**. GERD can lead to other health problems. You need to see a doctor if you have frequent heartburn and home treatment does not help.

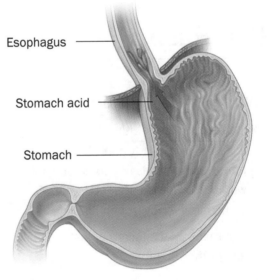

- Esophagus
- Stomach acid
- Stomach

You get heartburn when stomach acid flows up (refluxes) into the esophagus.

If you have GERD, go to the Web site on the back cover and enter **L457** in the search box to learn what you can do to control your symptoms.

**More**

## Home Treatment

◆ Eat smaller meals, and avoid late-night snacks. After eating, wait 2 to 3 hours before you lie down.

◆ Avoid foods that bring on heartburn. These may include citrus fruits and juices (orange, tomato), chocolate, fatty or fried foods, peppermint- or spearmint-flavored foods, alcohol, carbonated drinks, and coffee and other drinks with caffeine.

◆ Do not smoke or chew tobacco.

◆ If you get heartburn at night, raise the head of your bed 6 to 8 inches by putting the frame on blocks or placing a foam wedge under the head of your mattress. (Adding extra pillows does not work well.

◆ Take a nonprescription product for heartburn. For mild heartburn, an antacid, such as Maalox, Mylanta, or Tums, may help. Or try an acid reducer, such as Pepcid AC, Tagamet HB, or Zantac. You can also buy an acid blocker called Prilosec OTC without a prescription. Ask your pharmacist to help you choose one of these medicines.

◆ Do not wear tight clothing around your middle.

◆ Do not take aspirin, ibuprofen (Advil, Motrin), or naproxen (Aleve). These can cause heartburn or make it worse. If you need something for pain, try acetaminophen (Tylenol).

◆ Lose weight if you need to. Losing just 5 to 10 pounds can help.

# Heat Rash

### When to Call a Doctor

◆ Heat rash occurs with a fever of 100.4°F in a baby under 3 months, and the fever does not come down within 20 minutes after you take off some of the baby's clothing.

◆ The rash looks infected or lasts longer than 3 days.

◆ Your baby seems sick.

Heat rash is a rash of tiny red dots on a baby's head, neck, and shoulders. Some people call it prickly heat.

Heat rash often develops when parents dress their baby too warmly or when the weather is hot. Your baby needs, at the most, one more layer of clothing than you do. The skin should feel warm—not hot and not too cool. Place your hand between the baby's shoulder blades. If the skin is hot or moist, the baby is too warm.

## Home Treatment

◆ Keep the baby's skin cool and dry.

◆ Keep the baby's sleeping area comfortable—not too hot, not too cool.

◆ Dress your baby lightly during hot weather. Just a diaper may be fine. Be sure to protect the skin from sunburn.

# Heel Pain and Plantar Fasciitis

## When to Call a Doctor

- ◆ Heel pain occurs with fever, redness, or heat in your heel.

- ◆ You have numbness or tingling in your heel or foot.

- ◆ A heel injury causes pain when you put weight on your heel.

- ◆ You have pain when you are not putting any weight on your heel.

- ◆ Heel pain lasts more than 1 to 2 weeks, even with home treatment.

Heel pain is often caused by **plantar fasciitis**. The plantar fascia is a thick band of tissue that covers the bottom of your foot. If it gets irritated, it causes pain in your heel.

Plantar fasciitis is common in athletes, middle-aged people, and those who are overweight. It can result from:

- ◆ Standing for long periods of time.

- ◆ Doing repeated, high-impact movements such as running and jumping.

- ◆ "Overpronating" when you walk or run. This means the foot rolls inward too far when you take a step. Wearing shoes that are worn out or have poor arch support, having tight calf muscles, or running downhill or on uneven surfaces can make your foot roll inward even more.

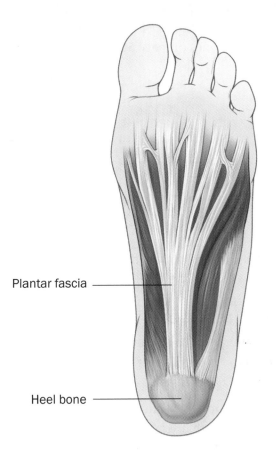

Heel pain is often caused by an irritated plantar fascia.

You may get a **heel spur** if calcium builds up where the plantar fascia attaches to the heel bone. Heel spurs usually do not cause pain and do not need to be treated. (Rarely, a painful heel spur may need to be removed.) The pain many people think is caused by heel spurs is in most cases caused by plantar fasciitis.

More

**Achilles tendinosis** can cause pain in the back of the heel. See Bursitis and Tendinosis on page 111. If you think you may have torn your Achilles tendon, see Strains, Sprains, and Broken Bones on page 50.

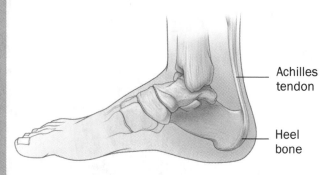

Problems with the Achilles tendon can cause pain in the back of the heel.

## Home Treatment

Start treating heel pain as soon as you feel it. If you ignore it until it gets bad, it may take a lot longer to get better.

◆ Cut back on all weight-bearing activities to the point that you do not have any pain. For exercise, try something that gets you off your feet, such as cycling or swimming. You may need to check with your doctor about when you can gradually get back to high-impact activities like running.

◆ Stretch your Achilles tendon and calf muscles several times a day. See page 314.

◆ Put ice on your heel at least once a day. See Ice and Cold Packs on page 243.

◆ Try nonprescription arch supports in your shoes.

◆ Don't go barefoot. Wear shoes or sandals with good cushioning and good arch support anytime you will be standing up or walking. If you get up at night to go to the bathroom, put on shoes. Replace shoes that are worn out.

◆ Take aspirin, ibuprofen (Advil, Motrin), or naproxen (Aleve) to relieve pain. Do not give aspirin to anyone younger than 20.

◆ For Achilles tendinosis or plantar fasciitis, try heel lifts or heel cups in both shoes. Use them only until the pain is gone.

If you have plantar fascia problems, there are special exercises and stretches that may help. To learn how to do them, go to the Web site on the back cover and enter **k148** in the search box.

Your doctor may also suggest other treatments for plantar fasciitis, such as taping, heel splints, shoe inserts, or steroid shots. Surgery is usually done only as a last resort when other treatments have not worked.

# Hemorrhoids and Rectal Problems

## When to Call a Doctor

**Call 911 if:**

◆ You pass very bloody or dark red stools, or there is a lot of blood in the toilet.

**Call your doctor if:**

◆ You have severe rectal pain.

◆ Your stools are black or tarry or have streaks of blood and you have a fever.

◆ Rectal bleeding occurs for no clear reason and is not related to passing stools.

◆ Rectal bleeding lasts for more than 1 week or happens more than once.

◆ Stools are narrower than usual (they may be no wider than a pencil).

◆ You still have rectal pain after a full week of home treatment.

◆ Any unusual material or tissue seeps or sticks out of the anus.

◆ A lump near the anus gets bigger or more painful and you get a fever.

## Hemorrhoids

Hemorrhoids are enlarged and inflamed veins that may form inside or outside the anus. Straining to pass hard stools, being overweight or pregnant, and sitting or standing for long periods can all cause hemorrhoids.

Hemorrhoids usually last several days and often come back. You may have:

◆ Bright red streaks of blood on stools or toilet paper, or blood dripping from the anus.

◆ Mucus leaking from the anus.

◆ Irritation or itching.

◆ The feeling that you cannot complete a bowel movement.

◆ Tissue or a lump sticking out of the anus.

Pain is not usually a symptom, unless a blood clot forms in a hemorrhoid or the blood flow to a hemorrhoid is cut off (strangulated). A clotted hemorrhoid may be extremely painful but is not dangerous. But a strangulated hemorrhoid may need emergency care.

Hemorrhoids may get better with home treatment. If you have hemorrhoids that bleed a lot, are painful, or make it hard to keep your anal area clean, you may want to  talk to your doctor about surgery or other procedures. For help deciding what treatment is right for you, go to the Web site on the back cover and enter **v666** in the search box.

## Other Rectal Problems

The rectum is the lower part of the large intestine (see the picture on page 171). At the end of the rectum is the anus, where stools pass out of the body.

Most people have rectal itching, pain, or bleeding at some time. These problems are often minor and will go away on their own or with home treatment.

**More**

**Anal itching** can have many causes.

◆ Skin around the anus may be irritated by stool. But trying to keep the area too clean by rubbing it with dry toilet paper or using harsh soap may damage the skin.

◆ Itching can be a sign of pinworms, especially in homes with children. See page 215.

◆ Caffeine and spicy foods can irritate the rectum.

An **anal fissure** may cause pain during bowel movements and streaks of blood on stools. A fissure is a long, narrow sore that may form when the tissue near the anus is torn during a bowel movement.

Rectal bleeding, recent changes in bowel habits, and rectal pain are also symptoms of **colorectal cancer**. If you have these symptoms, see your doctor to find out if you need tests (see page 127). This is especially important if you are over 50 and have a family history of colon cancer.

## Home Treatment

◆ Take warm baths. They are soothing and cleansing, especially after a bowel movement. Warm baths with just enough water to cover the anal area—called sitz baths—can help with hemorrhoids but may make anal itching worse.

◆ Wear cotton underwear and loose clothing to decrease moisture in the anal area.

◆ Put a cool, wet cloth on the anus for 10 minutes, 4 times a day.

◆ Ease itching and irritation with zinc oxide, petroleum jelly, or hydrocortisone (1%) cream. Use a suppository such as Preparation H to ease pain and moisten the anal canal. Ask your doctor before you use any product that has an anesthetic (these products have the suffix "-caine" in the name or ingredients). These products cause allergic reactions in some people.

◆ To keep your stool soft, drink plenty of water and eat lots of fresh fruits, vegetables, and whole grains. You may need to use a nonprescription stool softener until you are better. See Constipation on page 130.

◆ Try not to strain when passing stools. Never hold your breath.

◆ Avoid sitting or standing too much. Take short walks to increase blood flow in your pelvic region.

◆ Keep the anal area clean, but be gentle when you clean it. Use water and a mild soap, such as Ivory, or use baby wipes or Tucks pads.

# Hernia

## When to Call a Doctor

- A testicle swells and is painful, especially in a child or teen. This could be very serious. See page 246.

- You have a known hernia and you have sudden, severe pain in your groin or scrotum, along with nausea, vomiting, and fever.

- Mild groin pain or an unexplained bump or swelling in the groin lasts for more than 1 week.

- The skin over a hernia or bulge in the groin or belly turns red.

- You cannot push a hernia back into place with gentle pressure when you are lying down.

Most hernias occur when tissue bulges through a weak spot in the belly wall into the groin. These are called inguinal hernias. They are more common in men than in women. In men, inguinal hernias often bulge into the scrotum.

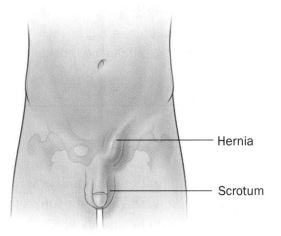

Hernia

Scrotum

A hernia can cause a bulge or lump in the groin or scrotum.

If you have a hernia:

- You may have the sense that something has "given way."

- You may have a tender bulge in your groin or scrotum. The bulge may appear slowly over time, or it may form suddenly after heavy lifting, coughing, or straining. The bulge may flatten when you lie down.

- You may have groin pain that extends into the scrotum. Pain may get worse with bending or lifting. But not all hernias cause pain.

A hernia can form anywhere there is a weakness in the belly wall. Besides the groin, common places for this are the belly button and the site of an incision from a past surgery. Some people are born with a weak spot in the belly wall.

Once in a while, tissue may get trapped in the hernia. If the blood supply to the tissue is cut off, the tissue will swell and die and then can get infected. Rapidly increasing pain in the groin or scrotum is a sign that this happened and that you need medical care now.

**More**

## Home Treatment

These tips will also help prevent hernias:

◆ Use proper lifting techniques. See page 90. Do not lift weights that are too heavy for you.

◆ Lose weight if you need to.

◆ Avoid constipation, and don't strain when you pass stools or urinate. See page 131 for tips on adding more fiber to your diet and avoiding constipation.

◆ Stop smoking, especially if you have a long-term cough.

### Hiatal Hernias

A hiatal hernia occurs when part of the stomach bulges into the chest cavity. Sometimes this will cause a backflow of stomach acid, which can cause heartburn and a sour taste in the mouth.

See Heartburn on page 183.

# High Blood Pressure

## When to Call a Doctor

**Call 911** if you have high blood pressure and get a sudden, severe headache.

**Call your doctor if:**

◆ Your high blood pressure is usually under control but suddenly rises much higher than normal.

◆ You take your blood pressure and it is 180/110 or higher.

◆ You have high blood pressure and get new chest pain or discomfort. See Chest Pain on page 119.

◆ Your blood pressure is higher than 140/90 on two or more occasions.

◆ You have any problems with your blood pressure medicine.

Blood pressure is a measure of the force of blood against the walls of your arteries. Blood pressure readings include two numbers, such as 130/80. (Say "130 over 80.")

◆ The first (or top) number in the reading is the systolic pressure. This is the force of blood when the heart beats.

◆ The second (or bottom) number is the diastolic pressure. This is the force of blood between heartbeats, when the heart is at rest.

| Blood Pressure Level | Systolic (Top Number) | Diastolic (Bottom Number) |
|---|---|---|
| Normal for adults | 119 or below | 79 or below |
| Borderline-high (prehypertension) | 120 to 139 | 80 to 89 |
| High (hypertension) | 140 or above | 90 or above |

If you have high or borderline-high blood pressure, changes in your lifestyle may help lower your blood pressure. Some people also need medicines to get their blood pressure under control.

Despite what a lot of people think, high blood pressure usually does not cause headaches or make you feel dizzy or faint. Often called the "silent killer," it usually has no symptoms.

But it does increase your risk for heart attack, stroke, and kidney and eye damage. Your risk goes up as your blood pressure goes up. The longer your blood pressure stays high, the higher your risk.

## Home Treatment

If your blood pressure is normal, the steps below will help you keep it that way. If you have borderline-high or high blood pressure, these steps may help you lower your blood pressure or keep it from getting worse.

◆ Try to reach and stay at a healthy weight. This is especially important if you put on weight around the waist rather than in the hips and thighs. Losing even 10 pounds can help lower your blood pressure. See page 300.

◆ Exercise for at least 30 minutes on most days of the week. You do not have to do all 30 minutes at once. Try three 10-minute walks. See Exercise and Health on page 311.

◆ Do not drink much alcohol.

◆ Limit salt. To learn how to reduce salt in your diet, see page 292.

◆ Make sure you get enough potassium, calcium, and magnesium. Eat plenty of fruits (such as bananas and oranges), vegetables, dried beans and peas, whole grains, and low-fat dairy products to get these minerals.

◆ Limit saturated fats. Saturated fat is found in animal products such as milk, cheese, and meat. Limiting these foods will help you lose weight and lower your risk for heart disease. See page 307 for tips on how to cut down on them.

◆ If you smoke, quit. Smoking increases your risk for heart attack and stroke. If you need help quitting, see page 316.

## Are You at Risk for High Blood Pressure?

You are more likely to have high blood pressure if:

◆ You smoke.

◆ You are overweight.

◆ Others in your family have high blood pressure.

◆ You are African American.

◆ You don't get regular exercise.

◆ You drink too much alcohol.

◆ You have a lot of salt or not enough potassium, calcium, or magnesium in your diet.

◆ You use decongestants, anti-inflammatory drugs (such as ibuprofen or naproxen), or steroids on a regular basis.

**More**

**If you know you have high blood pressure:**

◆ Take any prescribed blood pressure medicines as your doctor tells you. If you stop taking them, your blood pressure may quickly go back up.

◆ Talk to your doctor about taking an aspirin each day to reduce your risk of heart attack or stroke. Do not start taking aspirin before you have talked to your doctor about it.

◆ See your doctor at least once a year.

◆ If you take blood pressure medicine, talk to your doctor before you take decongestants or anti-inflammatory drugs, such as ibuprofen (Advil, Motrin) or naproxen (Aleve). Some of these can raise blood pressure.

◆ Learn how to check your blood pressure at home.

# High Cholesterol

## When to Call a Doctor

◆ Your cholesterol is over 200, and your doctor does not know about it (for instance, if you had a cholesterol test at a health fair or at a work-related event).

◆ You are over age 30 and have never had your cholesterol checked. This is especially important if your family has a history of heart disease, diabetes, or high cholesterol.

Cholesterol is a kind of fat your body makes. You also get it from foods that come from animals, such as meat, milk and dairy foods, eggs, chicken, and fish.

Your body needs some cholesterol. But when you have too much, it can build up in your arteries and make it harder for blood to flow through them. This problem is called **atherosclerosis**. It is the starting point for most heart and blood flow problems, including heart attacks and strokes.

### Good and Bad Cholesterol

Your body has a few kinds of cholesterol.

◆ **LDL** is the "bad" cholesterol. For LDL, a lower number is better. High LDL increases your risk for heart disease, heart attack, and stroke.

◆ **HDL** is the "good" cholesterol. It helps clear the bad cholesterol from the body. For HDL, a higher number is better. Raising your HDL may reduce your risk for heart disease, stroke, and a blood flow problem called peripheral artery disease.

◆ **Triglycerides** are another type of fat in the blood. High triglycerides may increase your risk of heart disease and stroke.

### What Do the Numbers Mean?

The numbers on page 193 are for people who are at average risk for heart disease. If you have diabetes or heart disease or are at higher risk for heart disease, your doctor may use different numbers for what your cholesterol should be.

**Total cholesterol**

Normal: Less than 200

Borderline-high: 200 to 239

High: 240 and above

**LDL ("bad" cholesterol)**

Best: Less than 100

Near-best: 100 to 129

Borderline-high: 130 to 159

High: 160 to 189

Very high: 190 and above

**HDL ("good" cholesterol)**

Best: Above 60

Too low: Less than 40

**Triglycerides**

Borderline-high: 150 to 199

High: 200 to 499

Very high: 500 and above

### When to Have Cholesterol Tests

You and your doctor can decide how often you should be tested based on your risk for heart disease. Most healthy adults who are not at high risk should have their cholesterol checked at least every 5 years.

It's a good idea to have your cholesterol checked more often if:

◆ Your total cholesterol was over 200 in a previous test.

◆ Your family has a history of early heart attack. Early means before age 55 in your father or brother or before age 65 in your mother or sister.

◆ You smoke.

◆ You have high blood pressure (over 140/90) or take blood pressure medicine.

◆ You have diabetes.

◆ Your HDL was below 40 or your triglycerides were over 150 in a previous test.

These all increase your risk for heart disease. That's why you need to have your cholesterol checked more often.

Basic cholesterol tests are easy, quick, and cheap. Call your local health department to find out where you can get a free or low-cost test.

## How to Reduce Your Cholesterol

◆ Eat a heart-healthy diet that is low in saturated fat and cholesterol.

❖ Eat less total fat, especially saturated fat. See the tips for eating less fat on page 307. Your total fat intake can be up to 35 percent of total calories, as long as most of it is unsaturated fat.

❖ Ask your doctor or a registered dietitian about the TLC (Therapeutic Lifestyle Changes) diet. This diet will help you lower saturated fat to 7 percent or less of your total calories and your cholesterol from food to less than 200 mg per day.

❖ Eat at least 2 servings of fruits and at least 3 servings of vegetables each day.

❖ Eat 2 to 3 servings (4 to 6 ounces) of baked or broiled fish per week. Talk to your doctor about whether you should take fish oil supplements and, if so, what kind and how much to take.

❖ Eat more fiber (fruit, beans and peas, whole grains). See page 308.

**More**

◆ Exercise for at least 30 minutes most days of the week. It increases your HDL level and may lower your LDL level. It can also help you lose weight and lower your blood pressure. If you need help getting started, see page 311.

◆ If you smoke, quit. Smoking increases your risk of heart attack and stroke.

◆ Lose weight if you need to. Losing even 5 to 10 pounds can lower triglycerides and raise HDL. Your LDL may fall as well. Exercise and a healthy diet can help you keep the weight off. See page 300.

Start with these changes. Regular exercise and a diet low in saturated fat are often enough to lower cholesterol.

Some people also need to take medicines. They may have very high cholesterol or diabetes, be at high risk for heart disease, or have other health problems. For help deciding whether you should take medicines for high cholesterol, go to the Web site on the back cover and enter **x194** in the search box.

You can do everything right and still have high cholesterol. Although a lot of cholesterol comes from food, your liver makes cholesterol too. Your cholesterol goes up as you age, no matter how healthy you are. But healthy habits can help you avoid some of the problems related to cholesterol, like heart attack, heart disease, and stroke.

# Hives

## When to Call a Doctor

**Call 911** if hives occur with dizziness, wheezing, trouble breathing, tightness in the chest, or swelling of the tongue, lips, or face.

**Call a doctor if:**

◆ You get hives soon after you start a new medicine.

◆ Hives cover all or most of your body.

◆ You still have hives after a full day of home treatment.

Hives are raised, red, itchy, often fluid-filled patches of skin that may come and go at random. Some people call them wheals or welts. Hives may last a few minutes or a few days. They can range in size from less than ¼ inch to more than 3 inches across.

An insect sting may cause a single hive. You may get many hives in response to a medicine, food, or infection. Other causes include plant allergies, inhaled allergens, stress, makeup, and exposure to heat, cold, sunlight, or rubber latex. Often you cannot find the cause.

## Home Treatment

◆ If you know what caused the hives, avoid it. If it was a food, don't eat it again. If it was makeup, don't wear it again. If it was a medicine, tell your doctor, and do not take it again.

◆ Use cool, moist cloths to help relieve itching. For more tips, see page 142.

◆ Take an oral antihistamine (such as Benadryl or Chlor-Trimeton) to treat the hives and relieve itching. Once the hives go away, decrease the dose of the medicine slowly over 5 to 7 days.

# Impetigo

## When to Call a Doctor

◆ Impetigo covers a total area more than 2 inches wide.

◆ Impetigo does not improve after 3 to 4 days of home treatment, or new sores appear. Your doctor may prescribe an antibiotic.

◆ Your face is swollen or tender, especially near the nose and lips or around the eyes.

◆ You get a fever, or you have increased pain, swelling, warmth, or redness near the sores.

Impetigo is an infection that causes oozing, honey-colored, crusty sores. It often appears between the upper lip and nose after a cold or at the corner of the mouth. Impetigo is much more common in children than in adults.

Small areas of impetigo may get better with prompt home treatment.

## Home Treatment

◆ Do not scratch. Scratching can spread impetigo to other areas.

◆ Soak the area in warm water for 15 to 20 minutes to remove crusts. For the face, put a warm, wet washcloth on the sores. Then scrub gently with a washcloth and antibacterial soap. Pat dry. Do this several times a day, using a clean washcloth each time.

◆ Apply an antibiotic ointment. Cover the area with gauze taped well away from the sores. This will help keep the infection from spreading and prevent scratching.

◆ Men should shave around the sores, not over them. Use a clean blade each day. Do not use a shaving brush.

◆ Do not share towels, washcloths, or bathwater.

◆ If your child has a runny nose, keep the area between the child's upper lip and nose clean.

# Ingrown Toenail

## When to Call a Doctor

◆ You have increasing pain, swelling, warmth, or redness around the nail; red streaks leading from the nail; pus; and fever.

◆ You have diabetes or blood flow problems and get an ingrown toenail.

You can get an ingrown toenail if:

◆ You cut your toenail so that the nail cuts into the skin at the edge of the nail. Always cut your toenails straight across, not curved.

◆ You wear shoes that are too tight.

Because the nail can easily get infected, it needs prompt care.

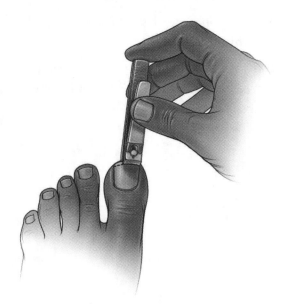

Cut toenails straight across.

## Home Treatment

◆ Soak your foot in warm water for 15 minutes each day to soften the skin around the nail. (This may also relieve swelling and pain while the nail grows out.) You may want to add Epsom salt to the water.

◆ To keep the nail from cutting the skin, wedge a small piece of wet cotton under the corner of the nail to cushion it and lift it slightly. Repeat each day until the nail has grown out and you can trim it.

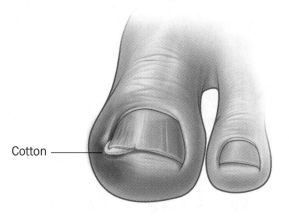

Cotton

Use a piece of wet cotton to cushion and lift the nail.

◆ Cut the toenail straight across. Leave it a little longer at the corners so that the sharp ends don't cut into the skin.

◆ Wear roomy shoes, and keep your feet clean and dry.

# Irritable Bowel Syndrome

## When to Call a Doctor

- Your symptoms get worse, start to disrupt your usual activities, or do not respond as usual to home treatment.

- You are more and more tired all the time.

- Your symptoms often wake you.

- Your pain gets worse when you move or cough.

- You have belly pain and a fever.

- You have belly pain that does not get better when you pass gas or stools.

- You are losing weight, and you don't know why.

- Your appetite has decreased.

- There is blood in your stools, or your stools look black and tarry.

Irritable bowel syndrome (IBS) is one of the most common problems of the digestive tract. Symptoms often increase with stress or after you eat and include:

- Bloating, belly pain, and gas.

- Mucus in the stool.

- The feeling that you cannot complete a bowel movement.

- Irregular bowel habits, with constipation, diarrhea, or both.

People can have IBS for many years. An episode may be worse than the one before it, but the disorder itself does not get worse over time or lead to more serious diseases such as cancer. Symptoms tend to get better over time.

If you have frequent digestive problems but have not been diagnosed with IBS, try to rule out other reasons for your stomach upset, such as new foods, stress, or the flu. Try home treatment for 1 to 2 weeks. If it does not help, call your doctor. Your doctor may prescribe medicine for you to take while you continue with home treatment.

There are no tests that can diagnose irritable bowel syndrome, but your doctor may want to do tests to rule out other problems. Be sure to think about and discuss how much testing is right for you. This may depend on your age, your symptoms, your response to treatment, and your chances of having a more serious problem.

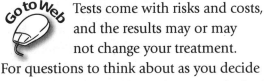 Tests come with risks and costs, and the results may or may not change your treatment. For questions to think about as you decide about testing, go to the Web site on the back cover and enter **h696** in the search box.

More

## Home Treatment

### If constipation is your main symptom:

◆ Eat more fruits, vegetables, beans, and whole grains. Add these fiber-rich foods to your diet slowly so they do not make gas or cramps worse.

◆ Add unprocessed wheat bran to your diet. Start by using 1 tablespoon a day, and slowly increase to 4 tablespoons a day. Sprinkle bran on cereal, soup, and casseroles. Drink extra water to avoid bloating.

◆ Try a product that contains a bulk-forming agent, such as Citrucel, FiberCon, or Metamucil. Start with 1 tablespoon or less each day, and drink extra water to prevent bloating.

◆ Use a laxative only if your doctor suggests it.

◆ Get some exercise every day. Exercise helps the digestive system work better.

### If diarrhea is your main symptom:

◆ Try the diet tips for relieving constipation. Fiber-rich foods and wheat bran can sometimes help relieve diarrhea.

◆ Avoid foods that make diarrhea worse. Try cutting out one food at a time; then add it back bit by bit. If a food does not seem to be related to symptoms, you do not need to avoid it. Many people find that the following foods or ingredients make their symptoms worse:

❖ Alcohol, caffeine, and nicotine

❖ Beans, broccoli, cabbage, and apples

❖ Spicy foods

❖ Foods high in acid, such as citrus fruit

❖ Fatty foods, including bacon, sausage, butter, oils, and anything deep-fried

◆ Avoid dairy products that have lactose (milk sugar) if they seem to make symptoms worse. But be sure to get enough calcium in your diet from other sources. See Lactose Intolerance on page 139.

◆ Avoid sorbitol, an artificial sweetener, and olestra, a fat substitute used in some processed foods.

◆ Add more starchy food (whole-grain breads, rice, potatoes, pasta) to your diet.

◆ If diarrhea does not stop, a nonprescription medicine such as loperamide (in products such as Imodium) may help. Check with your doctor if you are using loperamide more than 3 times a week.

### To reduce stress:

◆ Keep a record of the life events that occur with your symptoms. This may help you see any link between stress and your symptoms.

◆ Get regular, brisk exercise, such as swimming, cycling, or walking.

◆ Learn and use a relaxation technique. See page 320.

◆ Look for more tips in Dealing With Stress on page 318.

# Jaw Pain and Temporomandibular Disorder

## When to Call a Doctor

- Jaw pain is severe.
- You have jaw pain or other problems after an injury to the jaw.
- Your jaw locks.
- A jaw problem has not improved after 2 weeks of home treatment.
- You have noticed a change in the way your teeth fit together when you close your mouth.

The temporomandibular joint connects the lower jawbone to the skull. When you have pain in this joint and in the jaw muscles, you have a problem called **temporomandibular (TM) disorder**.

- You may feel pain in one or both jaws when you chew or yawn.
- You may have painful clicking, popping, or grating in the jaw joint.
- Your jaw may lock, or you may not be able to open your mouth wide.
- You may often have headaches or pain in your neck, face, or shoulders.

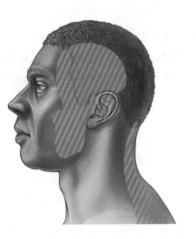

TM disorder causes pain in the shaded areas.

The most common cause of TM disorder is tension in the jaw, neck, and shoulder muscles. Stress or habits such as clenching or grinding your teeth can cause a lot of tension in these muscles. TM disorder can also occur if there is a problem in the jaw joint itself, such as arthritis.

Home treatment can relieve most TM problems. Your doctor may also suggest a plastic mouth plate or physical therapy. Surgery is rarely needed and may make things worse.

## Home Treatment

The key to treating TM disorder is to reduce tension in your jaw.

- Try not to clench or grind your teeth. Do not bite your nails or tuck the phone receiver between your shoulder and jaw.
- At the first sign of pain in your jaw muscles, stop chewing gum or tough foods. Eat softer foods, and use both sides of your mouth to chew.
- Use good posture. Poor posture may disturb the way the muscles and bones in your face work together.

**More**

◆ Rest your jaw, keeping your teeth apart and your lips closed. (Keep your tongue on the roof of your mouth, not between your teeth.) Do not open your mouth too wide.

◆ Put an ice pack on the joint for 10 minutes, 3 times a day. Gently open and close your mouth while the ice pack is on. If the jaw muscle is swollen, use ice 6 times a day.

◆ Take ibuprofen (Advil, Motrin) or naproxen (Aleve) to reduce swelling and pain.

◆ If there is no swelling, you can put moist heat on your jaw for 10 to 15 minutes, 3 times a day. Gently open and close your mouth while the heat is on. You can also alternate heat with cold.

◆ Relax. If you have a lot of stress in your life, try some relaxation techniques. See page 320. Get help if you are under severe stress or suffer from anxiety or depression.

# Kidney Stones

## When to Call a Doctor

◆ You think you have a kidney stone. Symptoms include:

❖ Sudden pain in your side, groin, or genital area that gets worse over 15 to 60 minutes until it is steady and severe.

❖ Nausea and vomiting.

❖ Blood in the urine.

❖ Feeling like you need to urinate often or having pain when you urinate.

❖ Diarrhea, constipation, or loss of appetite.

❖ Not being able to find a comfortable position.

◆ You have fever or chills and increasing pain in your back, just below your rib cage.

◆ You have blood in your urine.

◆ You pass a stone, even if there was little or no pain. Save the stone, and ask your doctor whether it needs to be tested.

Kidney stones can form from the minerals in urine. The most common cause is not drinking enough water.

As long as they stay in the kidneys, kidney stones usually cause no problems. But if a stone moves into the ureter, which is the tube that leads to the bladder (see the picture on page 251), it may block the flow of urine and cause severe pain. In fact, it may be the worst pain you have ever had.

When the stone moves into the bladder, the pain may vanish suddenly. But it can hurt again when the stone passes out of the body.

Most small kidney stones pass without you needing treatment other than pain medicine. In rare cases, you may need surgery or a procedure that uses sound waves to break the stones into small pieces.

## Home Treatment

◆ Drink extra water—2 cups every 2 hours. This will help the stone pass and can help prevent future stones.

◆ Take aspirin, acetaminophen (Tylenol), or ibuprofen (Advil, Motrin) to relieve pain. Do not take aspirin if you are under age 20.

◆ Use heat on sore areas in your back or belly for 20 minutes at a time. Moist heat (a hot pack or a hot bath or shower) works better than dry heat.

# Knee Problems

### When to Call a Doctor

◆ Your knee gives out or will not bear weight.

◆ You felt or heard a "pop" in your knee at the time of an injury.

◆ Your knee swells a lot within 30 minutes of an injury.

◆ You have signs of damage to the nerves or blood vessels, such as numbness, tingling, a pins-and-needles feeling, or pale or bluish skin below the injury.

◆ Your knee looks deformed.

◆ You cannot straighten or bend your knee, or the joint locks.

◆ Your knee is red, hot, swollen, or painful to touch.

◆ The pain is bad enough that you are limping, or it does not improve with 2 days of home treatment.

The knee is a joint that can get hurt easily. It is simply three long leg bones held together with ligaments and muscles. Problems can occur when you overstress your knee. Three common ones are:

◆ **Sprained knee ligaments.** (Ligaments connect bone to bone.) Sprains are usually the result of the knee bending or twisting too far in a direction that it's not supposed to go. Sometimes a ligament may tear. You can tear cartilage in the knee as well. Cartilage is tissue that cushions the joint.

◆ **Kneecap pain,** also known as patellofemoral pain. This is pain around or behind the kneecap. You may have it when you run downhill, when you go up or down stairs, or after you sit for long periods of time.

◆ **Jumper's knee,** also known as patellar tendinosis. This affects the tendon that attaches your kneecap to your shinbone and causes pain right below your knee. It's common in basketball and volleyball players.

**More**

201

Also see Strains, Sprains, and Broken Bones on page 50 and Bursitis and Tendinosis on page 111.

If knee pain is not related to exercise or a recent or past injury, see Arthritis on page 82.

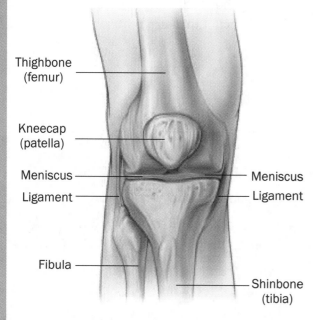

Thighbone
(femur)

Kneecap
(patella)

Meniscus

Ligament

Fibula

Meniscus

Ligament

Shinbone
(tibia)

You can have knee problems when the structures that support the joint are injured or inflamed.

## Home Treatment

◆ Rest and protect your knee. Take a break from anything that causes pain. After several days of rest, you can start gentle exercises and stretching.

◆ Put ice or a cold pack on your knee for 10 to 15 minutes at a time. See Ice and Cold Packs on page 243.

◆ Prop up your knee on a pillow when you ice it or anytime you sit or lie down for the next 3 days. Try to keep it above the level of your heart. This will help reduce swelling.

◆ Take ibuprofen (Advil, Motrin) or naproxen (Aleve) for pain and swelling.

◆ Ask your doctor about wearing a brace or an elastic or neoprene sleeve with a hole that holds the kneecap in place. This will help ease pain during activity. You can buy one at a pharmacy or sporting goods store.

## Preventing Knee Problems

◆ Strengthen and stretch the leg muscles evenly, especially those in the front of the thigh (called the quadriceps) and the back of the thigh (called the hamstrings). See page 314. This is the best way to prevent knee problems.

◆ Do not do deep knee bends. Imagine a line that starts at the tip of your toes and goes straight up. When you do knee bends, your knees should not jut past that line.

◆ Do not run downhill unless your muscles are well trained and strong enough for it.

◆ Wear shoes with good arch supports. Replace running shoes every 300 to 500 miles.

◆ Do not wear shoes with cleats when you play contact sports.

◆ Do not wear high-heeled shoes.

# Laryngitis

## When to Call a Doctor

◆ You have a high fever. See the fever guidelines on page 160.

◆ You have symptoms of a worse infection, such as fast or shallow breathing, a cough that brings up colored mucus from the lungs, or pain, fever, and fatigue that are getting a lot worse.

◆ You are hoarse for more than 2 to 3 weeks.

Laryngitis is an infection or irritation of the voice box (larynx). If you have laryngitis, you may be hoarse, lose your voice, and feel like you need to clear your throat a lot. You may also have fever, throat pain, and a cough and feel more tired than usual.

You can get laryngitis because of:

◆ A virus, such as a cold.

◆ Allergies.

◆ Lots of talking, singing, or yelling.

◆ Cigarette smoke.

◆ Backflow (reflux) of stomach acid into the throat.

Your voice box will usually heal in 5 to 10 days. Medicine does not help much.

If you drink a lot of alcohol or smoke, you may reach a point where your throat and voice box are irritated all the time.

## Home Treatment

◆ If a cold makes you hoarse, treat the cold (see page 124). You may be hoarse for up to a week after a cold goes away.

◆ Rest your voice. Try not to talk much or clear your throat.

◆ Do not smoke, and avoid other people's smoke. If you need help to quit smoking, see page 316.

◆ Use a humidifier in your bedroom or your whole house. Or try standing in the steam from a hot shower.

◆ Drink extra water and other fluids.

◆ To soothe your throat, gargle with warm salt water (1 teaspoon of salt in 8 ounces of water), or drink weak tea or hot water with honey or lemon juice in it. Do not give honey to children younger than 1 year.

◆ If you think that problems with stomach acid reflux may be the cause, reducing heartburn may help. See page 184.

# Leg Pain and Muscle Cramps

## When to Call a Doctor

- You have sudden leg pain, and the skin of your lower leg, foot, or toes is cold, pale, or blue-black. This could be a serious problem.

- You have swelling, redness, and pain in the leg or calf and have fever. These are signs of phlebitis (see the chart on page 205).

- Leg pain always starts after you walk a certain distance and then goes away when you stop walking. This is a sign of a blood flow problem.

- Home treatment does not relieve your muscle cramps.

Leg pain and muscle cramps ("charley horse" or "a stitch") are common. They often occur at night or during exercise, especially if the weather is hot or humid. Dehydration, low levels of potassium, or using a muscle that is not stretched well may cause cramps.

## Home Treatment

- If you have pain, swelling, or heaviness in the calf of only one of your legs, or if you have other symptoms that cause you to suspect phlebitis, call your doctor before you try home treatment.

- Warm up well and stretch before exercise. Also stretch after you exercise. If a muscle cramps, gently stretch and massage it.

- Drink plenty of fluids. Drink extra fluids before and during exercise, especially if the weather is hot or humid.

- Get plenty of potassium in your diet. Bananas, orange juice, and potatoes are good sources.

- If leg cramps wake you at night, take a warm bath and do some stretches before you go to bed. Keep your legs warm while sleeping.

- For shin splints, put a cold pack on your leg for 10 to 15 minutes at a time, and take acetaminophen (Tylenol) or ibuprofen (Advil, Motrin) for pain. Take 1 to 2 weeks of rest from high-impact activities like running. Return to exercise slowly.

- To avoid stomach muscle cramps ("side stitch") during exercise, do side stretches before you start. Try to take deep, even breaths.

## Growing Pains

Children age 6 to 12 often have harmless "growing pains" in their legs at night. Unless your child's pain is severe, you don't need to worry about these. A heating pad, acetaminophen (Tylenol), or gentle massage may help.

| Common Causes of Leg Pain | Symptoms | Comments |
| --- | --- | --- |
| Muscle cramps | Sudden cramping pain, usually in lower leg; leg may feel like it is in "knots" | Often happens at night or during exercise |
| Shin splints | Pain in front of lower leg | Often caused by overuse or high-impact exercise (such as running on a hard surface), especially if you are not used to it |
| Arthritis | Pain in leg joints (knees, ankles, toes) | See Arthritis, p. 82. |
| Sciatica (a back problem) | Leg pain that extends from buttocks down back of leg and into foot | See Sciatica, p. 88. |
| Phlebitis (an inflamed vein) | Pain and swelling in one calf; common after surgery, bed rest, and extended air travel | Can be serious if blood clot forms, breaks loose, and travels to lungs |
| Decreased blood flow (intermittent claudication) | Cramping pain in the calf that starts after you walk a certain distance and goes away when you rest; leg pain and cold, pale skin | |

# Lice and Scabies

## When to Call a Doctor

◆ You have severe nighttime itching that does not go away after a few days.

◆ You see live lice or new nits after you have used a nonprescription lice medicine. Your doctor can prescribe a stronger medicine.

Lice are tiny, white insects that may live on the skin, hair, or clothing. They feed by biting the skin and sucking blood. Scabies are tiny mites that dig under the skin and lay eggs.

Both cause an allergic rash and itching. And both are common in children who go to day care or school.

**More** ▶

| Common Questions | Lice | Scabies |
|---|---|---|
| Where are they found? | In hair on the head (head lice); on clothing (body lice); in groin area, underarms, and eyelashes (pubic lice) | Between folds of skin on fingers and toes, wrists, underarms, knees, elbows, and groin |
| How are they spread? | By close contact with an infested person or his or her clothing, hats, bedding, towels, brushes, or combs; pubic lice by sexual contact | By close contact with an infested person or his or her bedding, clothing, or towels |
| How do you get rid of them? | Medicine for head lice. Wash clothing, bedding, and towels. | Medicine applied to the entire body and left on overnight. Wash clothing, bedding, and towels. Itching may last for several weeks. |

## Home Treatment

◆ To get rid of lice, try a nonprescription medicine such as Nix or RID. Follow the directions on the label exactly. After you use the medicine, comb the hair well with a fine-toothed nit comb to remove all lice eggs, called nits. You can buy nit combs at most drugstores and supermarkets.

◆ To get rid of scabies, you will need prescription medicine. Call your doctor.

◆ On the day you start treatment for lice or scabies, wash all dirty clothing, bedding, and towels in hot water. Iron or dry-clean items that cannot be washed, or freeze them for 24 hours.

◆ Call your pharmacist or health department for more information about treatment and prevention.

### When Can My Child Go Back to School?

Some schools have a "no nits" policy stating that children may not return to school until they are free of lice nits.

Children who have scabies can go back to school as soon as they complete the prescription medicine.

# Menopause

## When to Call a Doctor

◆ Your periods are longer, heavier, or harder to predict than usual.

◆ You have new bleeding between periods.

◆ You have bleeding after your periods have stopped for 6 months.

◆ You have vaginal dryness, and a lubricant does not help. Your doctor may prescribe an estrogen cream or suppository.

◆ Your symptoms are disrupting your life, even with home treatment.

◆ You have unexplained bleeding (different from what your doctor told you to expect) while you are taking hormones.

Menopause occurs when the body starts making less of the female hormones estrogen and progesterone. This happens between ages 45 and 55 for most women and may take several years to complete.

Having both ovaries removed (oopherec-tomy) also causes menopause, though you can take hormones to delay it.

Hormone changes may cause:

◆ **Irregular periods.** Your flow may be lighter or heavier than usual. The time between periods may get shorter or longer. You may have spotting. Some women have regular periods until their periods stop suddenly. Others have irregular periods for a long time.

◆ **Hot flashes.** These cause intense heat, sweating, and flushing that can last from a few minutes to an hour. A hot flash usually starts in the chest and spreads out to the neck, face, and arms. If hot flashes often wake you up at night, you may feel tired and distracted because you're not sleeping enough.

◆ **Vaginal dryness.** Your vagina may become drier, thinner, and less stretchy. These changes can make sex hurt. And they may increase your risk for infections (see page 255) and bladder control problems (see page 100).

◆ **Mood changes.** Some women feel nervous, moody, or depressed as they go through menopause. You may lack energy or have trouble sleeping.

You may also need to think about some other issues:

◆ **Osteoporosis.** Loss of estrogen may weaken your bones and make them more likely to break. Hormone therapy can help prevent this but may cause other health problems. To learn more, see page 214. Be sure to get plenty of calcium and vitamin D.

◆ **Birth control.** Until you have finished menopause, your body will continue to release eggs (ovulate). This means you could get pregnant. If you don't want to get pregnant, use birth control until your doctor confirms that you have finished menopause or until you have not had a period for 12 months.

◆ **Heart disease.** Women who are at the age to start menopause are more likely to get heart disease. Work with your doctor to learn what you can do to prevent it.

**More**

# Hormone Therapy

Your doctor may prescribe hormone therapy to treat symptoms of menopause. There are two types:

◆ Estrogen replacement therapy (ERT). ERT is estrogen alone. Because ERT may increase the risk of uterine cancer, it is usually used only for women who have had their uterus removed.

◆ Hormone replacement therapy (HRT). HRT is estrogen and progestin, another female hormone. Progestin helps protect against uterine cancer.

Hormone pills are taken every day. You can get some forms of hormone therapy as skin patches, vaginal creams, or vaginal rings.

## Benefits of therapy

◆ Reduces hot flashes and vaginal dryness.

◆ Helps keep bones strong and lowers your risk of osteoporosis. But there are other medicines that can help with this too.

## Risks of therapy

◆ Increases your risk of breast cancer, stroke, and heart problems over time.

◆ May cause bloating, sore breasts, vaginal bleeding, and other side effects.

◆ Not advised for women who have had breast cancer, uterine cancer, blood clots, heart attack, stroke, liver disease, or undiagnosed uterine bleeding.

For some women, the short-term benefit of reducing menopause symptoms may outweigh the risks. Using hormone therapy for 1 to 2 years may help with symptoms while they are at their worst without causing the long-term side effects.

 Talk with your doctor about whether hormone therapy is a good idea for you. For help with your decision, go to the Web site on the back cover and enter **t747** in the search box.

If you already take hormones, talk with your doctor each year about whether it is still the right thing for you.

# Home Treatment

◆ For hot flashes:

  ❖ Keep your home and workplace cool, or use a fan.

  ❖ Dress in layers that are easy to take off. Wear natural fibers like cotton and silk.

  ❖ Drink cold drinks, not hot ones.

  ❖ Limit caffeine and alcohol, and do not smoke.

  ❖ Eat lots of small meals rather than three big ones. Your body has to produce a lot of heat to digest a large meal.

  ❖ Try a relaxation technique. See page 320.

◆ For vaginal dryness and pain during sex, use a water-soluble lubricant, such as Astroglide or Replens. Do not use Vaseline or other oil-based products.

◆ Keep a written record of your periods. You may need to discuss them with your doctor.

◆ Get regular exercise. It can ease stress and reduce your risk of heart disease and other health problems.

◆ Get support if you need it. Talking with other women may help.

◆ Try to stay relaxed about menopause. Being tense may make you feel worse.

# Menstrual Cramps

## When to Call a Doctor

◆ You have sudden, severe pain in your pelvis or belly, with or without menstrual bleeding.

◆ You have cramps and a fever.

◆ Menstrual cramps have recently gotten worse.

◆ Pelvic pain does not seem related to your menstrual cycle.

◆ Cramps start 5 to 7 days before your period or continue after your period stops.

◆ Cramps do not respond to home treatment for 3 cycles, or they keep you from your normal activities.

◆ You think your copper IUD is causing cramps, and the pain is more than you can stand or worse than what your doctor told you to expect.

Many women have painful periods. It's common to have:

◆ Cramping in the lower belly, back, or thighs.

◆ Headaches.

◆ Diarrhea, constipation, or nausea.

◆ Dizziness.

These problems are often caused by normal hormone changes. Pain and cramps can also be related to endometriosis (a problem with the uterus), pelvic infections, or noncancerous growths (fibroids) in the uterus.

If you tend to get symptoms other than cramping (such as weight gain, headache, and tension) before your period starts, you may have PMS. See page 219.

### IUDs and Cramps

If you get a copper IUD (intrauterine device) for birth control, you may have bad cramps for the first few months of use.

If cramping does not stop, you may need to have the IUD removed and use other birth control. See page 96. Birth control pills or the levonorgestrel IUD (Mirena) can reduce cramping.

## Home Treatment

◆ Take ibuprofen (Advil, Motrin) or naproxen (Aleve) the day before your period starts, or at the first sign of pain. These medicines may ease cramps better than aspirin or acetaminophen (Tylenol).

◆ Exercise. It makes cramps less severe.

◆ Use a heating pad or take a hot bath to relax tense muscles and relieve cramps.

◆ Try herbal teas, such as ginger, chamomile, or mint. These may help soothe tense muscles and anxious moods.

# Missed or Irregular Periods

## When to Call a Doctor

◆ You have lower belly pain and think you could be pregnant.

◆ A home pregnancy test says you are pregnant, or you think you're pregnant even though the test says you are not.

◆ You have missed 2 regular periods and don't know why.

◆ You miss 2 or 3 periods while taking birth control pills, and you have not skipped any pills.

◆ You have not had your first period by age 16.

Many women miss periods now and then. Missed or irregular periods have many possible causes.

◆ Pregnancy. This is usually the first thing to consider.

◆ Stress or travel.

◆ Weight loss or weight gain.

◆ Increased exercise. Missed periods are common in endurance athletes.

◆ Birth control pills or Depo-Provera shots. These may cause lighter, less frequent, or skipped periods.

◆ Menopause. See page 207.

◆ Medicines, including steroids, tranquilizers, diet pills, and illegal drugs.

◆ Menarche (the start of menstrual periods). Periods may be irregular for the first few years.

◆ Hormone imbalance or problems in the pelvic organs.

◆ Breast-feeding.

◆ An untreated thyroid problem.

If you have skipped a period, try to relax. Unless you're pregnant, chances are your cycle will return to normal next month.

If you are sexually active and don't want to get pregnant, you need to use birth control. You may also want to get a prescription for emergency birth control in case you need it. See page 97.

## Home Pregnancy Tests

If you get pregnant, it's important to find out right away so you can take good care of yourself and your baby. The quickest way to know is with a home pregnancy test. Some tests can tell that you are pregnant within a few days of your first missed period.

Tests are cheap and very accurate when you use them right. Choose a test that has simple instructions, and follow them exactly. Mistakes can cause false results.

If the test shows that you are pregnant, see your doctor to confirm it. Even if the test says you are not pregnant, it's a good idea to see your doctor to be certain.

## Home Treatment

◆ If you had sex during the past month, take a home pregnancy test. See page 210. Treat yourself like you are pregnant until you know for sure.

◆ Avoid fad diets that greatly restrict calories and food variety, and avoid quick weight loss.

◆ Increase exercise slowly. If you are an endurance athlete, cut back on training, and talk with a doctor about hormone and calcium supplements to protect against bone loss.

◆ Try relaxation techniques to deal with stress. See page 320.

# Neck Pain

## When to Call a Doctor

**Call 911** if neck pain occurs with chest pain or other symptoms of a heart attack (see page 38).

**Call your doctor if:**

◆ A stiff neck occurs with fever and a bad headache. You may have a serious illness. See page 161.

◆ You have severe neck pain after an injury or fall. See page 49.

◆ You have new weakness or constant numbness in your arms or legs.

◆ Neck pain goes down one arm, or you have numbness or tingling in your hands.

◆ A blow or injury to your neck (whiplash) causes new pain.

◆ You cannot control your pain with home treatment.

◆ Pain has not gotten better after 2 weeks of home treatment.

Most people have pain, stiffness, or a kink in the neck from time to time. Neck pain is most often caused by tension, strain, or spasm in the neck muscles or inflammation of the ligaments, tendons, or joints in the neck. This can happen when:

◆ You stay too long in a position that stresses the neck. Some examples are cradling the phone between your ear and shoulder, sleeping on your stomach or with your neck twisted, or looking up or down at a computer screen all day.

◆ You repeat movements that stress the neck. You might do this during exercise or sports, on the job, or at home.

Arthritis or damage to the discs in the neck can cause a pinched nerve. With this problem, the pain usually spreads down one arm. Your arm or hand may tingle or feel numb or weak. If you have symptoms of a pinched nerve, you need to see your doctor.

**More**

# Neck Exercises

These exercises make your neck stronger and more flexible and help you avoid neck problems. You do not need to do every exercise. Do the ones that help the most. Go slow, and stop any exercise that hurts. Do the exercises twice a day.

### Dorsal glide

Sit or stand tall, looking straight ahead (a "palace guard" posture). Slowly tuck your chin as you glide your head backward over your body. Hold for a count of 5; then relax. Repeat 6 to 10 times. This stretches the back of the neck. If you feel pain, do not glide so far back.

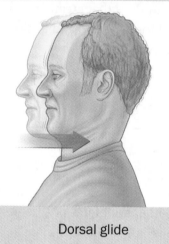

Dorsal glide

### Shoulder lifts

Lie facedown with your arms beside your body. Lift your shoulders straight up from the floor as high as you can without pain. Keep your chin down and face the floor. Keep your belly and hips pressed to the floor. Repeat 6 to 10 times. See the picture on page 92.

### Chest and shoulder stretch

Sit or stand tall, and glide your head backward as in the dorsal glide. Raise both arms so that your hands are next to your ears. As you exhale, lower your elbows down and back. Feel your shoulder blades slide down and together. Hold for a few seconds and then relax. Repeat 6 to 10 times.

### Hands on head

Move your head backward, forward, and side to side against gentle pressure from your hands. Hold each position for several seconds. Repeat 6 to 10 times.

Chest and shoulder stretch

## Home Treatment

Much of the home treatment for back pain also works for neck pain. See page 86. These tips may also help:

◆ Put ice or a cold pack on your neck for 10 to 15 minutes several times a day for the next 2 to 3 days. This will reduce pain and speed healing. If the problem is near your shoulder or upper back, it often helps more to ice the back of your neck.

◆ After the first 72 hours (or if you have chronic neck pain), you may put heat on the sore area for 20 minutes at a time.

◆ Take aspirin, ibuprofen (Advil, Motrin), or acetaminophen (Tylenol) to help relieve pain. Do not give aspirin to anyone younger than 20.

◆ Take some easy walks. The gentle swinging motion of your arms often relieves pain. Start with short walks of 5 to 10 minutes, 3 to 4 times a day.

◆ If neck pain occurs with a headache, see page 176.

◆ Once the pain starts to get better, try the neck exercises on page 212.

## Preventing Neck Pain

You can prevent most neck pain by using good posture, getting regular exercise, and not stressing your neck too much or too often. You can strengthen and protect your neck by doing neck exercises. See page 212.

Reducing stress may help too. See the relaxation exercises on page 320.

To avoid pain at the end of the day, be careful how you sit, stand, and move during the day.

◆ Sit straight in your chair with your lower back supported. Do not sit for long periods without getting up or changing positions. Take mini-breaks several times each hour to stretch your neck.

◆ If you work at a computer, have the top of the screen at eye level. Use a document holder that puts the copy at the same level as the screen.

◆ If you use the phone a lot, use a headset or speakerphone.

To avoid neck stiffness in the morning, you may need better neck support when you sleep. (Morning neck pain may also be the result of things you did the day before.)

◆ Fold a towel lengthwise into a 4-inch-wide pad and wrap it around your neck. Pin the ends together for good support.

◆ You may need a special neck support pillow. Look for a pillow that supports your neck comfortably when you lie on your back and on your side (try before buying). Do not use pillows that push your head forward when you are on your back.

◆ Do not sleep on your stomach with your neck twisted or bent.

# Osteoporosis

## When to Call a Doctor

◆ You think you have a broken bone, or you cannot move a part of your body.

◆ You have sudden, severe pain or cannot bear weight on a body part.

◆ One of your arms or legs is not its normal shape. This may mean you have a broken bone.

◆ You are concerned about your risk for osteoporosis.

Also see Strains, Sprains, and Broken Bones on page 50.

Osteoporosis means that your bones are thin and weak and can break easily. The problem affects millions of older adults, especially older women.

Osteoporosis is more common after menopause, when the body makes less estrogen. Too much thyroid hormone can also weaken your bones.

You are at highest risk for osteoporosis if:

◆ Other people in your family have had it.

◆ You do not get much exercise and have not gotten much in the past.

◆ You have a slender body frame.

◆ You smoke, or you drink a lot of alcohol.

◆ You are of Asian or European heritage.

Osteoporosis usually develops over many years without symptoms. The first sign may be a broken bone, loss of height, a slowly forming curve or hump in the upper back, or back pain.

A special X-ray called a **DEXA scan** measures bone thickness (density) and can tell you how much bone loss you have. If you are at high risk for osteoporosis, or if you are a woman over 65, a bone density test may give you and your doctor information that can help you decide whether you need treatment. For help deciding whether you are at risk and need this test, go to the Web site on the back cover and enter **m508** in the search box.

## What You Can Do

Weakening bones are a natural part of growing older. But if you start healthy habits early in life, you may be able to delay the problem. If you already have osteoporosis, these same habits can help slow the disease process and may reduce your risk of broken bones.

◆ Get plenty of exercise. Walking, jogging, dancing, lifting weights, and other exercises make bones stronger.

◆ Eat a healthy diet with lots of calcium and vitamin D. You need both of these to build strong, healthy bones.

  ❖ Get calcium from yogurt, cheese, milk, and dark green vegetables.

  ❖ Get vitamin D from eggs, fatty fish, and fortified cereal and milk.

  ❖ Talk to your doctor about taking a calcium and vitamin D supplement if you think you might need one. Many people don't get enough calcium. This is especially true after age 35, when your need for calcium goes up.

- If you smoke, quit. If you need help quitting, see page 316.

- Limit alcohol to 1 drink a day or less.

- Cut down on caffeine. Caffeine makes your body lose calcium faster.

There are medicines that can help prevent osteoporosis. Estrogen is one choice, but there are others. Talk with your doctor about what's right for you. Also see Hormone Therapy on page 208.

If you know your bones are weak, be extra careful to avoid falls. See page 332 for tips on how to make your home safer.

# Pinworms

## When to Call a Doctor

- You or your child has itching in the anal area (especially at night), but you have not seen any worms. If this is the first infection, see a doctor to make sure that pinworms are the problem.

- You or your child vomits or has pain after taking pinworm medicine.

- You or your child still has anal itching after treatment. You may need another round of treatment or a stronger medicine.

- You or your child has pinworms and has any of these symptoms:

  - Fever or belly pain

  - Redness, tenderness, swelling, or itching in the genital area

  - Pain when urinating

Pinworms are tiny worms that infect the digestive tract. They are most common in school-age children, but anyone can get them.

Pinworms lay their eggs just outside the anus. This makes the area itch. Itching is often worse at night. When a child scratches and then later sucks a thumb or puts a finger in his or her mouth, the child swallows the eggs, and the cycle starts again.

Pinworms are hard to avoid if you have young children. The problem spreads easily, and the eggs can survive on clothing, bedding, and toys for days. Teach children to wash their hands after they use the toilet and before they eat.

## Home Treatment

- Ask your pharmacist for a nonprescription medicine for pinworms. Do not take the medicine if you are pregnant, and do not give it to a child under 2 years unless your doctor tells you to.

**More**

◆ Treat every child in the house between the ages of 2 and 10. If there is still a pinworm problem, you may need to treat everyone else in the house as well.

◆ On the first day of treatment, wash all underwear, pajamas, bedding, and towels in hot water and detergent to get rid of any eggs. Clean toys with disinfectant, or wash them. Clean bathrooms and sleeping areas with a strong disinfectant.

◆ Trim your child's fingernails and keep them short.

◆ Wash hands often. Take morning showers, and change and wash pajamas and underwear every day until you finish the treatment.

# Pneumonia

## When to Call a Doctor

◆ You have fever and a cough that brings up yellow, green, rust-colored, or bloody mucus from your lungs.

◆ You have new pain in your chest that gets worse when you take a deep breath or cough.

◆ You have had a cold, bronchitis, or other viral illness and get worse instead of better.

◆ Fast, shallow breathing.

◆ Pain in the chest muscles (chest-wall pain) that is worse when you cough or take a deep breath.

◆ Fast heartbeat.

◆ Fatigue that is worse than you would get from a cold.

Pneumonia can be a serious problem for babies, older adults, and people who have long-term health problems. It's important for these groups to get the pneumococcal vaccine. See page 324.

Good home care for colds and flu can help prevent pneumonia.

## Home Treatment

◆ If your doctor prescribes any medicines, take them as you are told.

◆ Drink extra fluids. This will help thin the mucus in your lungs.

◆ Take acetaminophen (Tylenol), aspirin, or ibuprofen (Advil, Motrin) to reduce fever and pain. Do not take aspirin if you have asthma, and do not give aspirin to anyone under 20.

◆ Get lots of rest. It takes time to get well.

Pneumonia is an infection or inflammation in the lungs. It sometimes follows a viral illness like a cold, the flu, or bronchitis. Having bronchitis and another lung disease, such as asthma, may make you more likely to get pneumonia.

Pneumonia is usually caused by bacteria, but it can be caused by viruses and other things too. A person who has bacterial pneumonia is usually very sick, with:

◆ A bad cough that brings up yellow, green, rust-colored, or bloody mucus (sputum) from the lungs.

◆ Fever and shaking chills.

# Pregnancy Problems

## When to Call a Doctor

### Call 911 if:

◆ You have severe vaginal bleeding. When you are pregnant, severe means soaking through more than 1 pad in less than an hour.

◆ You have severe pain in your belly or pelvis.

◆ You faint.

◆ Fluid gushes or leaks from your vagina and you know or think the umbilical cord is bulging into your vagina. If this happens, get on your hands and knees, and keep your rear end higher than your head. This will decrease the pressure on the cord until help arrives.

### Call your doctor if:

◆ You have sudden swelling of your face, hands, or feet; a severe headache; or new vision problems (dimness, blurring).

◆ You have pain, cramping, or any vaginal bleeding.

◆ You have a fever.

◆ You have regular contractions (5 to 6 minutes apart, lasting at least 45 seconds each).

◆ You have a sudden release of fluid from your vagina.

◆ You have low back pain or pelvic pressure.

◆ You notice that your baby has stopped moving or is moving much less than normal.

◆ You vomit more than 3 times a day, or you are too sick to eat or drink.

◆ You itch all over your body. You may also have dark urine or pale stools, or your skin or eyes may turn yellow.

Problems can happen during pregnancy no matter how careful you are. But you can increase the chances that your baby will be healthy by following some basic guidelines.

## Work With Your Doctor

◆ Go to all your prenatal appointments. At each visit, your doctor will check your blood pressure and check your urine for protein. High blood pressure and protein in the urine are signs of preeclampsia. This problem can be dangerous for you and your baby.

◆ Follow your doctor's advice about activity. Your doctor will let you know how much exercise is safe for you. This may change as you get closer to the end of your pregnancy.

◆ Ask your doctor whether you can have sex. If you are at risk for preterm labor, your doctor may ask you to not have sex after a certain point.

◆ If you take medicine for another health problem, talk with your doctor about whether you can continue your treatment or need to change it.

More

## Morning Sickness

Many women have nausea and vomiting during the first few months they are pregnant. This is called morning sickness, though it can occur at any time of day. It is normal but unpleasant.

To avoid or at least reduce morning sickness:

◆ Eat five or six small meals a day so your stomach is never empty. Eat some protein in each of the meals.

◆ Eat crackers or dry toast as soon as you get up in the morning.

◆ Sip a sports drink when you have trouble with solid food.

◆ Get more vitamin $B_6$ by eating more whole grains and cereals, wheat germ, nuts, seeds, and legumes. But talk with your doctor before you take any vitamin supplements.

◆ Try ginger tea or ginger candy.

◆ Avoid foods or smells that make you sick.

◆ Get plenty of rest.

Call your doctor if you cannot hold down food or liquids, if you are vomiting more than 3 times a day, or if you are losing weight.

## Get Good Nutrition

◆ Eat a balanced diet that has plenty of calcium- and iron-rich foods. Foods high in calcium include milk, cheese, yogurt, almonds, and broccoli. Iron-rich foods include beef, shellfish, chicken and turkey, eggs, beans, raisins, whole-grain bread, and leafy green vegetables.

◆ If you need help paying for food, call your local WIC (Women, Infants, and Children) agency to learn whether you are eligible for help. WIC provides vouchers for nutritious food, nutrition education, and breast-feeding support to pregnant women, women with new babies, and children younger than 5.

◆ Take a daily multivitamin that contains 0.4 mg of folic acid (folate). Folic acid helps prevent certain birth defects. Other good sources of folic acid are fortified cereal and whole wheat bread.

◆ Drink plenty of fluids. Dehydration can cause contractions.

◆ If you drink coffee or soda with caffeine, cut back to 2 cups or less a day.

## Protect Your Baby

◆ Do not smoke.

◆ Do not drink alcohol or use illegal drugs.

◆ If you have a cat, have someone else clean the litter box. Avoid cat feces.

◆ Wash your hands well after you handle raw meat. Fully cook all meat before you eat it.

◆ Avoid all chemical vapors, paint fumes, and poisons.

◆ Avoid getting very hot. Do not use saunas or hot tubs. Don't stay out in the sun in hot weather for long periods. Take acetaminophen (Tylenol) for a high fever.

◆ Do not take any prescription or over-the-counter medicines, herbal supplements, or vitamins (other than your prenatal vitamins) without talking to your doctor or pharmacist first.

◆ Take care to prevent falls. During pregnancy, your joints are loose, and your balance is off. After your 25th week, avoid sports with a high risk of falls, such as bicycling, skiing, in-line skating, and horseback or motorcycle riding. Do not dive or scuba dive.

## Prepare for Childbirth

Late in your pregnancy, it's a good idea to start getting ready for the birth itself.

◆ Take childbirth classes with your partner or the person you choose to be your "coach."

◆ Learn about early signs of labor so you know what to watch for.

◆ If you have other children, talk to them about the new baby and help them adjust to the idea.

◆ Learn a relaxation exercise or two (see page 320). They can help while you are in labor.

◆ Think about creating a birth plan with your doctor that states what you want and what you expect to happen during labor and delivery. This can cover things like who you want there for the birth and whether you want medicine to help with the pain. But keep in mind that some things may be out of your and your doctor's control.

◆ Learn about breast-feeding and find resources that can help (such as La Leche League or the Nursing Mothers Counsel). See page 106.

◆ Get plenty of rest, eat well, and be nice to yourself.

# Premenstrual Syndrome (PMS)

### When to Call a Doctor

◆ You do not feel better within a few days after your period starts.

◆ PMS often keeps you away from work, school, and your normal activities.

◆ You feel out of control because of PMS.

Many women have cramps, tender breasts, and other mild symptoms just before and during the first few days of their periods. This is normal. When the symptoms are so bad that they disrupt your life or affect your relationships, they are called premenstrual syndrome, or PMS.

PMS symptoms are different for each woman. Some of the common ones include:

◆ Breast swelling, bloating, weight gain, and acne.

◆ Mood changes, food cravings, and decreased sex drive.

◆ Cramps, headaches, breast pain, and muscle aches.

◆ Sleep problems and lack of energy.

You may be able to prevent or reduce your symptoms with some of the diet and lifestyle changes and other tips in the Home Treatment section. But it may take a couple of periods before things improve.

**More**

If PMS is severely disrupting your life, see your doctor. Your doctor can prescribe medicines that may help. For help deciding whether these are right for you, go to the Web site on the back cover and enter **z963** in the search box.

A small number of women have premenstrual dysphoric disorder (PMDD), a severe form of PMS that can make you angry or even violent and upset your relationships at work and home. Prescription medicines and self-care can help you get back in control.

## Home Treatment

◆ Keep a daily record of your symptoms—what they are, how bad they are, and when you have them. By helping you see patterns in your cycle, this record may help you prevent, reduce, or better cope with PMS. For example, if you know when your cramps usually start, you can start taking medicine just before they begin. This works better than waiting until you are in pain.

◆ Eat small meals every 3 to 4 hours. Include plenty of whole grains, fruits, and vegetables. Limit fats and sweets.

◆ Reduce salt to help limit bloating.

◆ Do not smoke, and reduce alcohol and caffeine.

◆ Exercise.

◆ Try nonprescription PMS medicines such as Midol or Pamprin. These contain several drugs to help relieve cramps, bloating, and headache.

◆ Take calcium (1,200 mg daily), vitamin $B_6$ (50 to 100 mg daily), or magnesium (400 mg daily). These may improve your mood, reduce bloating and pain, and help with other PMS symptoms.

◆ Reduce stress as much as you can. Try yoga or other relaxation techniques. See page 320.

◆ Find support. Talk with your family, friends, and any others who may be affected by your symptoms. Or join a PMS support group.

# Prostate Cancer

## When to Call a Doctor

◆ You have blood or pus in your urine.

◆ You have urinary symptoms that come on quickly, bother you enough that you want help, or last longer than 2 months. (Also see Prostate Enlargement on page 222.)

◆ You already have prostate problems and you develop back or bone pain.

Prostate cancer is the second leading cause of cancer deaths in men. (See pictures of the prostate on pages 222 and 224.) When found early, before it has spread to other organs, it can often be cured. And it tends to grow slowly. Many older men with prostate cancer die of another cause (like heart disease) before the cancer has grown enough to cause problems.

Most men with prostate cancer have no symptoms. In a few cases, the cancer can cause urinary symptoms like those of prostate enlargement. See page 222. If it spreads to bones or other organs, it can cause pain and other symptoms.

Any man can get prostate cancer. But the risk is highest for:

◆ Older men. Most men who get prostate cancer are over 65.

◆ African-American men.

◆ Men who have a family history of prostate cancer.

◆ Men who eat a high-fat diet.

## Should You Be Tested?

Doctors can use one of two simple tests to look for prostate cancer:

◆ Digital rectal exam, in which the doctor puts a gloved finger in your rectum and feels the prostate

◆ PSA blood test

Many experts are not sure that routine testing is right for men without symptoms. Finding prostate cancer early can save lives in some cases. But for men who are older and do not have symptoms, knowing they have prostate cancer may not extend or improve their lives.

 To help decide whether testing is right for you, go to the Web site on the back cover and enter **t951** in the search box. Then talk to your doctor.

## Should You Be Treated?

If you have prostate cancer, here are a few things you should know:

◆ You may not die any sooner than you would have without the cancer. Prostate cancer tends to occur later in life and usually grows slowly.

◆ If the cancer does not cause symptoms, it may not affect your quality of life.

◆ The younger you are and the larger or more advanced the cancer is, the more serious the disease may be.

◆ Treatment can be painful and can cause lasting problems with bladder control or erections.

Learn all you can about your treatment options—which may include not treating the cancer. You need to consider your age, your health, and the nature of the cancer itself when you make treatment decisions. For example, if you are older and the cancer is not growing much, it may make sense to take a wait-and-see approach.

To help decide what approach you want to take, go to the Web site on the back cover and enter **r808** in the search box. Your doctor can help you with the decision.

# Prostate Enlargement

## When to Call a Doctor

- You cannot urinate at all.

- You feel like you cannot empty your bladder completely.

- You have urinary problems along with fever, chills, vomiting, or pain in your back or belly.

- It hurts or burns when you urinate.

- There is blood or pus in your urine.

- You have new or worse urination problems after you start a new medicine.

As a man ages, his prostate gland may get bigger. This is called **benign prostatic hyperplasia,** or **BPH**. As the gland gets bigger, it may squeeze or partly block the urethra. This can cause problems with urine flow, such as:

- Trouble getting the urine stream started or fully stopped. This may cause dribbling. (But dribbling is very common. It may not mean you have BPH.)

- Needing to urinate more often, especially at night.

- A weak urine stream.

- Feeling like you cannot empty your bladder all the way.

BPH is not a serious problem unless you have a lot of trouble urinating or unless backed-up urine causes bladder or kidney problems.

Many men find that they can manage their symptoms with self-care. Sometimes symptoms clear up on their own. In these cases, the best treatment may be no treatment at all.

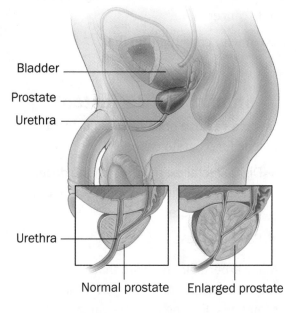

As the prostate gets bigger, it may squeeze the urethra.

Some men decide to try one of the medicines that can help with symptoms. For help deciding whether these are right for you, go to the Web site on the back cover and enter **s204** in the search box. Then talk to your doctor. Surgery may also be an option.

222

## Home Treatment

◆ Avoid allergy and cold medicines (antihistamines, decongestants, and nasal sprays). They can make urinary problems worse.

◆ If having to get up at night to urinate bothers you, cut down on fluids before bed, especially those with alcohol or caffeine. But drink plenty of water and other fluids during the day.

◆ Take plenty of time to urinate. Turn on a faucet, or try to picture running water. Some men find this helps. Read or think of other things while you wait.

◆ Sit on the toilet to urinate.

◆ Try "double voiding." Urinate as much as you can, relax for a few moments, and then try again.

◆ Herbal products such as saw palmetto help some men with BPH. Talk to your doctor before you take this or any herbal product.

Also see the tips in Bladder Control on page 100.

# Prostatitis

## When to Call a Doctor

◆ You have urinary problems along with fever, chills, vomiting, or pain in your back or belly.

◆ Your urine is bloody, red, or pink for no clear reason (see page 67).

◆ Pelvic pain or urinary problems last more than 5 days, even with home treatment.

◆ Pelvic pain or urinary problems suddenly change or get worse.

◆ It hurts when you urinate, ejaculate, or pass stool.

◆ There is a strange discharge from your penis. Also see Sexually Transmitted Diseases on page 229.

Prostatitis is any painful inflammation or infection of the prostate. If you have this problem:

◆ You may often feel the urge to urinate but can pass only a little urine each time.

◆ It may burn when you urinate.

◆ You may feel like you can't empty your bladder all the way.

◆ You may have trouble starting to urinate or have a weak urine flow.

◆ You may have to urinate a lot at night.

◆ You may have pelvic pain. You may feel it in your lower back or belly, your scrotum, the area between your scrotum and anus, your upper thighs, or the pubic area.

◆ It may hurt when you ejaculate.

**More**

A prostate infection caused by bacteria usually gets better with home treatment and antibiotics. If the infection comes back, you may need to take more antibiotics.

But most men with prostatitis do not have a bacterial infection. In these cases, home treatment tends to be the best approach.

## Home Treatment

◆ Avoid alcohol, caffeine, and spicy foods. They may make your symptoms worse.

◆ Take hot baths to help soothe pain and reduce stress.

◆ Eat plenty of high-fiber foods, and drink plenty of water. This will help you avoid constipation. Straining can hurt a lot when you have prostatitis.

◆ Take acetaminophen (Tylenol) or ibuprofen (Advil, Motrin) for pain.

◆ If your doctor gives you antibiotics for a prostate infection, take them as you are told.

Seminal vesicle

Vas deferens

Bladder

Prostate

Urethra

Penis

Testicle

Rectum

Epididymis

Male pelvic organs
(the prostate is just under the bladder)

# Psoriasis

### When to Call a Doctor

◆ Psoriasis covers much of your body or is very red. Severe cases often need medical care.

◆ You have signs of skin infection. These may include pain, swelling, warmth, or redness; red streaks leading from the area; pus; and fever.

Psoriasis is a long-term skin problem that causes raised, red patches topped with silvery, scaling skin. The patches are most often on the knees, elbows, scalp, hands,

feet, or lower back. If the problem is severe, your skin may be itchy and tender.

You can treat psoriasis with good care at home and, sometimes, with medicine from your doctor. Your doctor also may suggest ultraviolet light treatments.

Psoriasis does not spread from person to person.

## Home Treatment

◆ Keep your skin moist. Use a very mild soap when you bathe. After you bathe, use a moisturizing ointment, cream, or lotion while your skin is still damp. This seals in moisture.

- Use hydrocortisone cream on small patches. Other products for psoriasis (lotions, gels, shampoos) may also help, but they may make your skin more sensitive to the sun.

- Try to prevent sunburn. Short periods of sunlight reduce psoriasis in most people. But sunburn injures the skin and may make psoriasis worse or cause it to appear in new areas. Use sunscreen on areas that do not have psoriasis.

- Avoid harsh chemicals and skin products, such as those that contain alcohol.

- Use a cool-mist vaporizer or humidifier to add moisture to your bedroom.

- Try to reduce stress. See page 319. Stress may make psoriasis worse in some people.

# Rashes

## When to Call a Doctor

- You have a rash that develops quickly and looks like bruises or tiny purple or red blood spots under the skin. You may have a serious illness. See page 161.

- You have a rash with signs of infection. These may include increased pain, redness, swelling or warmth; red streaks leading from the rash; pus; and fever.

- You get a rash after being bitten by a tick. See page 14.

- You get a rash after you start a new medicine.

- You have a rash with fever and joint pain.

- A rash occurs with a sore throat. See information about scarlet fever on page 239.

- You are not sure what's causing a rash.

- A rash does not clear up after 2 to 3 weeks of home treatment.

Rashes can be caused by lots of things—illness, allergy, bacteria, heat, and stress, to name a few.

When you first get a rash, ask yourself these questions to help find the cause:

- Do you have a rash in an area that came in contact with something new? This could be a plant; soaps, detergents, or shampoos; perfumes, makeup, or lotions; jewelry or fabric; or a new tool, an appliance, or latex gloves. Any of these could irritate your skin.

- Have you eaten anything new that you may be allergic to?

- Are you taking any new medicines?

- Have you lately been more stressed or upset than usual?

- Have you been sick?

- Is the rash spreading?

- Does it itch?

Also see the Skin Problems chart on page 61. If your child has a rash, the Rashes in Children chart on page 227 may help.

**More**

## Poison Ivy, Oak, and Sumac

The leaves of poison ivy, oak, and sumac have an oil that many people are allergic to. If you touch the leaves or the oil, you may get a red, blistered, and very itchy rash. The rash often appears in lines where the leaves brushed against the skin.

You may be able to prevent or reduce the rash if you act fast.

◆ Wash your skin with rubbing alcohol or lots of water within 10 to 15 minutes to get the oil off your skin.

◆ Use soap only after using lots of water.

◆ Wash your clothes, your dog, and anything else that may have touched the plant.

If you get a rash anyway, follow the tips in Home Treatment.

# Home Treatment

◆ Wash the area with water. Soap may irritate the rash. Pat dry.

◆ Use cold, wet cloths to reduce itching. Also see Relief From Itching on page 142.

◆ Keep cool, and stay out of the sun.

◆ Leave the rash open to the air. Baby powder can help keep it dry.

◆ If you have a plant rash, calamine lotion may help. Use it 3 or 4 times a day. A mild lotion like Cetaphil may soothe some rashes.

◆ Use hydrocortisone cream to provide short-term relief from itching. Do not use it on the face or the genital area.

◆ Do not use products that have caused a rash in the past, such as detergents, skin care products, makeup, clothing, or jewelry.

◆ Use fragrance-free or hypoallergenic soaps, detergents, lotions, and makeup if you often have rashes.

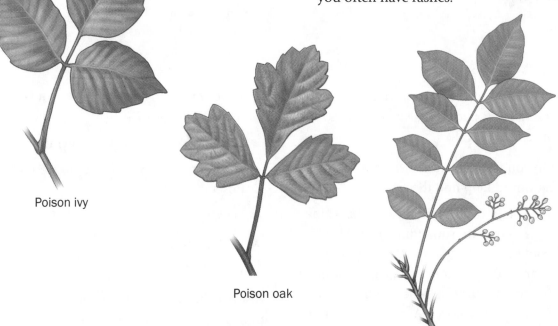

Poison ivy

Poison oak

Poison sumac

Learn what poison ivy, oak, and sumac look like so you can avoid them.

| Rashes in Children | |
|---|---|
| **Symptoms** | **Possible Causes** |
| Red spots like pimples that turn to blisters; fever | Chickenpox, p. 121 |
| Rash in diaper area only | Diaper rash, p. 135<br>Yeast infection, p. 255 |
| Red rash on face that looks like slapped cheeks; pink rash on torso that comes and goes; possible fever | Fifth disease, p. 164 |
| Red or pink dots on head, neck, shoulders; more common in babies | Heat rash, p. 184. |
| Sudden high fever for 2 to 3 days followed by rosy pink rash on torso, arms, and neck after fever goes down | Roseola, p. 228 |
| Fine pink rash that starts on face and covers whole body; swollen glands behind ears | Rubella (rare) |
| Fever, runny nose, hacking cough; red eyes 2 to 3 days before spotty red rash covers whole body | Measles (rare) |
| High fever, sore throat, sandpapery rash, and raspberry-textured tongue | Scarlet fever, p. 239 |
| Blisters on mouth and tongue appearing 1 to 2 days after onset of fever and sore mouth or throat; painless, blistering rash on fingers, hands, feet | Hand-foot-and-mouth disease, p. 175 |

# Rosacea

## When to Call a Doctor

- You think you may have rosacea.
- Redness, pimples, and eye irritation get worse even with treatment.

Rosacea is a long-term skin problem that causes:

- Red patches, red lines (tiny blood vessels), and small pimples on the face. You may think you have acne.

- Burning and soreness in the eyes or eyelids. Rosacea can lead to more serious eye problems if you do not treat it.

- Large bumps on the nose and face in severe cases.

You are more likely to get rosacea if you have fair skin and blush easily or if your face stays red and flushed longer than most people's. The problem tends to run in families.

The sooner you start to treat rosacea, the better. If it stays mild, you may be able to control it well. Prescription medicines may help if home treatment is not enough.

**More**

## Home Treatment

- Find out what triggers redness and pimples for you, and try to avoid those things. They may include:

  - ❖ Very cold or hot weather. In winter, wear a hat and scarf to shield your face from cold and wind. Use a face moisturizer.

  - ❖ Stress. Eat a healthy diet, and get plenty of exercise and sleep.

  - ❖ Alcohol, spicy foods, or very hot drinks.

  - ❖ Getting too hot when you exercise. Try working out for a shorter time. In the summer, exercise during the cool morning hours or in an air-conditioned gym.

  - ❖ Hot showers. Take warm or cool ones instead. Don't use hot tubs or saunas.

- Always wear sunscreen on exposed skin.

- Use soaps, lotions, and makeup made for sensitive skin that don't contain alcohol, are not abrasive, and won't clog pores.

- If you have rosacea on your eyelids, gently wash your eyelids with a product made for the eyes. Use artificial tears if your eyes feel dry.

- Talk to your doctor about antibiotic creams and other medicines that can help with pimples and redness. In advanced cases, laser treatment can reduce redness.

# Roseola

## When to Call a Doctor

See the fever guidelines on page 158.

Roseola is a mild viral illness in young children that often starts with a sudden high fever (103°F to 105°F). The fever lasts 2 to 3 days. As the fever drops, a rosy pink rash appears on the torso, neck, and arms. The rash may last 1 to 2 days. Most babies feel fine when they have roseola.

Since the fever is quite high and comes on quickly, some children may have fever seizures. See page 161.

Roseola is most common in children from 6 months to 2 years old. It's rare after age 4.

## Home Treatment

- If your child has a fever over 102°F and feels bad, give acetaminophen (Tylenol). Do not give your child aspirin.

- Give your child plenty of liquids.

# Sexually Transmitted Diseases (STDs)

## When to Call a Doctor

All sexually transmitted diseases (STDs) need to be diagnosed and treated. Your doctor or a health professional at your local health department can help with testing and treatment.

**Call your doctor if:**

◆ You think you may have been exposed to an STD. Your sex partner(s) may also need to be treated, even if they have no symptoms. Without treatment, you and your partner(s) may reinfect each other or have serious complications.

◆ You have any unusual discharge from your vagina or penis; burning when you urinate; or any sores, redness, or growths on your genitals.

◆ Your behavior or your partner's puts you at risk for HIV.

◆ You are pregnant and have any reason to think you may have been exposed to an STD, especially HIV.

◆ You have symptoms such as fatigue, weight loss, fever, diarrhea, cough, or swollen lymph nodes that do not go away after a short time and do not seem to be related to any illness.

◆ You are HIV-positive and you have:

❖ Fever over 103°F.

❖ Fever over 101°F that lasts 3 days or longer.

❖ Increased outbreaks of cold sores or any unusual skin or mouth sores.

❖ Severe numbness or pain in your hands and feet.

❖ Unexplained weight loss.

❖ Unexplained fever and night sweats.

❖ Severe fatigue.

❖ Diarrhea or other bowel changes.

❖ Shortness of breath and a frequent dry cough.

❖ Swollen lymph nodes in your neck, armpits, or groin.

❖ Personality changes, trouble concentrating, confusion, or severe headache.

Sexually transmitted diseases, also called STDs, are infections passed from person to person through sex, genital contact, and contact with fluids such as semen, vaginal fluids, and blood (including menstrual blood). Some of these infections can also be spread by sharing drug needles, razors, and other items that may have infected blood or fluids on them.

You can get an STD from any kind of sexual contact. This includes:

◆ Vaginal sex.

◆ Anal sex.

◆ Oral sex.

**More**

Preventing STDs is a lot easier than treating them or living with them. To learn how to protect yourself, see Safe Sex on page 322.

## Sexually Transmitted Diseases

| Symptoms | Disease | Treatment | Other Concerns |
|---|---|---|---|
| Discharge from vagina or penis; pain or burning when you urinate; for women, pain and bleeding during or after sex | **Chlamydia, gonorrhea, trichomoniasis** | Antibiotics for all partners. Do not have sex until you and your partner(s) have finished treatment and have no symptoms. | If not treated, can lead to pelvic inflammatory disease and fertility problems.<br><br>Gonorrhea can spread to joints, causing arthritis. |
| Red, painless sore in genital or rectal area or on mouth about 3 weeks after exposure<br><br>Two months later: Rash, patchy hair loss, fever, flu-like symptoms | **Syphilis** | Antibiotics for all partners. Do not have sex until you and your partner(s) have finished treatment and have no symptoms. | If not treated, can cause serious health problems and death. |
| Painful sores or blisters in genital or anal area 2 to 7 days after exposure; fever, swollen lymph nodes, headache, and muscle aches | **Genital herpes** | No cure. Medicine can reduce pain and speed healing during an outbreak. | Those with frequent or severe outbreaks may take medicine daily to help prevent them. Couples should avoid sex during an outbreak. Pregnant women should tell their doctor immediately if they have an outbreak. |
| Small, fleshy bumps or flat, white patches in genital or anal area | **Genital warts and HPV (human papillomavirus)** | No cure for HPV. Warts can be removed but may return. Infection may go away on its own. | HPV can increase a woman's risk for cervical cancer. |
| Yellowing of skin and whites of eyes; flu-like symptoms; steady pain in upper right belly, under rib cage; diarrhea or constipation; muscle aches and joint pain; skin rash | **Hepatitis B virus** | No treatment for short-term (acute) hepatitis; most people get better in 6 to 8 weeks.<br><br>Medicine for long-term (chronic) hepatitis, but no cure. | Can become chronic and lead to liver damage or cancer.<br><br>If you are at risk for hepatitis B, get the vaccine. See page 326. |
| Flu-like symptoms soon after infection; then no symptoms for years until disease progresses | **HIV (human immunodeficiency virus)** | No cure. Medicine slows progress of disease, delays AIDS, and prolongs life. | Weakens immune system, leading to AIDS and in many cases death. See page 231. |

Some of the most common STDs are described in the chart on page 230. If you think you may have been exposed to any of them, use the chart to check your symptoms and learn more.

## HIV: Should You Get Tested?

HIV (human immunodeficiency virus) is a virus that attacks your immune system. This makes it hard for your body to fight infection and disease. AIDS is the last and most severe stage of HIV infection.

### Are You at Risk?

All kinds of people get HIV—men and women, gay and straight, all ages, all races. If you or your partner does things that could expose you to HIV, you are at risk.

HIV spreads through contact with body fluids such as semen, vaginal fluids, and blood (including menstrual blood). The behaviors that spread HIV include:

- Having more than one sex partner.
- Having unprotected sex. Unprotected sex means having sex without properly using a condom. This is especially risky if you are a man who has sex with men, but it is a risk for everyone. Sex without condoms is not safe unless both you and your partner are sure that neither of you has HIV and that neither of you is having sex with anyone else.
- Sharing needles or other drug supplies with someone who is HIV-positive.
- Having a sex partner who does any of the above.

## STDs During Pregnancy

Many STDs can be spread from an infected mother to her unborn baby. These include chlamydia, gonorrhea, hepatitis B, herpes, HIV, and syphilis.

The good news is that getting treated while you are pregnant can prevent the spread of many of these diseases to your child.

If you are infected with or think you may have been exposed to an STD, talk to your doctor about how you can protect your baby before and after he or she is born.

You will not get HIV from touching, hugging, or lightly kissing someone who is HIV-positive. HIV is not spread by mosquitoes, toilet seats, donating blood, or being touched or coughed on by someone who is HIV-positive or who has AIDS.

### Getting Tested

If you do things that put you at risk for HIV infection, be sure to have an HIV test every 6 months. Here's why:

- Medicine for HIV can help delay or prevent AIDS and helps you live longer and better. The sooner you find out whether you have HIV and start getting checked, the better your chances of staying healthy. Regular checks of your immune system will help you and your doctor know when you need to start medicine.
- A blood test is the only way to know whether you have HIV. You may not feel sick or notice any symptoms for years, but inside your body, the virus is growing.

**More**

◆ If you have HIV and do not know it, you may spread the disease to others.

◆ If you are pregnant, getting tested is the most important thing you can do for yourself and your baby. If you are HIV-positive, medicine during pregnancy can greatly reduce the chance that your baby will be born with HIV.

All it takes is a simple, cheap blood test. The test checks for HIV antibodies in your blood. If HIV antibodies are found, you are considered HIV-positive. If HIV antibodies are not found, you may need to be tested again. This is to make sure HIV antibodies do not appear at a later time, since it can take up to 6 months after you are first exposed to HIV for antibodies to appear.

You can have the test in your doctor's office or at the local health department.

If you find out you are HIV-positive, work with your doctor to get the right treatment and stay as healthy as you can. Many people live with HIV for years or even decades before they develop AIDS.

If you need help dealing with HIV or AIDS, or if you just want to learn more, call the CDC-INFO hotline at 1-800-232-4636.

# Sinusitis

## When to Call a Doctor

◆ Cold symptoms last longer than 10 to 14 days or get worse after the first 7 days.

◆ You have a severe headache that is different from a "normal" headache, and nonprescription medicines do not help.

◆ You have swelling in your face, or your vision changes or gets blurry.

◆ Nasal discharge changes from clear to yellow or green after 5 to 7 days of a cold, and pain and fever get worse. If nasal discharge is colored from the start of a cold, call if it lasts longer than 7 to 10 days.

◆ You have facial pain (especially in one sinus area or along the ridge between the nose and lower eyelid) after 2 days of home treatment.

◆ You have finished your antibiotics and still have symptoms.

Sinusitis is an inflammation or infection of the sinuses and nasal passages. The sinuses become blocked, which causes pain and pressure in the face.

Sinusitis most often follows a cold. Sinus problems can also be related to allergies, an infected tooth, air pollution, and other things.

### Is It Sinusitis or a Cold?

Colds and sinusitis have some of the same symptoms, like a stuffy nose and cough. But if you have a sinus problem, you may also have:

◆ Pain over your cheekbones and upper teeth.

◆ Pain in your forehead over your eyebrows.

◆ Pain around or behind your eyes.

Along with the pain you may have a headache, swelling around your eyes, fever, or mucus draining down the back of your throat. Facial pain and these other symptoms are not likely with just a cold.

In children, coughing and nasal discharge that last more than 7 to 10 days along with headache and facial pain are signs that the problem may be sinusitis.

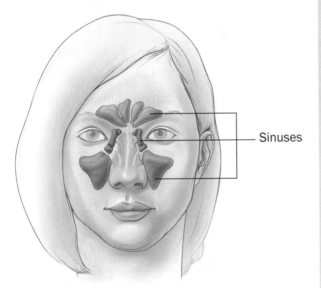

Sinuses

The sinuses are hollow spaces in the head.

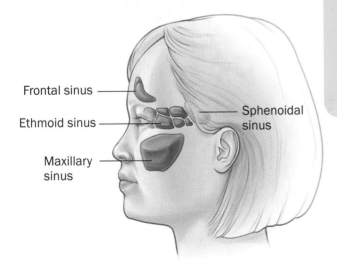

Frontal sinus

Ethmoid sinus

Maxillary sinus

Sphenoidal sinus

## Do You Need Antibiotics?

Sinusitis usually gets better with good self-care. If you try the tips in Home Treatment, you may be able to avoid antibiotics and a trip to the doctor.

But if your symptoms are severe or last more than 10 to 14 days, you may need antibiotics. If you do not treat a bad sinus infection or it does not respond to treatment, it can lead to long-term sinus problems that are harder to treat.

There are good reasons not to use antibiotics unless you really need them:

◆ Antibiotics can cost a lot.

◆ You will probably have to see the doctor to get a prescription. This costs you time and money.

◆ Antibiotics can have harmful side effects, such as diarrhea, vomiting, and skin rashes.

◆ The most important reason of all: If you take antibiotics when you don't need them, they may not work when you do need them. Each time you take antibiotics you are more likely to carry some bacteria that were not killed by the medicine. Over time, these bacteria get tougher and can cause longer and more serious infections. To treat them you may need different, stronger, and more costly antibiotics

More

# Home Treatment

- Drink plenty of water and other fluids to keep mucus thin.

- Put a warm, damp towel or gel pack on your face several times a day for 5 to 10 minutes at a time.

- Breathe warm, moist air from a steamy shower, a hot bath, or a sink filled with hot water.

- Use a humidifier in your home, or at least in your bedroom. Avoid cold, dry air.

- Use an oral decongestant, a decongestant nasal spray, or a cough medicine that has guaifenesin. Do not use a nasal decongestant spray for more than 3 days in a row.

- Do not take antihistamines unless your symptoms may also be caused by allergies.

- Take aspirin, acetaminophen (Tylenol), or ibuprofen (Advil, Motrin) to relieve facial pain and headache. Do not give aspirin to anyone younger than 20.

- Do not smoke, and avoid other people's smoke.

- If you see streaks of mucus in the back of your throat, gargle with warm water.

- Blow your nose gently. Do not block one nostril when you blow your nose.

- A saltwater (saline) wash can help clear out mucus and bacteria. You can use nonprescription saline nose drops or a homemade saltwater mix.

  - Use a bulb syringe to gently squirt the liquid into your nose. Or snuff it from the palm of your hand, one nostril at a time.

  - Blow your nose gently when you are done.

  - Repeat 2 to 4 times a day.

## Saline Nose Drops

Nonprescription saline nasal sprays (such as NaSal and Ocean) are cheap and easy to use. They will keep nasal tissues moist and help clean out mucus and bacteria. Unlike other kinds of nasal sprays, they do not cause swelling inside the nose.

You can also make saline nose drops at home. Mix ¼ teaspoon salt with 1 cup of warm water in a clean bottle with a dropper. After 3 days, throw out the mix and make a fresh one.

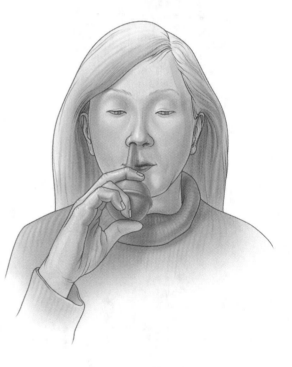

Using a bulb syringe

# Skin Cancer

## When to Call a Doctor

- A mole is itchy, tender, or painful.

- A mole starts to get bigger or changes color or shape.

- A mole scales, oozes, or bleeds, or its color spreads into surrounding skin.

- You notice a new bump or nodule on a mole, or any change in how the mole looks.

- You have a sore that does not heal.

- You have any irritated or unusual skin growth.

If your moles do not change over time, there is little reason to worry about them. If you have a family history of malignant melanoma, let your doctor know. You may be at greater risk.

Skin cancer is the most common type of cancer. Most skin cancer is caused by sun damage, so it tends to occur on areas that get the most sun, such as the face, neck, and arms. Light-skinned, blue-eyed people are more likely to get skin cancer. Dark-skinned people have less risk.

Most of a person's harmful sun exposure occurs by age 20, so keep your children protected. (See Don't Get Sunburned on page 56.) Repeated sun exposure (including sunlamps) and severe sunburns can greatly increase your risk of skin cancer.

Most skin cancers are **nonmelanoma** skin cancers. These include basal cell and squamous cell carcinomas. Nonmelanoma skin cancer is rarely life-threatening. But it is still best to find and treat it promptly. It is usually easy to treat.

**Melanoma** is a more serious type of skin cancer. It may affect only the skin, or it may spread to other organs and bones. Melanoma can be deadly if it is not found and treated early. Early removal of thin melanomas can cure the disease in most cases.

### Watch for Skin Changes

Once a month, examine all areas of your skin with a mirror (or have someone help you). Look for odd moles, spots, bumps, or sores that will not heal. Pay extra attention to areas that get a lot of sun: hands, arms, back, chest, back of the neck, face, and ears. Report any changes to your doctor.

Skin cancers differ from other skin growths in these ways:

- They tend to bleed more and are often open sores that do not heal.

- They tend to grow slowly. But melanoma may appear suddenly and grow quickly.

More

Also watch for any of these **ABCD changes** in a mole or other growth:

◆ **A**symmetry: One half does not match the other half.

◆ **B**order: The edges are ragged, notched, or blurred.

◆ **C**olor: The mole changes color, has shades of red and black, or has a red, white, and blue blotchy appearance.

◆ **D**iameter (size): A mole grows larger than a pencil eraser.

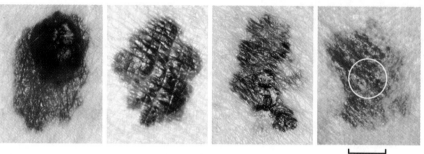

| Asymmetry | Border irregularity | Color | 6 mm Diameter |

Watch for these "ABCD" mole changes.

# Sleep Problems

## When to Call a Doctor

◆ You regularly take sleeping pills and cannot stop taking them.

◆ You think a medicine or a health problem is causing sleep problems.

◆ You or your partner snores loudly and often feels extremely sleepy during the day.

◆ You, your partner, or your child often stops breathing, gasps, and chokes during sleep.

◆ Your child snores, has trouble breathing while asleep, sleeps restlessly and wakes up often, or is very sleepy during the day.

◆ You often wake up because your legs move or get cramps.

◆ A full month of self-care does not solve your sleep problem.

**Insomnia** can mean:

◆ Having trouble getting to sleep (taking more than 45 minutes to fall asleep).

◆ Waking up often and not being able to fall back asleep.

◆ Waking up too early in the morning when you do not want to.

None of these are problems unless you feel tired all the time. If you are less sleepy at night or wake up early in the morning but still feel rested and alert, there is little need to worry.

Short-term insomnia, lasting from a few nights to a few weeks, is usually caused by worry or stress. Long-term insomnia, which can last months or even years, is often caused by frequent or constant anxiety, medicines, long-term pain, depression, or other health problems.

**Sleep apnea** is a problem usually caused by a blockage in your airways. When airflow through the nose and mouth is blocked, you repeatedly stop breathing for 10 to 15 seconds or longer while you are asleep. People who have sleep apnea often snore loudly and are very tired during the day. They are not aware of waking up at night but do have very restless sleep.

Changing some of your pre-bedtime habits may help cure mild insomnia or sleep apnea. More severe insomnia or sleep apnea may need medical treatment.

## Tips for Better Sleep

Try this seven-step formula for 2 weeks:

1. Do relaxing activities in the evening. Read (but not in bed). Take a warm bath. Or do some slow, easy stretches.

2. Use your bed for sleeping and sex only. Do not eat, watch TV, read, or work in bed.

3. Sleep only at bedtime. Do not take naps, especially in the late afternoon and evening.

## Snoring

Up to half of all adults snore once in a while; about 1 in 4 adults snores regularly. Snoring is caused by blockage of the airways in the back of the mouth and nose. The airways can be blocked for many reasons, such as excess neck tissue caused by being overweight or a stuffy nose caused by allergies or a cold. Some people who snore have sleep apnea.

Snoring can disrupt your sleep patterns, which may leave you sleepy and less alert during the day. It can also disrupt the sleep of family members or roommates.

### Tips for people who snore

◆ Exercise daily to maintain a healthy weight and improve muscle tone. Don't exercise within 2 hours of bedtime (it may make it harder to fall asleep).

◆ Avoid heavy meals, alcohol, sleeping pills, and antihistamines before bedtime.

◆ Try to sleep on your side instead of your back. (Sew a pocket onto the back of your pajama top, and put a tennis ball in the pocket. This will keep you off your back.)

◆ Go to bed at the same time every night, even on weekends.

◆ Let a bedmate or roommate who does not snore fall asleep first.

If snoring is a problem for you or affects your household, see a doctor. You may need an exam of your nose, mouth, and neck.

 Treatment will depend on what is making you snore. Your doctor may want to do a sleep study to see if sleep apnea is one of the reasons why you snore. For help deciding whether you want this kind of testing, go to the Web site on the back cover and enter **y240** in the search box.

**More**

4. Go to bed only when you feel sleepy.

5. If you lie awake for more than 15 minutes, get up, leave the room, and do something relaxing.

6. Repeat steps 4 and 5 until it is time to get up.

7. Get up at the same time every day, even on weekends.

These tips may help too:

◆ Keep your bedroom dark, quiet, and cool. Try using a sleep mask and earplugs. Or try a noise machine that makes relaxing sounds like waterfalls or the ocean.

◆ Get regular exercise. But don't do a hard workout within 2 hours of going to bed.

◆ Avoid alcohol and smoking before bedtime. Limit caffeine, and avoid it after noon.

◆ Avoid foods that upset your stomach.

◆ Drink a glass of warm milk at bedtime. But don't drink more than one glass of fluid before you go to bed, or you may have to get up in the night.

◆ Review all your prescription and nonprescription medicines with a pharmacist to rule out side effects that affect your sleep.

You may want to read about anxiety on page 80 or depression on page 156. Either problem can upset your sleep.

## What About Sleeping Pills?

Prescription and nonprescription sleep medicines may give you fast relief from insomnia. However, it is best to use these only for a short time and to stop taking them as soon as you can. They can cause daytime confusion, memory loss, and dizziness. You can also get addicted to some of them.

Continued use of sleeping pills actually makes sleep problems worse in many people.

## Sleep Habits in Babies

Babies go through sleep cycles that have periods of light sleep or deep or heavy sleep. In each sleep cycle, there may be about 60 minutes of light sleep, 60 to 90 minutes of deep sleep, and another 30 minutes of light sleep. At the end of this cycle, the baby is semi-alert and can be wakened easily.

You can help your baby sleep through the night by helping the baby learn to soothe himself or herself back to sleep during periods of light sleep.

For babies age 4 to 6 months:

◆ Put the baby in the crib when he or she is drowsy but still awake.

◆ Make middle-of-the-night feedings short. Do not turn them into playtime.

◆ As the baby gets older, delay the middle-of-the-night feeding, and stop it sometime after age 6 months.

Always put your baby to sleep on his or her back. This is the best choice for preventing sudden infant death syndrome (SIDS).

# Sore Throat

## When to Call a Doctor

◆ You have trouble breathing or swallowing because of a sore throat, or you drool a lot because you cannot swallow.

◆ You get a severe sore throat after being exposed to someone with strep throat.

◆ You have a sore throat with at least 2 of these 3 symptoms of strep throat:

❖ Fever of 101°F or higher

❖ White or yellow coating on the tonsils

❖ Swollen lymph nodes in the neck, armpits, or groin (see the picture on page 245)

◆ A rash occurs with a sore throat. Scarlet fever is a rash you may get because of strep throat. Like strep throat, scarlet fever is treated with antibiotics.

◆ You have a sore throat that's not related to a cold, allergies, smoking, overuse of your voice, or any other clear reason.

◆ A mild sore throat lasts longer than 2 weeks.

◆ Your child has had at least 4 to 6 episodes of tonsillitis in the past year, even with treatment with antibiotics.

◆ Your child breathes through his or her mouth a lot of the time, often snores, or has a very nasal- or muffled-sounding voice a lot of the time. These are signs of a problem with the adenoids.

Most sore throats are minor and go away with home treatment. You may get a sore throat because of:

◆ A cold or other virus.

◆ Smoking, air pollution, or dry air.

◆ Yelling.

◆ Breathing through your mouth when you sleep. People who have stuffy noses from allergies or colds often do this.

◆ Backflow (reflux) of stomach acid into the throat. If you think this may be the cause of your throat pain, see Heartburn on page 183.

## Tonsillitis

In children, sore throats are often caused by inflammation of the tonsils (tonsillitis) or adenoids (adenoiditis). This is usually caused by a virus.

Along with a sore throat, your child may have fever, swollen lymph nodes, tiredness, and symptoms like a cold, such as a runny nose and cough. It may hurt to swallow. The tonsils are often bright red, spotted with pus, and swollen.

**More**

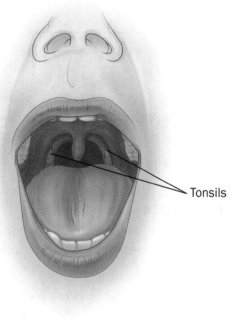

Location of tonsils

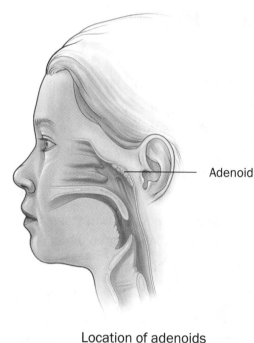

Location of adenoids

Adenoiditis can also cause headache and vomiting. If the adenoids are inflamed a lot of the time, they can swell and block the tubes that connect the throat and the ears. This can lead to ear infections. See page 145.

## Strep Throat

Strep throat is a sore throat caused by strep-tococcal bacteria. It is most common in children 3 to 15 years old. You can get strep throat even if you have had your tonsils taken out.

Most sore throats are not strep throat. The more you feel like you have a cold, the less likely it is that you have strep. Strep throat causes some or all of these symptoms:

- Severe and sudden sore throat
- Fever of 101 °F or higher
- Swollen lymph nodes
- White or yellow coating on the tonsils

Antibiotics are used to treat strep throat and prevent rheumatic fever, a rare but serious problem that can occur if strep is not treated.

## Mono

Mono (mononucleosis) is a viral illness that can cause a severe, long-lasting sore throat. It is most common in older teens and young adults.

Mono may also cause fever, body aches, and swollen lymph nodes in the neck, armpits, and groin. You may feel tired and weak. The upper left part of your belly may hurt (because your spleen is enlarged).

Most people recover from mono after several weeks. But it may take a few months to get your energy back, and lymph nodes may stay swollen for up to a month (see page 245).

There is no treatment for mono except rest, plenty of fluids, saltwater gargles for throat pain, and aspirin or acetaminophen (Tylenol) for body aches. Do not give aspirin to anyone younger than 20.

## Home Treatment

◆ Gargle with warm salt water several times a day to reduce throat swelling and pain. Mix 1 teaspoon of salt in 8 ounces of water.

◆ Drink extra fluids to soothe your throat. Honey and lemon in hot water or in weak tea may help. Do not give honey to children younger than 1 year.

◆ Do not smoke, and avoid other people's smoke. If you need help quitting, see page 316.

◆ Take acetaminophen (Tylenol), aspirin, or ibuprofen (Advil, Motrin) to relieve pain and reduce fever. Do not give aspirin to anyone younger than 20.

◆ Try nonprescription throat lozenges that have a painkiller to numb your throat, such as Sucrets Maximum Strength. Cough drops or hard candy may also help. But do not give them to children, who may choke on them.

◆ If you have strep, stay home from work or school until 24 hours after you have started antibiotics.

◆ If you have mono, do not share eating or drinking utensils; do not kiss anyone; and do not donate blood while you have symptoms.

## Tonsils and Adenoids: Should They Be Taken Out?

Your child may need to have his or her **tonsils** removed if:

◆ Your child has had severe tonsillitis caused by strep at least 4 to 6 times in the past year, even after treatment with at least two antibiotics.

◆ Your child has breathing or sleep problems because of swollen tonsils.

◆ There are deep pockets of infection in the tonsils that have not gotten better after treatment with medicine.

Your child may need to have his or her **adenoids** removed if:

◆ The adenoids block the airway and cause breathing trouble and sleep problems.

◆ Your doctor thinks an adenoid problem is causing frequent ear infections that are hard to treat.

If your doctor recommends surgery but your child does not have the problems described above, you may want to get a second opinion to be sure. The benefits need to greatly outweigh the costs, risks, and pain.

# Sports Injuries

## When to Call a Doctor

◆ You cannot use a limb or joint at all because of an injury.

◆ A limb or joint has an odd shape.

◆ You do not get better with home treatment.

For a sudden injury like an ankle sprain or broken bone, see page 50.

Sports injuries are common among active people. Most are caused by either accidents or overuse. Accidents are hard to avoid if you play a sport. But you can avoid overuse injuries if you train properly and use the right equipment.

You can find information on specific injuries on the following pages:

◆ Bursitis and tendinosis, page 111

◆ Tennis elbow and golfer's elbow, page 112

◆ Knee problems, page 201

◆ Achilles tendon problems, page 186

◆ Heel pain and plantar fasciitis, page 185

◆ Shin splints, page 205

◆ Strains, sprains, broken bones, and dislocations, page 50

◆ Stress fractures, page 50

## Preventing Injuries

◆ Warm up before you exercise. Cold, stiff muscles and ligaments are more likely to get hurt. Cool down and stretch when you are done.

◆ Do not make sudden increases in how hard or how long you exercise. Slow buildups are better. As you get more fit, you will be able to exercise harder without hurting yourself.

◆ Use proper sports techniques and equipment. For example, wear supportive, well-cushioned shoes for running, aerobics, and walking. Use a two-handed tennis backhand stroke. Wear knee pads and wrist guards for in-line skating. Make sure that your bike is adjusted properly for your body. Wear the right kind of helmet for your sport.

◆ Switch between hard workouts and easier ones to let your body rest. For example, if you run, alternate long or hard runs with shorter or easier ones. If you lift weights, do not work the same muscles 2 days in a row.

◆ Try cross-training. This means you do several activities instead of the same one all the time. Cross-training lets you work different muscle groups while the others rest. For example, rotate days of walking or running with biking or swimming.

◆ Do not ignore aches and pains. When you feel the first twinge of pain, rest or reduce your activity for a few days. Taking care of the problem early with ice and other home treatment may help you avoid a more serious injury.

# Ice and Cold Packs

Ice can relieve pain, swelling, and inflammation from injuries and problems like bursitis and arthritis. You can use any of these items to "ice" an area:

◆ A cold pack you buy at the drugstore or grocery store. Store the pack in the freezer.

◆ A homemade cold pack. Seal 1 pint of rubbing alcohol and 3 pints of water in a 1-gallon, heavy-duty, plastic freezer bag. Seal that bag inside a second bag. Mark it "Cold pack: Do not eat," and store it in the freezer.

◆ A bag of frozen vegetables. Peas or corn work well. Do not eat them once you have used them as a cold pack. Label the bag "do not eat." You can reuse it several times.

◆ An ice towel. Wet a towel with cold water, and squeeze it until it is just damp. Fold the towel, place it in a plastic bag, and freeze it for 15 minutes. Take the towel out of the bag, and use it like a cold pack

◆ An ice pack. Put about a pound of ice in a plastic bag. Add water to barely cover the ice. Squeeze the air out of the bag, and seal it. Wrap the bag in a damp towel and put it on the sore area.

Ice the area at least 3 times a day. For the first 48 hours, ice for 10 to 15 minutes once an hour. After that, a good pattern is to ice for 10 to 15 minutes, 3 times a day: in the morning, in the late afternoon after work or school, and about half an hour before you go to bed. Also ice after any long periods of activity or hard exercise.

Always keep a damp cloth between your skin and the cold pack so that the cold does not damage your skin. Press the pack firmly so that it touches all parts of the affected area.

Do not use cold for longer than 10 to 15 minutes at a time, and do not fall asleep with ice on your skin.

More ➤

## Home Treatment

The biggest challenge for most people with sports injuries is to get enough rest and heal without losing their overall fitness.

◆ Stay fit by cross-training with activities that do not stress the injury. If you have sore knees, try swimming. If you have sore feet or ankles, get on a bike. If your elbows or shoulders hurt, try walking. Do not return too fast to the activity that caused the injury.

◆ Get back to your regular activity gradually. Start with a slow, easy pace, and do the activity for shorter periods of time than usual. If you are lifting weights, use less weight and do fewer reps. Increase the pace, time, and intensity only if you have no pain.

◆ Break down your sport into small steps. Once you can throw a ball a short distance without pain, try throwing it a little farther. If you can walk without pain, try slow jogging. Once you can jog slowly without pain, try running a little faster.

# Styes

## When to Call a Doctor

◆ Redness and swelling spread to the entire eyelid or the eyeball.

◆ The stye hurts a lot, grows larger quickly, or does not stop draining.

◆ The stye blocks your vision.

◆ The stye gets worse even with home treatment or does not improve within 1 week.

A stye is an infection of the eyelash follicle. It looks like a small, red bump or pimple either in the eyelid or on the edge of the lid. Styes come to a head and break open after a few days.

Styes are very common and are not a serious problem. But they can hurt, and they may blur your vision. Most will go away with home treatment.

## Home Treatment

◆ Do not rub your eye, and do not squeeze or open the stye.

◆ Apply a warm, moist cloth for 10 minutes, 3 to 6 times a day, until the stye comes to a head and drains.

◆ Do not wear eye makeup or contact lenses until the stye heals.

# Swollen Lymph Nodes

The lymph nodes are small glands found all through the body. They swell as the body fights minor infections from colds, insect bites, or small cuts. More serious infections and some types of cancer can make lymph nodes hard, sore, and quite large.

The lymph nodes in the neck are the ones people most often notice. They may swell when you have a cold or sore throat. The lymph nodes in the groin may swell if you have a vaginal or other pelvic infection or if you have a cut or sore on your leg or foot.

## Home Treatment

Treat the cold or other infection that is making the lymph nodes large. Use the index in the back of the book or the symptom charts on pages 61 to 67 to find what you need.

Lymph nodes may stay swollen or hard for several weeks after the infection goes away. This is very common in children. If the lymph nodes near the site of the infection are not sore and are not getting larger, you can watch them at home and report them at the child's next doctor visit.

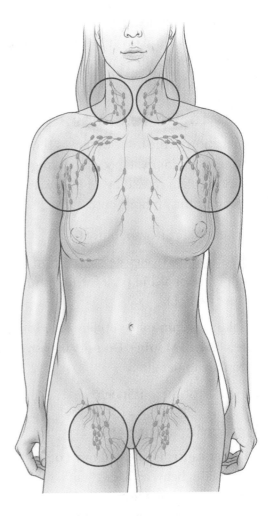

Swollen lymph nodes in the neck, armpits, and groin are usually easy to feel.

# Testicle Problems

## When to Call a Doctor

- You have sudden, severe pain in a testicle or the scrotum. This may be a sign of testicular torsion, which needs urgent medical care.

- Pain or swelling in a testicle or the scrotum gets worse over a period of several hours or days or does not go away after a few days.

- Pain or swelling occurs with fever.

- Pain or swelling starts after exposure to the mumps virus.

- You find a lump.

- You have a change in the shape, size or feel of a testicle.

- One testicle feels very heavy.

The testicles produce sperm and male hormones. Males normally have two testicles, which are behind the penis inside a sac of skin called the scrotum.

## Injury to the Testicles

The location of the testicles makes them an easy target for injury, especially during contact sports. Pain caused by an injury should go away within an hour or so.

To relieve pain after an injury:

- Use a pillow to elevate the scrotum, and apply ice or a cold pack for 10 minutes, once an hour.

- Take acetaminophen (Tylenol) or ibuprofen (Advil, Motrin). Do not take aspirin if you are under 20.

- Wear a jockstrap if it helps.

## Testicular Cancer

Testicular cancer is rare and most often affects males between ages 15 and 35. It usually affects only one testicle and responds well to treatment if found early.

Symptoms may include a painless lump or swelling that men find on their own. The testicle may also feel heavier than normal.

### How to Do a Self-Exam

After taking a warm bath or shower:

- Stand with your right leg on the side of the tub or the toilet seat.

- Gently roll your right testicle between the thumb and fingers of both hands. Feel for any hard lumps or swelling. The testicle should feel round and smooth.

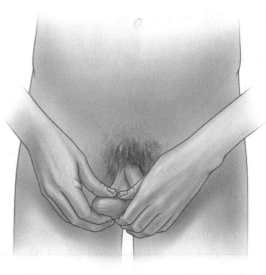

Feel each testicle for hard lumps or swelling.

246

◆ Look for any changes in the size, shape, or feel of the testicle. It is normal for one testicle to be slightly larger than the other.

◆ Repeat the exam on your left testicle.

◆ Tell your doctor about any lumps, swelling, major size differences, or changes in feeling or appearance.

| Other Testicle Problems | | | |
|---|---|---|---|
| **Problem** | **Symptoms** | **Cause** | **Comments** |
| Epididymitis (inflammation of tube at top of testicle; see picture on page 224) | Pain and swelling in scrotum that slowly gets worse; scrotum feels hot and tender; fever | Sexually transmitted disease; irritation from bladder infection or injury | Call your doctor. You may need antibiotics. |
| Orchitis (inflammation of a testicle) | Pain and swelling in the scrotum; scrotum feels heavy | Mumps virus; bacterial infection of prostate or epididymis (see picture on page 224) | Call your doctor. If not treated, orchitis can cause infertility. Make sure your son gets the MMR vaccine to prevent mumps. See page 325. |
| Torsion (testicle rotates on its spermatic cord, cutting off blood flow) | Sudden, severe pain in the scrotum that may spread to the belly; nausea and vomiting; fever | Unknown. May occur during sleep or after heavy exercise. Most common in teenage boys. | **This may be an emergency.** You may need surgery within hours to restore blood flow and prevent permanent damage. |

# Toilet Training

Every child has his or her own schedule for becoming toilet-trained. Most children are ready to start between 24 and 30 months of age.

Your child may be ready if he or she:

◆ Passes stools at about the same time each day.

◆ Is able to have a dry diaper for at least 2 hours at a time during the day.

◆ Makes certain faces when urinating or passing stools.

◆ Lets you know when a diaper is dirty and asks to have it changed.

◆ Seems eager to please and can follow simple instructions.

◆ Tells you that he or she wants to use the toilet or wear "big kids" underwear.

If you think your child is ready to start toilet training, some of these tips may make it go more smoothly:

◆ Get your child a potty chair. Give him or her time to get used to it. Have your child sit on the chair with a diaper on when he or she is passing stools or urinating.

◆ Let your child watch you or a sibling of the same sex use the toilet. Talk with your child about what you're doing.

◆ Choose clothing for your child that's easy to take off. Elastic waistbands and Velcro or snaps work best. Pull-on diapers can help too.

◆ Reward every success with hugs and praise. Expect some accidents in the first few weeks, and don't get mad when they happen. Keep a relaxed attitude.

# Toothache

## When to Call a Dentist

◆ You have signs of a tooth or gum infection, such as:

❖ Increased pain, swelling, warmth, or redness.

❖ Red streaks on the skin over the area.

❖ Pus or blood that drains into the mouth.

❖ Swollen lymph nodes in the neck.

◆ You have a severe toothache that does not improve after 2 hours of home treatment.

◆ You have facial pain or swelling.

◆ You have a painful bump near the sore tooth.

◆ A toothache keeps you from sleeping or doing your usual activities.

◆ You have had a toothache off and on for 2 weeks or longer.

You may have teeth that ache or tingle when you touch them or when you eat or drink something hot, cold, sweet, or sour. The pain may come from a worn-down tooth or from gums that have pulled away from the teeth and exposed the roots and inner parts of the teeth.

If you have sharp pain, you may have tooth decay or infection, have lost a filling, or have a crack in the tooth. Another cause is damage from nervous grinding of your teeth. A tooth that is coming in but cannot break through the gum also can cause a toothache.

A dentist can help find the cause of your toothache and keep your tooth alive.

## Home Treatment

◆ Put ice or a cold pack on the outside of your cheek for 10 to 15 minutes at a time. Put a thin cloth between the ice and your skin. Do not use heat.

◆ Take aspirin, ibuprofen (Advil, Motrin) or naproxen (Aleve) to relieve pain and swelling. Do not give aspirin to anyone younger than 20.

◆ Avoid very hot, cold, or sweet foods and drinks if they make the pain worse.

◆ Talk to your dentist about special tooth-paste for sensitive teeth. Brush with this toothpaste regularly, or rub a small amount of it on the sensitive area with a clean finger 2 or 3 times a day. Floss gently.

◆ Do not smoke or chew tobacco. It can make gum problems worse and makes you less able to fight infection in your gums. If you need help quitting, see page 316.

# Ulcers

## When to Call a Doctor

**Call 911 if:**

◆ You have pain in your upper belly with chest pain or pressure or other symptoms of a heart attack. See page 38.

◆ You have been diagnosed with an ulcer and:

❖ You have severe, nonstop belly pain.

❖ You have severe vomiting.

❖ You vomit blood or what looks like coffee grounds.

❖ You pass very bloody or dark red stools.

❖ Your belly is hard and swollen.

❖ You faint.

**Call your doctor if:**

◆ Mild symptoms of an ulcer do not improve after 10 to 14 days of home treatment.

◆ You are losing weight and you don't know why.

◆ You often vomit or feel nauseated right after you eat.

◆ Belly pain wakes you from sleep.

◆ It often hurts to swallow, or you have trouble swallowing.

**More**

A peptic ulcer is a sore or crater in the lining of the digestive tract. Without treatment, ulcers can cause dangerous health problems, such as bleeding in the stomach and small intestine.

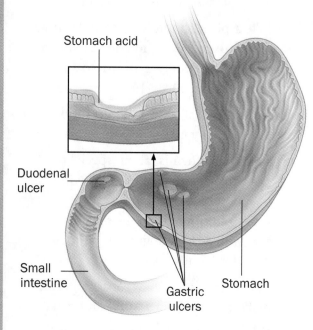

Stomach acid

Duodenal ulcer

Small intestine

Gastric ulcers

Stomach

Most ulcers form in the stomach (gastric ulcers) or in the opening to the small intestine (duodenal ulcers).

The two most common causes of ulcers are:

◆ Infection with *H. pylori* bacteria. Most people who have *H. pylori* in their stomachs do not get ulcers, but it does increase your risk.

◆ Frequent or long-term use of aspirin, ibuprofen (Advil, Motrin), naproxen (Aleve), and other anti-inflammatory medicines. This can damage the digestive tract.

Your risk of an ulcer is higher if you smoke or drink a lot of alcohol.

Symptoms of an ulcer may include a burning or gnawing pain between your belly button and breastbone. The pain often occurs between meals and may wake you

during the night. Eating something or taking an antacid usually relieves the pain. Ulcers may also cause bloating, nausea, or vomiting after meals.

## Home Treatment

◆ Avoid foods that seem to bring on symptoms. Spicy or greasy foods are a problem for many people with ulcers. You don't need to avoid a food if it doesn't cause problems.

◆ Avoid coffee, tea, cola, and other sources of caffeine. Many people find that caffeine makes their pain worse.

◆ Try eating smaller, more frequent meals.

◆ If you smoke, quit. Smoking slows healing of ulcers and increases the chance that they will come back.

◆ Limit alcohol. Large amounts may slow healing and make symptoms worse.

◆ Do not take aspirin, ibuprofen (Advil, Motrin), or naproxen (Aleve). Try acetaminophen (Tylenol) if you need something for pain.

◆ Try a nonprescription antacid, such as Tums, Maalox, or Mylanta, or an acid reducer, such as Pepcid AC, Tagamet HB, or Zantac 75. You can also buy an acid blocker called Prilosec OTC without a prescription.

  ❖ If you take antacids, you may need frequent, large doses to do the job. Talk with your doctor about the best dose.

  ❖ Your doctor may also suggest that you take a prescription medicine such as Prevacid, Prilosec, or Nexium. These drugs greatly reduce the production of stomach acid, which can help your ulcer heal.

◆ Learn to relax and cope better with stress. See page 318.

# Urinary Tract Infections

## When to Call a Doctor

◆ Painful urination occurs with:

  ❖ Fever and chills.

  ❖ Not being able to urinate when you feel the urge.

  ❖ Pain in the back, side, groin, or genital area.

  ❖ Blood or pus in the urine.

  ❖ Unusual discharge from the vagina or penis.

  ❖ Nausea and vomiting.

◆ Urinary symptoms do not improve after 1 or 2 days, or they get worse even with home treatment. Untreated urinary tract infections (UTIs) can spread, which may lead to kidney infections and other serious problems.

◆ You are pregnant or have diabetes and you have symptoms of a UTI.

◆ You think that your child may have a UTI. See page 252.

Urinary tract infections, or UTIs, are usually caused by bacteria that live in the body all the time. Infection can occur in any part of the urinary tract.

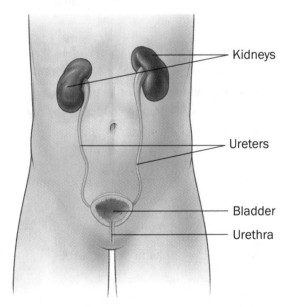

Kidneys

Ureters

Bladder

Urethra

The kidneys filter the blood, and the waste products from the blood become urine. Urine travels through the ureters to the bladder and then leaves the body through the urethra.

Symptoms of a UTI may include:

◆ Burning or pain when you urinate, as well as itching or pain in the urethra.

◆ Cloudy or reddish urine with a strange odor.

◆ Pain in the lower belly or back.

◆ Often having the urge to urinate but not being able to pass much urine.

◆ Fever and chills if the infection is bad, especially if it has spread to the kidneys.

Urinary pain or burning may also be a symptom of a sexually transmitted disease. See page 230.

Men with symptoms like those of a UTI may have a prostate infection (see page 223) or epididymitis (see page 247).

**More**

# Home Treatment

Start home treatment at the first sign of a UTI. A day or two of self-care may clear up a minor infection.

- Drink extra fluids (think in terms of gallons) as soon as you notice symptoms and for the next 24 hours.

- Urinate often, and follow the other tips in Preventing UTIs.

- Watch for fever. A fever may mean you have a more serious infection.

- Use a heating pad or take a hot bath to help relieve pain. Do not use bubble bath or harsh soaps.

- Do not have sex until symptoms improve.

### Cost-saving tip

If you get UTIs often, ask your doctor whether it would be okay to get an extra prescription to have on hand for the future. That way, the next time you get a UTI, you can start the medicine without having to wait for an appointment.

If your doctor agrees that this is a safe option for you, it may save you time and money. It also lets you treat your UTI right away.

## Preventing UTIs

The tips below may be especially useful if you tend to get UTIs.

- Drink plenty of water and other fluids.

- Urinate often.

- Females should wipe from front to back after using the toilet. This will reduce the spread of bacteria from the anus to the urethra. Teach young girls this habit when you toilet train them.

- Do not use douches, vaginal deodorants, or perfumed feminine hygiene products. Avoid bubble baths.

- Do not use a diaphragm for birth control. Choose another method.

- Wash your genitals once a day with water and a mild soap. Rinse and dry well.

- Drink extra water before you have sex, and urinate right afterward.

- Wear cotton underwear, cotton-lined panty hose, and loose clothing.

- Avoid alcohol, caffeine, and carbonated drinks. These can irritate the bladder.

- Drink cranberry and blueberry juice.

## UTIs in Children

UTIs in children are of special concern because they can easily spread to the kidneys and cause damage and scarring. Repeated scarring can lead to high blood pressure and kidney problems, including kidney failure. Babies and young children seem to be more likely to have scarring.

UTIs in children usually clear up fast if you treat them right away. But it can be hard to tell that your baby or young child has a UTI. Young children may not have the usual symptoms, and they cannot tell you how they feel.

The only signs of UTI in a baby or young child may be:

- Unexplained fever.

- Urine that looks or smells odd.

- Not eating.

- Vomiting.

- Being extremely fussy.

Call your child's doctor today if you suspect your child has a UTI.

# Vaginal Bleeding

## When to Call a Doctor

**Call 911** if you have severe vaginal bleeding and you faint or feel lightheaded. (Severe means soaking at least 2 pads or 2 super tampons in 2 hours.)

**Call a doctor if:**

◆ You are pregnant and have any vaginal bleeding.

◆ You have pain in your lower belly with unexpected vaginal bleeding.

◆ You have unexpected bleeding and a fever.

◆ Bleeding is heavy.

◆ Bleeding between periods lasts longer than 1 week or happens 3 months in a row.

◆ You bleed after you have sex or douche.

◆ You are over 35 and have any bleeding between periods.

◆ You are over 35 and your periods last longer than 10 days.

◆ You use a hormonal form of birth control (pills, shots, the patch) and your periods are not like what your doctor told you to expect.

◆ You have any bleeding after menopause.

## Bleeding Between Periods

Many women have bleeding or spotting between periods. It does not always mean you have a health problem.

Common causes of bleeding or spotting include:

◆ Ovulation (when the ovary releases an egg each cycle).

◆ Birth control pills or Depo-Provera shots.

◆ Using an IUD (intrauterine device).

◆ Breast-feeding.

◆ Stress.

In all these cases, if the bleeding is not heavy and occurs only once in a while, you probably don't need to worry. Do not take aspirin. It may make the bleeding last longer.

Less common causes of bleeding are:

◆ Uterine fibroids. These growths are not cancer.

◆ Miscarriage or a problem with a pregnancy (see page 217).

◆ Ectopic pregnancy. This means a fertilized egg has attached somewhere other than the uterus.

◆ Pelvic infection. You may also have fever, cramping, pain during sex, and a smelly vaginal discharge. See page 255.

◆ A problem with the cervix (the opening of the uterus).

◆ Cervical or uterine cancer (rarely).

**More**

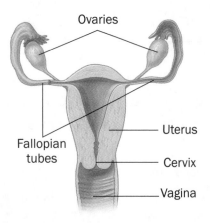

The female pelvic organs

## Bleeding After Menopause

If you have gone through menopause (see page 207) and are not taking hormones, you should not have any vaginal bleeding. If you do, you may have an abnormal growth in your uterus and should see a doctor.

If you are taking hormones, a little bleeding after menopause may be normal. But be sure to tell your doctor about it.

## Normal Menstrual Bleeding

The menstrual cycle is the series of changes a woman's body goes through to prepare for a possible pregnancy.

About once a month, the uterus grows a new, thickened lining (endometrium) so that it is ready to receive a fertilized egg. The ovaries release an egg. If the egg does not get fertilized or does not implant in the uterus, the uterus sheds its lining.

The bleeding that results is your monthly period. For most women, the bleeding lasts from 2 to 7 days. It may be heavy or light. Each woman is different. Learn what's normal for you, and watch for changes.

Also see Missed or Irregular Periods on page 210.

# Vaginitis and Yeast Infections

## When to Call a Doctor

- You have lower belly or pelvic pain, fever, and unusual vaginal discharge.

- You have pain or bleeding during or after sex, and a lubricant does not help.

- Your vaginal discharge smells bad or does not look normal.

- You think you have a yeast infection but are not sure.

- You know you have a yeast infection and nonprescription medicine does not clear it up in 3 or 4 days.

- You think you may have a sexually transmitted disease. See page 230. Your sex partner(s) may need to be treated too.

- You get yeast infections often and are not taking antibiotics. This can be a sign of diabetes or other problems.

- You are or may be pregnant and have symptoms of a vaginal infection (pain, redness, itching, smelly discharge).

- You have symptoms of a urinary tract infection (pain or burning, frequent urge to urinate). See page 251.

If you plan to see a doctor, do not douche, use vaginal creams, or have sex for 48 hours before your appointment.

Vaginitis is any infection, inflammation, or irritation of the vagina that changes your normal vaginal discharge.

If it hurts or burns when you urinate and you feel the need to urinate often, you may have a urinary tract infection. See page 251.

## Home Treatment

- Follow the tips in Preventing Vaginal Problems on page 256.

- Do not have sex until your symptoms have gone away.

- Do not scratch. Relieve itching with a cold pack or cool bath.

- Make sure the cause of vaginitis is not a forgotten tampon or other object.

- If you think you may be pregnant, do a home pregnancy test. See page 210. Infection can be more serious if you are pregnant.

- If you know that you have a yeast infection, try a nonprescription medicine such as Monistat or Gyne-Lotrimin. If you're pregnant, talk with your doctor first.

- Use pads instead of tampons if you are using a vaginal cream or suppository. The tampons can absorb the medicine.

Vaginitis may clear up in a few days. If your symptoms do not go away, be sure to call your doctor.

**More**

## Vaginal Problems

| Common Causes | Symptoms | What to Do |
|---|---|---|
| Yeast infection | Itching and redness; white, odor-free discharge that looks like cottage cheese; burning when you urinate or have sex | Infection may clear on its own; try nonprescription medicine for yeast infection (Monistat, Gyne-Lotrimin). |
| Bacterial vaginosis | Thin gray or yellow discharge that smells fishy; pain when you urinate or have sex | Call doctor for treatment, especially if you are pregnant. |
| Trichomoniasis and other sexually transmitted diseases (see page 230) | Redness and irritation; bad odor; a lot of foamy, white or colored discharge; pain during sex | Call doctor for treatment. Any partner(s) need treatment too. |
| Atrophic vaginitis (happens during menopause) | Burning, pain, and dryness when you have sex | Try vaginal lubricant (Astroglide, Replens). Ask doctor about estrogen cream. |

## Preventing Vaginal Problems

◆ Do not take antibiotics unless you really need to.

◆ Wash your vaginal area once a day with plain water or a mild, unscented soap. Rinse and dry well.

◆ Do not douche.

◆ Do not use feminine deodorant sprays and other perfumed products. They irritate and dry tender skin.

◆ During your period, change tampons at least 3 times a day, or switch between tampons and pads. Don't leave tampons in for more than 8 hours. And be sure to remove the last tampon you use.

◆ Wipe from front to back after you use the toilet.

◆ Limit how many sex partners you have. Use condoms.

◆ If you think problems may be related to your birth control (diaphragm, spermicide, condoms), discuss other options with your doctor. See page 96.

◆ Do not wear panty hose or tight nylon underwear.

◆ Try a vaginal lubricant during sex if you have a problem with dryness.

# Varicose Veins

## When to Call a Doctor

◆ You have sudden pain or swelling in your leg. You may have a clot in a deep vein, which could be serious.

◆ The skin over a varicose vein bleeds heavily on its own or after an injury, and you cannot stop the bleeding.

◆ You have an open sore on your leg or foot.

◆ A tender lump appears on your leg for no clear reason (you have not bumped or bruised your leg).

Varicose veins are large, twisted veins near the surface of the skin. They are most common in the legs and ankles.

You get a varicose vein when a vein becomes weak and stretched and can no longer help move blood up and back to the heart. (This is not harmful, because there are so many other veins in the body.) Blood pools in the weak vein, causing it to swell.

Obesity, pregnancy, or standing for long periods of time can cause varicose veins. They also tend to run in the family.

◆ Varicose veins may not cause any symptoms. The blue color of the veins may be the only reason you notice them.

◆ Your legs, feet, or ankles may ache, swell a little, and feel tired.

◆ If the veins get worse, they can cause dry, itchy skin and may break open and bleed, causing open sores.

Some people have tiny varicose veins on the surface of the skin. These are called spider veins. They are not a health problem, but you may not like the way they look if you have them.

 Varicose veins usually do not need treatment other than self-care. If they bother you or cause bleeding or skin problems, you may want to think about treatments such as sclerotherapy or surgery. For help deciding whether you want or need treatment, go to the Web site on the back cover and enter **d904** in the search box.

## Home Treatment

◆ Wear supportive, full-length elastic stockings. Do not wear knee-highs. For mild symptoms, regular support panty hose may work. Or your doctor can give you a prescription for compression stockings, which you can buy at a drugstore or medical supply store.

◆ Do not wear socks or stockings that leave red marks around your legs. Do not wear tight belts or pants that are tight in the waist or thighs.

◆ Put your feet up when you sit. If you cannot put your feet up, then sit with your feet flat on the floor or crossed at the ankles. Do not cross your legs at the knee. At the end of the day, lie down and prop your legs above heart level.

◆ If you have to sit a lot (at work, for example), get up and walk around often. If you have to stand a lot, move around often, or sit down and put your feet up when you can.

◆ Get regular exercise, such as walking, cycling, swimming, or dancing. Working your leg muscles keeps blood from pooling in the legs.

◆ Lose weight if you need to. See page 300.

# Vomiting, Age 3 and Younger

## When to Call a Doctor

### Call 911 if:

◆ Your child faints, or you cannot wake your child.

◆ Your child has signs of severe dehydration. These include sunken eyes, no tears, and a dry mouth and tongue; a sunken soft spot on your baby's head; little or no urine for 8 hours; skin that sags when you pinch it; and fast breathing and a fast heartbeat.

◆ Your child vomits blood or what looks like coffee grounds.

### Call a doctor if:

◆ Vomiting occurs with severe headache, a stiff neck, not acting alert, or having trouble waking up. Your child may have a serious illness. See page 161.

◆ Your child refuses to drink or cannot take in enough liquid to replace lost fluids.

◆ Severe vomiting (vomiting most or all clear liquids and feedings) occurs in a baby younger than 3 months. For older children, call if severe vomiting goes on:

❖ Longer than 4 hours in a baby 3 to 12 months old.

❖ Longer than 8 hours in a child 1 to 3 years old.

◆ Your child vomits now and then, has no other symptoms, and can keep fluids down between vomiting. Call if this goes on longer than:

❖ 1 to 2 days in a baby younger than 3 months.

❖ 2 to 4 days in a baby 3 to 6 months old.

❖ 1 to 2 weeks in a child 7 months to 3 years old.

◆ Your child has severe belly pain.

◆ Your child has belly pain and vomiting for more than 12 hours but has little or no diarrhea.

◆ Belly pain started several hours before the vomiting and seems like more than just stomach cramps.

◆ Your child has pain in just one part of the belly, especially the lower right belly. See the picture on page 69. It may be hard to tell where the pain is in a small child.

Vomiting in children is often caused by:

◆ Viral stomach flu. Stomach flu often starts with vomiting that is followed in a few hours (sometimes 8 to 12 hours or longer) by diarrhea. Sometimes there is no diarrhea.

◆ Eating unusual kinds or amounts of food. A baby's digestive system sometimes cannot handle large amounts of juice, fruit, or even milk.

Vomiting can also be caused by serious illness, though this is not common. In these cases, vomiting will usually occur with other signs of illness, such as stiff neck, constant crying, and not being alert or active.

Babies and young children need special care when they are vomiting, because they can quickly get dehydrated. This means the body has lost too much fluid. Keep a close watch on how your child looks and acts, and make sure he or she gets enough fluids.

## Home Treatment

### Age up to 6 months

◆ Do not feed your baby anything for 30 to 60 minutes after he or she has vomited. Watch your baby closely for signs of dehydration (see When to Call a Doctor).

◆ If your baby is breast-fed, offer short but frequent feedings.

◆ If your baby is formula-fed, switch to an oral electrolyte solution, such as Pedialyte or Infalyte. Offer 1 tablespoon every 10 minutes for the first hour. After the first hour, slowly increase the amount you offer your baby. You can go back to regular feedings after 6 hours have passed without your baby vomiting.

◆ Do not give your baby plain water.

### Age 7 months to 3 years

◆ After 1 hour has passed since your child last vomited, give 1 ounce of a clear liquid every 20 minutes for 1 hour. Safe choices are children's oral rehydration solution, clear broth, Jell-O, and fruit juice mixed to half strength with water.

◆ Increase the amount by 1 ounce an hour as long as your child does not vomit.

◆ Do not use sports drinks (such as Gatorade or All Sport), soda, or full-strength fruit juice. These drinks have too much sugar. Do not offer plain water or diet soda. These lack the calories and minerals your child needs.

◆ After 6 hours with no vomiting, offer your child regular foods. Avoid high-fiber foods (such as beans) and foods with a lot of sugar, such as candy or ice cream.

# Vomiting and Nausea, Age 4 and Older

## When to Call a Doctor

### Call 911 if:

◆ Vomiting occurs with chest pain or pressure or other signs of a heart attack. See page 38.

◆ You have signs of severe dehydration. These include little or no urine for 8 hours; sunken eyes, no tears, and a dry mouth and tongue; skin that sags when you pinch it; feeling very dizzy or lightheaded; fast breathing and heartbeat; and not feeling or acting alert.

◆ You vomit a lot of blood or what looks like coffee grounds.

### Call a doctor if:

◆ You vomit after a head injury. See page 37.

◆ Symptoms of mild dehydration (dry mouth, dark urine, not much urine) get worse even with home treatment.

◆ Vomiting occurs with any of these signs of serious illness:

❖ Severe headache, sleepiness, or stiff neck. See page 161.

❖ Fever and increasing pain in the lower right belly. See page 69.

❖ Fever and shaking chills.

❖ Swelling in the belly.

❖ Pain in the upper right or upper left belly.

◆ Vomiting and fever last longer than 48 hours.

◆ You think that a medicine may be causing the problem.

◆ Any vomiting lasts longer than 1 week.

For vomiting in a child 3 years or younger, see page 258.

Nausea is a very unpleasant feeling in the pit of your stomach. You may feel weak and sweaty and produce lots of spit. Intense nausea often leads to vomiting, or "throwing up." Good home treatment will help you feel better and avoid dehydration.

Common causes of nausea and vomiting are:

◆ Viral stomach flu or food poisoning. See page 167.

◆ Stress or nervousness.

◆ Medicines, especially antibiotics, aspirin, ibuprofen (Advil, Motrin), and naproxen (Aleve).

◆ Pregnancy and morning sickness. See page 217.

◆ Diabetes.

◆ Migraine headaches. See page 176.

◆ Head injury. See page 37.

Nausea and vomiting can also be signs of other serious problems. Be sure to check the Digestive Problems chart on page 66 if this topic does not meet your needs.

## Home Treatment

◆ Watch for and treat early signs of dehydration. See page 31. Older adults and young children who are vomiting can quickly get dehydrated.

◆ After vomiting has stopped for 1 hour, take small sips of a clear liquid every 10 to 15 minutes. Drink more as you feel better and your body can handle it. Clear liquids include apple or grape juice mixed to half strength with water; rehydration drinks (see page 33); weak tea with sugar; clear broth; and Jell-O. Avoid orange juice and grapefruit juice.

◆ If vomiting lasts longer than 24 hours, sip a rehydration drink to restore lost fluids and nutrients. See page 33.

◆ When you feel better, try clear soups and liquids and mild foods. Jell-O, bananas, rice, applesauce, dry toast, and crackers are good choices. Stick with these mild foods until all symptoms have been gone for 12 to 48 hours.

◆ Rest in bed until you feel better.

# Warts

### When to Call a Doctor

◆ A wart looks infected.

◆ A plantar wart hurts when you walk, and foam pads do not help.

◆ You have warts in the anal or genital area. See page 230.

◆ You have a wart on your face that you want removed.

◆ You have diabetes or peripheral artery disease and get a wart on your foot.

Warts are skin growths caused by a virus. They can appear anywhere on the body. Plantar warts are on the soles of the feet. Most of the wart lies under the skin surface and may make you feel like you are walking on a pebble.

Warts come and go for no clear reason. They can last a week, a month, or even years.

There are several ways to deal with warts:

◆ Do not treat them. If warts don't bother you, there is no reason to spend time and money treating them.

◆ Use home treatment to remove them. There are three methods for this: salicylic acid, tape, and cryotherapy. See Home Treatment on page 262. Home treatment works a lot of the time but not always.

◆ Have surgery to remove them. If you have a very painful wart that will not go away, or if you have enough warts to bother you, you may want to think about surgery. But you should know that warts may come back after surgery.

 Talk with your doctor about your treatment choices and their pros and cons. For help deciding what's right for you, go to the Web site on the back cover and enter **v098** in the search box.

# Home Treatment

- Do not try to remove genital warts. See page 230.

- Do not pick at a wart. It may spread to the skin under your nails.

- Do not try to cut or burn off a wart.

- Do not try to remove a wart if you have diabetes or peripheral artery disease. Talk to your doctor.

## To Remove Warts

Try the least costly method first. You may save a trip to your doctor. If you find a treatment that works, stick with it.

If you are sure that your skin growth is a wart, you can treat it with one of three methods:

- **Method 1:** Use a nonprescription salicylic acid product. Over time, this will soften the wart so that you can rub or file it off. Follow the instructions on the label. Salicylic acid works as well as or better than any other treatment for warts. It may take 2 to 3 months to work.

- **Method 2:** Cover the wart with a piece of waterproof tape (such as duct tape), and leave it on for 6 days. After 6 days, remove the tape and soak the wart in water. Then gently rub it with a nail file or pumice stone. (You will need to clean or replace the nail file or pumice stone often.) Leave the tape off overnight. Repeat the process until the wart is gone, but not longer than 2 months. This method is very cheap and works for most people who do it right.

- **Method 3:** Use a nonprescription cryotherapy product. You spray medicine into a foam applicator and then hold the applicator to the wart for a few seconds. This "freezes" the wart off. Pregnant or breast-feeding women and children younger than 4 should not use this treatment.

If treatment irritates the area, take a 2- to 3-day break from it.

If you rub the wart with a pumice stone or file to remove dead tissue, do not use the item for any other purpose. It can spread the wart-causing virus. Wash your hands with soap after you touch the debris from the wart or the pumice stone or file.

## To Reduce Pain From a Plantar Wart

- Wear comfortable shoes and socks. Don't wear high heels or shoes that put pressure on your foot.

- Cushion the wart with a doughnut-shaped pad or a moleskin patch you can buy at a drugstore. Place the pad around the plantar wart. You may also want to place pads or cushions in your shoes.

# Living Better With Chronic Disease

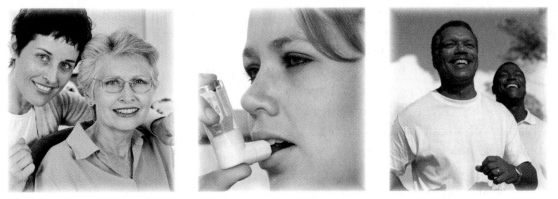

# How to Live Better With Chronic Disease

Chronic diseases are long-term health problems. They can last for months or years. Often they last a lifetime.

A minor chronic health problem may not have much of an impact on your life. But for millions of people, coping with a chronic disease is part of their daily lives. The good news is that even if chronic disease is part of your life, it doesn't have to be the only part. No matter what your health problem is, there are things you can do to help control your disease and live better.

**1. Get informed.** Good information can help you make good health decisions. If this book does not address the health problem you have—or even if it does—go to the Web site on the back cover to start learning about your disease.

Don't be afraid to use your doctor as a teacher. See page 2 for tips on how to get the most out of your partnership with your doctor.

**2. Get support.** For major health problems, support can make a big difference in how well you do and how good you feel. Look for support from:

◆ Family and friends. Let them know how they can help, even if all you need is someone to talk to.

◆ Support groups. People who have the same disease you do can be a great source of emotional and practical help. Look for a support group in your area or online. There are online groups and chat rooms for nearly every health problem. (Be careful with what you learn online, and talk to your doctor before you change your treatment or try any new medicines, vitamins, or herbal products.)

◆ Large organizations focused on specific diseases, like the American Diabetes Association or the American Heart Association.

◆ Counselors and therapists. Living with a chronic disease can be overwhelming at times. If you're feeling depressed or don't feel like you are coping well, talking with an expert might help.

**3. Follow your treatment plan.** Your doctor can guide your treatment, but whether you stick to the plan is up to you. Depending on the disease, treatment may include things like:

◆ Taking medicines every day, on time and in the right amount.

◆ Changing your diet. (Maybe you need to eat a low-sodium diet or avoid certain foods.)

◆ Making changes in your lifestyle, like being more active, quitting smoking, or getting more rest. For some health problems, changes like these are not just healthy habits. They're vital to treating the disease.

◆ Doing physical therapy.

◆ Having treatments like radiation, dialysis, or chemotherapy.

Following your treatment plan may be hard sometimes, but it can make a big difference. Talk with your doctor if you have any problems with your treatment. There may be ways to make it easier.

**4. Avoid "triggers" when you can.** Triggers are things that make your symptoms or disease worse. For example, smoke, dust, and pollution are common triggers for people with breathing problems. For someone with kidney disease, a high-protein meal or certain over-the-counter medicines might trigger symptoms. Stress and lack of sleep are triggers for some health problems.

If you're not sure what your triggers are, it may help to keep a record of your symptoms. Write down when you have them, how bad they are, and what seems to make them worse or better. With time, you may start to see patterns that can help you recognize your triggers. Then you can try to avoid them.

**5. Monitor your health.** Part of your self-care job may be to regularly test and keep track of some aspect of your disease. People with diabetes need to check their blood sugar every day. People with asthma have to check their peak flow, which measures how well they are breathing. If you have high blood pressure, you may need to check your own blood pressure often.

Doing these "self-tests" can help you:

◆ Know when there's a problem before it becomes severe. You may be able to stop the problem before it gets worse.

◆ Know when to call your doctor right away rather than wait for your next visit.

◆ Know how well your treatment is working. Your records can help your doctor track your health over time.

**6. Know what problems to watch for.** Sometimes there may be warning signs that your disease is about to flare up. Or you may need to watch for early signs of complications.

Talk to your doctor about what symptoms you should watch for, and have a plan for how to handle them. Should you go to the hospital? Is there medicine you can take? Get instructions for what to do if you suddenly get worse.

**7. See your doctor regularly.** Regular visits and, in some cases, tests let you and your doctor check in on your health and know whether your treatment needs to be changed. They can also help your doctor find problems early, when they may be easier to correct.

Agree on a schedule for visits and tests. Once a year? Every 3 months? Work with your doctor to decide what's best for you.

**8. Stay as healthy as you can.** Chronic disease can become harder to manage when you start to have other health problems too. For most people, healthy lifestyle choices—eating right, not smoking, being active, reducing stress—can make a difference. Remember to take care of your whole self.

## Where to Go From Here

The rest of this section covers six common chronic diseases: asthma, COPD, coronary artery disease, depression, diabetes, and heart failure. If you have one of these conditions, read on to learn the basics of how to manage your disease.

If you have a different health problem, check the index at the back of the book or go to the Web site on the back cover. With the right information and a little coaching, you can start living better with your disease today.

# Living Better With Asthma

If you have asthma, it may help to know just what it is and what it does to your body. Asthma causes inflammation and swelling in the airways (bronchial tubes) that lead to the lungs. This makes the airways narrower, which makes it harder for you to breathe.

How often you have trouble breathing depends on how bad your asthma is and what triggers it. Some people breathe normally most of the time, while others feel as if they are always short of breath. Other people may have trouble breathing only at night or when they exercise.

When you have a lot of trouble breathing, you are having an asthma attack.

Your airways are very swollen, and it's hard to get air through them.

Along with the symptoms asthma can cause from day to day, it also can damage your airways and lungs. Even mild asthma can cause long-term problems. Asthma can make illnesses like bronchitis and pneumonia worse. And it can lead to COPD (chronic obstructive pulmonary disease), a long-term lung disease.

But asthma does not have to control your life or your future. There are things you can do today and every day to prevent these kinds of problems and to live better with asthma.

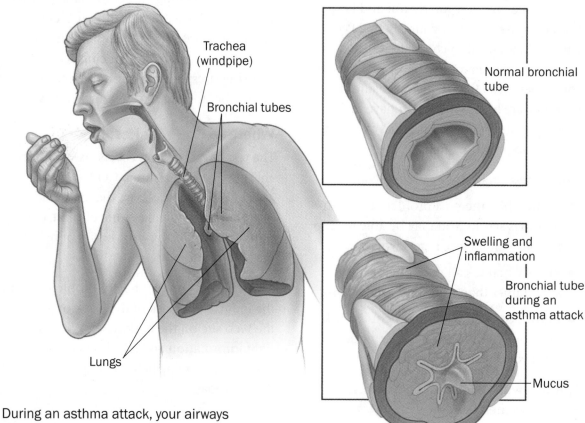

Trachea (windpipe)

Bronchial tubes

Lungs

Normal bronchial tube

Swelling and inflammation

Bronchial tube during an asthma attack

Mucus

During an asthma attack, your airways (bronchial tubes) are very swollen and inflamed. This is why it's hard to breathe.

266

### What You Can Do

◆ Have a plan! A daily treatment plan and an asthma action plan can give you much of what you need to manage your asthma. See Your Asthma Plans on this page.

◆ Take your asthma medicines. If you are not sure how or when to take them, talk to your doctor. See page 268.

◆ Take part in your care. Check your peak flow (see page 269). Keep track of your symptoms. Do not ignore your asthma just because you feel good.

◆ Learn what things make your asthma worse or lead to asthma attacks. Avoid these triggers when you can. See page 269.

◆ See your doctor regularly. How often depends on how bad your asthma is. If you have mild asthma, you may need a checkup every 6 to 12 months. If your asthma is out of control, you may need one every 2 months.

◆ If you smoke, quit. Smoking makes your asthma worse, and it raises your risk for lung cancer and other problems. If you need help quitting, see page 316.

## Your Asthma Plans

An important part of living well with asthma is using a daily treatment plan and an asthma action plan.

### Daily treatment plan

This plan tells you:

◆ Which medicines to take every day.

◆ How often to check your peak flow (see page 269).

◆ What else you need to do each day to manage your asthma.

Your daily treatment plan is focused on controlling your asthma over the long term. It can help you avoid symptoms and attacks and help prevent long-term problems from your asthma.

### Asthma action plan

An action plan tells you how to treat an asthma attack. It will help you make good, quick decisions about what to do when your asthma gets worse. It may even save your life.

To use an asthma action plan, you need to know a few things.

◆ Your peak flow. Peak flow is how fast you breathe out when you try your hardest. It tells you how well your airways and lungs are working. Checking your peak flow is easy. See page 269 to learn how.

◆ Your personal best peak flow. This number is a baseline for knowing whether you are doing well or getting worse. You find your personal best by taking peak flow readings over 2 to 3 weeks when your asthma is under control.

◆ Your asthma zones. There are three zones: green, yellow, and red. Your action plan tells you what to do when you are in each zone. The zones are based on your peak flow and your symptoms.

 These plans can help you feel better and avoid serious health problems. If you don't have a plan now, ask your doctor to help you make one. For help getting started, go to the Web site on the back cover and enter **f384** in the search box.

**More**

## Take Your Medicines

Asthma medicine helps prevent your symptoms and makes you more able to do the things you want to do. It helps you control your asthma instead of your asthma controlling you.

Most people need two types of asthma medicine:

◆ Controller medicine. Take your controller medicine every day, even when you do not have symptoms. It prevents lung damage and asthma attacks and helps stop problems before they occur.

◆ Quick-relief medicine. Use this when you have symptoms of an asthma attack. It acts fast to treat an attack before it gets bad. Always have some of this medicine with you.

### Using Your Inhaler

Asthma medicine usually comes in an inhaler, a device that lets you breathe the medicine in through your mouth so it goes right to your airways and lungs.

 To get the best results from your medicine, be sure to use the inhaler correctly. For a step-by-step guide (with pictures!), go to the Web site on the back cover and enter **n247** in the search box. You can also ask your doctor or pharmacist for help.

Your doctor may suggest that you use a spacer. A spacer is a piece you attach to the inhaler. It makes using an inhaler easier for many people.

If you still have trouble, tell your doctor. There may be another way you can take your medicine.

### Quick-Relief Medicine: For Attacks, Not Daily Use

Since quick-relief medicine helps your breathing problems so fast, you may be tempted to use it often to control your asthma instead of taking your controller medicine.

This is not a good idea. Quick-relief medicine is for times when you cannot prevent symptoms and need to treat them. It is not intended as the daily medicine you take to control your asthma—just like controller medicine is not used to treat an attack (it acts too slowly).

#### Why does it matter?

◆ The goal is to prevent symptoms before they start and prevent long-term damage. This is the job of controller medicine. Quick-relief medicine does not help as well with this.

◆ Using quick-relief medicine too often can make your asthma worse or cause your heart to beat too fast or in an odd rhythm. It can also make your medicine not work as well as it should.

Talk to your doctor if you are using quick-relief medicine more than twice a week or you go through more than one canister in 3 months.

Note: Some people with asthma need to take quick-relief medicine before they exercise. If your doctor has advised this, it is okay to take it as often as you exercise.

## Check Your Peak Flow

Peak flow (peak expiratory flow, or PEF) is how fast you can breathe out when you try your hardest. Checking your peak flow regularly can help you:

◆ Know when an asthma attack is coming and treat it before it gets bad. This helps you stay healthy and stay out of the hospital.

◆ Know how well your lungs are working, even if you don't have symptoms.

◆ Find out what things make your asthma worse. For example, if your peak flow is always worse when you are under stress or when you let your dog sleep in your bedroom, it's a good clue that these things are not good for your asthma.

Checking your peak flow is quick and easy. You can do it at home with a simple, low-cost device called a peak flow meter. Here's how:

◆ Take a breath and blow into the tube on the meter as hard and as fast as you can.

◆ Write down the number on the meter. Use a notebook or calendar where you can keep track of your peak flow and asthma symptoms over time.

◆ Do what your asthma action plan (see page 267) says to do based on your peak flow.

Work with your doctor to find out what your peak flow should be and how often to check it. Bring your records of your peak flow readings and symptoms whenever you have a checkup. These can help your doctor know whether you need to change your treatment.

Checking your peak flow is an easy, low-cost step to help you control your asthma and avoid severe attacks. For a complete, step-by-step guide to checking your peak flow, go to the Web site on the back cover and enter **r703** in the search box.

## Avoid Asthma Triggers

A trigger is anything that makes your asthma worse and can cause an attack. Smoke, pollution, pollen, pet dander, colds, stress, and cold air are triggers for many people.

You can learn what triggers an asthma attack for you by keeping track of your peak flow and your symptoms. When you get worse or better, think about what may have caused it. Is the pollen count high? Did you spend the evening in a smoky bar? Did you go for a jog in the cold air?

Once you know what your triggers are, try to prevent or avoid them. These tips may help with the most common triggers:

◆ If you smoke, quit. See page 316 if you need help quitting. Stay out of smoky places. Do not use a wood-burning stove or fireplace in your home.

◆ Reduce dust, dust mites, pollen, and mold in your home—especially your bedroom. See page 77 for lots of ideas that can help.

◆ Do not exercise outside when the air is cold and dry. Try an indoor workout at the gym. Walk at the mall. Get an exercise video you can do at home. (Check with your doctor if you are not sure whether it's safe for you to exercise.)

**More** ➤

◆ Keep pets out of the house or at least out of your bedroom. Have your pet stay in areas that have hard floors. They are easier to clean than carpeted ones.

 Avoiding your triggers can help prevent asthma attacks and keep you healthy and out of the hospital. For more help finding out what your triggers are and how to deal with them, go to the Web site on the back cover and enter **z654** in the search box.

## If Your Child Has Asthma

Many children have asthma and handle it very well. You can help your child feel better, do more, and avoid emergencies and long-term problems.

◆ Make sure your child takes his or her asthma medicines. This means taking controller medicines every day (or as prescribed) and using quick-relief medicine at the right times. Your child may need some help using an inhaler properly.

◆ Tell teachers, coaches, and the school nurse that your child has asthma. Talk about what to do if your child has an asthma attack.

◆ Make sure your child has quick-relief medicine available at all times.

◆ Help your child check and keep track of his or her peak flow. With a little support, many older children can do this on their own.

◆ Encourage your child to be active, play, and do what other kids do. Asthma does not have to hold your child back.

### For parents of teens with asthma

Teens may feel like asthma cuts into their freedom or sets them apart from their friends. There are ways you can help your teen stick with treatment and feel better about it.

◆ Let your teen meet with the doctor alone. This helps your teen take charge of his or her care.

◆ Work out a daily treatment plan that lets your teen do what he or she likes to do (sports, music, school activities).

◆ Help your teen see that treatment will help him or her lead an active, normal life.

◆ Talk with your teen about the dangers of smoking. Smoking is bad for all teens. It's especially bad for teens with asthma.

◆ Help your teen meet other teens with asthma so they can support each other.

## When to Call a Doctor

### Call 911 if:

◆ You have severe trouble breathing and do not have your asthma medicine with you.

◆ You have taken your quick-relief medicine and after 20 to 30 minutes you do not feel better.

◆ You measure your peak flow and it is less than 50 percent of your personal best.

### Call your doctor if:

◆ Your symptoms do not get better after you have followed your asthma action plan.

◆ You cough up yellow, dark brown, or bloody mucus.

◆ You do not have an asthma action plan and want one.

◆ You need to use quick-relief medicine more than twice a week (for reasons other than exercise).

◆ You have any problems with your asthma medicine.

# Living Better With COPD

COPD (chronic obstructive pulmonary disease) is a long-term illness that makes it hard to breathe. When you have COPD, air does not flow easily out of your lungs. You may be short of breath, cough a lot, and have a lot of mucus in your airways.

If you have emphysema or chronic bronchitis, you have a form of COPD.

With time, breathing problems get worse, and it gets harder to do everyday activities. COPD can lead to heart problems and to death.

But you can make a difference in your health. Good self-care can help you stay healthier for a longer time. For example, regular exercise, special breathing techniques, and rest breaks during the day may help you feel better from day to day. Taking the medicines your doctor prescribes may help with your breathing.

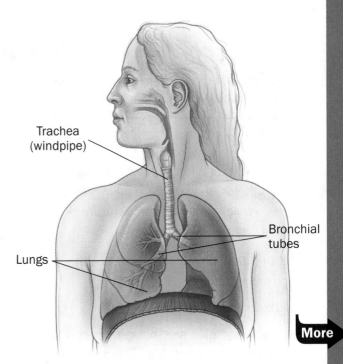

Trachea (windpipe)

Bronchial tubes

Lungs

**More**

When you have COPD, the airways (trachea and bronchial tubes) leading to the lungs may be blocked by swelling, damage, and mucus. This makes it hard to breathe.

**The best thing you can do is stop smoking.** This is the only sure way to slow the disease. But it may also be the hardest step to take when you have COPD.

Talk to your doctor about stop-smoking programs and medicines that can help. Also see Quitting Smoking on page 316.

## Take Your Medicines

COPD medicines reduce shortness of breath, control coughing and wheezing, and can prevent or reduce a flare-up. Most people with COPD find that medicine makes breathing easier.

COPD medicines usually come as an inhaler—a device that lets you breathe the medicine in through your mouth so it goes right to your airways and lungs.

 Be sure you are using your inhaler correctly. For a step-by-step guide (with pictures!), go to the Web site on the back cover and enter **e492** in the search box. You can also ask your doctor or pharmacist for help.

If you still have trouble using an inhaler, talk to your doctor. There may be another way you can take your medicine.

## Breathe Clean Air at Home

Many things can make your symptoms worse or cause flare-ups—smoke, poor air quality, dust, pollen, even the weather. Some of these COPD "triggers" are out of your control. But you can make your home a place where you can breathe easier.

◆ Do not let anyone smoke in your home. That means you too.

---

## COPD Flare-Ups

Sometimes your usual shortness of breath will suddenly get worse. You may start coughing more and have more mucus. This is called a COPD flare-up or exacerbation.

Air pollution or a lung infection can cause a flare-up. Sometimes a flare-up may happen after a quick change in temperature or being around chemicals.

A COPD flare-up can be life-threatening. If you have one:

◆ Use your inhaler medicine first.

◆ If your symptoms do not get better after you use your medicine, have someone take you to the emergency room. Call 911 if you have to.

You may need to be treated in a hospital until you can breathe better on your own. With the right treatment, most people recover from a flare-up, and their breathing is no worse than it was before.

Do everything you can do to avoid flare-ups and stay out of the hospital:

◆ Take your medicines.

◆ Avoid "triggers" like smoke, poor air quality, and chemicals.

◆ Stay as healthy as you can.

◆ Use air-conditioning so you don't have to open the windows. Fresh air may seem like a good idea, but pollen, mold, air pollution, and other outdoor irritants can make your COPD worse.

◆ Use an air conditioner or air purifier with a HEPA filter.

◆ Make sure gas appliances are vented well and have tight-fitting doors. Check flues and chimneys for cracks that could let in fumes. Don't use an open fireplace or wood-burning stove; wood smoke is bad for your breathing.

◆ Do not use strong chemicals or aerosol sprays in your home, and do not mix cleaning products. Try natural cleaners like vinegar, lemon juice, boric acid, or baking soda.

◆ Do not keep items for recycling indoors. Newspapers, rags, cans, or bottles can give off fumes.

◆ Reduce the dust in your house as much as you can. See page 77 for tips.

◆ Make sure outdoor fresh-air intake vents for heating and air-conditioning systems are above ground. Keep cars, trucks, and other sources of pollution away from the vents.

**More**

# Breathing Lessons

People with COPD tend to take quick, short breaths. Breathing this way makes it harder to get air into your lungs. But you can learn some other ways to breathe that make it easier.

Use these methods when you are more short of breath than normal. Practice them every day so you can do them well.

### Pursed-lip breathing

Breathe in through your nose and out through your mouth while almost closing your lips. Breathe in for about 4 seconds, and breathe out for 6 to 8 seconds.

Pursed-lip breathing helps you breathe more air out so that your next breath can be deeper. It makes you less short of breath and lets you exercise more.

### Breathing while bending

Bending forward at the waist may make it easier for you to breathe. It can reduce shortness of breath while you are exercising or resting.

### Breathing with your diaphragm

◆ Breathing with your diaphragm helps your lungs expand so that they take in more air.

◆ Lie on your back or prop yourself up on several pillows.

◆ With one hand on your belly and the other on your chest, breathe in. Push your belly out as far as you can. You should feel the hand on your belly move out, while the hand on your chest should not move. When you breathe out, the hand on your belly should move in.

◆ Once you can do this while you are lying down, you can learn to do it while sitting or standing.

## Stay Healthy, Feel Better

There are things you can do that will help you be able to do more and give you more energy.

- Stop smoking. This is the most important step you can take to feel better and live longer. See page 316 to get started.

- Avoid colds and the flu.

    ❖ Get a flu shot each fall. Ask those you live or work with to do the same, so they don't get the flu and infect you.

    ❖ Wash your hands often, especially during cold and flu season.

    ❖ Get a pneumococcal vaccine shot every 5 to 10 years or as advised by your doctor.

- Avoid smoke; cold, dry air; hot, humid air; and high altitudes. Stay inside with the windows closed when air pollution is bad.

- Exercise most days of the week. Walking is a great way to be more active. To learn what other kinds of exercise are great for  people with COPD, go to the Web site on the back cover and enter **L228** in the search box.

- Ask your doctor whether a pulmonary rehab program would be good for you. Rehab includes exercise programs, education about your disease and how to manage it, help with diet and other changes, and emotional support. Many people with COPD find these programs  helpful. To learn more, go to the Web site on the back cover and enter **m096** in the search box.

- Take short rest breaks when you are doing chores and other activities. This will help your breathing and help you avoid getting too tired.

- Eat regular, healthy meals. People with COPD often find it hard to eat because of their breathing problems, but there are some simple ways to make  it easier. Go to the Web site on the back cover and enter **k820** in the search box.

### What About Oxygen Therapy?

At some point you may need oxygen therapy. By boosting the oxygen in your blood, this treatment helps you breathe easier and gives you more energy. It may also help you live longer and stay out of the hospital.

You can use oxygen therapy while you move around and do daily tasks. You may breathe the oxygen through a flexible plastic tube in your nostrils (nasal cannula), a face mask, or a tube put into your windpipe.

The oxygen can be supplied in several ways. For example, you can get an oxygen gas tank, or you can get liquid oxygen that comes in a small container. Each has its pros and cons in terms of weight, cost, how much oxygen it holds, and how dangerous it is. (There is a risk of fire if you use oxygen around a lit cigarette or an open flame.)

You may need oxygen only when you exercise or when you are asleep. Or you may need it all the time. If you and your doctor decide that you need oxygen to prolong your life, work together to decide what is best for you.

## Planning for the Future

Over time, your breathing and your over-all health are probably going to get worse no matter what you do. It's normal to feel frightened, angry, hopeless, or even guilty. Talk to your family, friends, or a therapist about how you feel, or join a support group. Talking about your feelings can help you cope.

You may also feel a little more at peace with the future if you plan for it. Talk to your doctor and your family about what you want to happen when your health gets worse. Write out advance directives and a living will so that you get to decide what kind of treatment you have at the end of your life.

For help with end-of-life planning, see page 295.

### When to Call a Doctor

**Call 911** if you have severe trouble breathing.

**Call your doctor if:**

◆ You have shortness of breath or wheezing that is quickly getting worse.

◆ You are coughing more deeply or more often than usual.

◆ You cough up blood.

◆ Swelling in your legs or belly gets worse.

◆ You have a fever.

◆ Your medicine does not seem to be working as well as it had been.

# Living Better With Coronary Artery Disease

Coronary artery disease (CAD) means that the blood vessels that bring blood to the heart have become narrow or blocked. They usually get blocked by **plaque**, which is a buildup of fat and other substances.

When you have CAD, your blood vessels cannot bring as much blood and oxygen to your heart. Poor blood flow can cause **angina** (chest pain) when you force your heart to work harder. If the blood flow gets completely blocked, you may have a heart attack.

With poor blood flow over time, your heart may get weaker and not pump as well as it should. This can lead to dangerous heartbeat problems and heart failure.

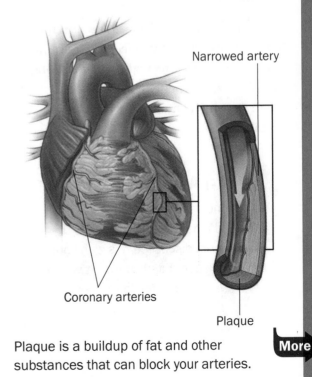

Narrowed artery

Coronary arteries

Plaque

Plaque is a buildup of fat and other substances that can block your arteries.

**More**

# How to Avoid a Heart Attack

For many people with CAD, their biggest fear is a heart attack. To avoid a heart attack and live longer and better, you will need to take steps to improve your health. The good news is that you are in control.

Here are things you can do now to get healthy and stay that way:

◆ If you smoke, quit. See page 278.

◆ Eat healthy food. Eat more fiber, and cut down on cholesterol, saturated fat, and salt. See page 277.

◆ Get some exercise most days of the week. Start with short walks or any other activity you enjoy. See page 278.

◆ Take any medicines your doctor prescribes.

You may not feel sick at all until your heart disease gets a lot worse. Some people have CAD for years without having chest pain or any other symptoms. This may make it hard to feel like you need to pay attention to the problem.

But try not to ignore the fact that you have heart disease, even if you feel fine right now. The goal is to keep feeling good for a long time. You have a better chance of doing that if you start living healthier today. What you do can make a big difference.

## An Aspirin a Day?

Taking one aspirin a day may help you avoid a heart attack or stroke. If you have not discussed this with your doctor, ask about it at your next visit to make sure it's safe for you.

# Dealing With Angina

Many people with CAD have no symptoms. But others may feel chest pain or pressure when they do things that make their heart work harder. This type of chest pain is called angina.

Angina is a signal that your heart is not getting enough oxygen. The pain usually is mild at first and gets worse over several minutes. It may spread to your belly, upper back, shoulders, neck, jaws, or arms.

If you have had angina for a while, you may be able to predict almost exactly how much activity will cause pain. You know what things cause your angina, and you know what to expect and what to do when it happens. This is called stable angina.

Watch for changes in your angina. If your angina is worse or lasts longer than usual, or you starting getting it more often, it could mean that your heart disease is getting worse. Call your doctor right away. You may need a checkup or tests, or your doctor may need to change your treatment.

### What to do when you have chest pain

◆ Stop what you are doing. Sit down and rest.

◆ If your doctor has prescribed a medicine like nitroglycerin, take one dose.

◆ If you are not feeling better within 5 minutes, **call 911**. Take a second dose of nitroglycerin while you wait for help to arrive. If you are not better 3 to 5 minutes after that dose, take a third dose. Do not take more than 3 doses in 15 minutes.

### If you take nitroglycerin

Nitroglycerin is a medicine that opens blood vessels to improve blood flow. This relieves chest pain and reduces how hard the heart has to work.

Your doctor will tell you when to use your nitroglycerin. You may need to take it:

◆ To relieve sudden angina.

◆ Before stressful activities that can cause angina, such as exercise or sex.

Do not take erection-producing medicines such as Viagra, Levitra, or Cialis if you are taking nitroglycerin. Taking any of them with nitroglycerin can be very dangerous. If you get chest pain and have taken one of these erection-producing medicines, tell your doctor so that you are not given nitroglycerin or a similar medicine.

## Eat a Heart-Healthy Diet

Most experts agree that the best diet for your heart is high in fiber, low in cholesterol and saturated fat, and low in salt.

The tips in the chart below can help you get started. (See page 305 for more about healthy eating.) Your doctor may suggest that you follow the DASH (Dietary Approaches to Stop Hypertension) diet or something similar. To learn what this diet  is and how it can help you, go to the Web site on the back cover and enter **s309** in the search box.

| Eating a Heart-Healthy Diet | |
|---|---|
| **Instead of:** | **Try this:** |
| Frying your food | Bake, broil, steam, poach, or grill your food. |
| Eating convenience foods (canned soups, TV dinners, frozen pizza) | Eat fresh fish, skinless chicken, fruits, and vegetables. |
| Using butter or oil high in saturated fat | Use products low in saturated fat, such as olive oil, vegetable oil, canola oil, or chicken broth. |
| Using salt, soy sauce, or barbecue sauce | Use salt-free spices. |
| Eating all of the meat product | Trim fat from meat and skin from chicken. |
| Eating egg yolks | Eat egg whites or egg substitutes. |

**More** ➤

## What Is Angioplasty?

Angioplasty is a way to widen a narrow or blocked coronary artery and improve blood flow to your heart without surgery. It is often used during or soon after a heart attack. It can also help prevent a heart attack for some people with coronary artery disease.

During angioplasty, your doctor threads a tiny tube called a catheter into the blocked or narrow artery. At the end of the catheter is a tiny balloon. The doctor inflates the balloon inside the artery to open the blocked area.

The doctor may also put a stent in the artery. A stent is a small, wire-mesh tube that expands and pushes out against the walls of the artery to keep it open. Some stents also release a drug that helps keep the artery open.

Whether you need angioplasty depends on how many blocked arteries you have, how badly they are blocked, other problems you may have, and other issues.

## Stop Smoking

Quitting smoking is one of the best things you can do if you do not want to die of heart disease. Your risk of dying from heart attack or stroke will start to go down very soon after you quit. Within several years, your risk will be no higher than someone who has never smoked.

If you have had angioplasty or bypass surgery to fix blocked arteries, those arteries will be less likely to get blocked again if you quit smoking.

You will also feel better once you quit smoking. Your angina may get better. You will have more energy and breathe easier. And you may feel more hopeful about your future and have less fear of getting sick or dying suddenly from heart disease.

Smoking is bad for everyone, but it is even worse for people with coronary artery disease.

◆ It makes your blood cells more likely to form clots. This can cause a heart attack or stroke.

◆ It can cause spasms in your coronary arteries, which can reduce the blood flow to your heart.

◆ It can make your heart beat in an odd rhythm.

◆ It lowers "good" cholesterol and lets "bad" cholesterol build up in your arteries more easily.

◆ It reduces how much oxygen your blood can carry. This means your heart (and the rest of your body) may not get enough oxygen.

Quitting smoking is not easy. Many people have to try several times before they quit for good. But the point is that they do finally succeed. And with the right help, so can you.

See Quitting Smoking on page 316 to learn how to get started.

## Exercise Your Heart

If you are not active right now, starting to exercise may seem hard. But it is worth it. You do not have to do a lot to make a difference.

Being more active can:

◆ Help you control your weight, blood pressure, and cholesterol.

◆ Make your heart stronger and reduce symptoms like chest pain.

◆ Help you avoid heart attack and stroke and live longer.

◆ Reduce stress and give you more energy.

Walking is a great, easy way to get exercise. If your doctor says it's safe, start out with some short walks. Make the walks a little bit longer until you are walking 20 to 30 minutes at a time.

If you don't enjoy walking, you might try swimming, biking, or water aerobics. Your doctor can help you make a plan.

The important thing is to try to get some exercise several days a week. Even a little bit of exercise can help if you have not been

 active at all. For some ideas that might work for you, go to the Web site on the back cover and enter **x762** in the search box.

You might also ask your doctor about joining a cardiac rehab program. Many people with heart disease find this type of program  helpful. To learn more about whether cardiac rehab might be right for you, go to the Web site on the back cover and enter **x867** in the search box.

### Be safe when you exercise

See your doctor before you start exercising. He or she may want to do a test to see how much activity your heart can handle.

If your doctor has prescribed nitroglycerin for you, be sure to have it with you whenever you exercise. Stop what you are doing right away if you have any chest pain or start to feel bad.

## When to Call a Doctor

**Call 911 if:**

◆ You have chest pain or pressure with other signs of a heart attack. These may include:

❖ Sweating.

❖ Shortness of breath.

❖ Nausea or vomiting.

❖ Pain in your upper back, belly, neck, jaw, or arms.

❖ Feeling dizzy or lightheaded.

❖ A fast or uneven heartbeat.

After calling 911, chew and swallow an adult aspirin unless you are allergic to aspirin. Do not try to drive yourself to the hospital.

◆ You have been diagnosed with angina, and you have chest pain or pressure that does not go away with rest or within 5 minutes of taking nitroglycerin.

◆ You faint.

**Call your doctor if:**

◆ You have chest pain (angina) more often than usual, or the pain is worse or different than usual.

◆ You have had any chest pain, even if it has gone away.

◆ You have any problems with your medicines.

# Living Better With Depression

Depression is a medical problem, not a character flaw or weakness. Many people do not get help because they're embarrassed or think they'll get over depression on their own.

If you are depressed, there is no reason for you to suffer. Treatment works very well for most people. With counseling, medicines, good self-care, and a little time, you can feel a lot better. Treatment can also help you avoid future problems with depression.

## Counseling Can Help

The words "counseling" or "therapy" may make you think of lying on a leather couch and talking about your childhood. But the most common kind of counseling does not look for hidden feelings or memories. It deals with how you think about things and how you act each day. It helps you replace thoughts or behaviors that make you feel bad with ones that make you feel better. Over time, these changes turn into habits.

To treat depression, you may need to see a counselor regularly for several months or longer. Keep going to the appointments even if it seems like they aren't helping. Sometimes it takes many meetings before you start to feel better.

### Choosing a counselor

Your counselor may be a psychiatrist (a medical doctor), a psychologist, or a licensed counselor. When you choose a counselor:

◆ Be sure the person has experience and training in treating depression. Also make sure that he or she has a license in your state. Some states have strict rules about who can work as a counselor.

◆ Choose someone you like and trust. For counseling to work, you have to talk honestly about your feelings. Having a counselor you feel comfortable with makes this easier. If you meet with someone and don't feel good about it, try someone else.

## What About St. John's Wort?

St. John's wort is an herbal supplement sold in health food stores and pharmacies. Europeans have used it for centuries to treat depression. But in the United States, it is still being tested.

High-quality St. John's wort may help with mild or moderate depression. After talking to your doctor about it, you may want to see if it works for you. Go to  the Web site on the back cover and enter **d183** in the search box to learn more.

Do not take St. John's wort with antidepressants or any other medicines unless your doctor has told you it's safe. It can cause dangerous reactions when you use it with other medicines.

Keep in mind that herbal supplements are not regulated the way medicines are. Always tell your doctor if you're using an herbal product. You could have serious side effects.

## Antidepressant Medicines

Antidepressant medicines help many people with depression get better. They can help keep the chemicals in your brain in balance. They do not change your personality.

There are many medicines that can help, and there is no evidence that one works better than another. But they have different side effects.

Your doctor will consider many things when deciding which drug to give you:

◆ How did you respond to medicines used in the past?

◆ Are you taking medicine for other health problems? Your doctor will not give you a drug that will react badly with any other drugs you're taking.

◆ Will the drug make any other illness you have worse or harder to treat?

◆ How old are you? How is your overall health? Older adults may need lower doses.

◆ How much are the side effects likely to bother you?

You may need to take antidepressants for as long as 2 months before you feel completely well. But you may start to feel better in 2 or 3 weeks. Here are things to keep in mind:

◆ Most antidepressants take 4 to 8 weeks to start working.

◆ Often the first drug the doctor prescribes will work well. If not, there are other choices. You may need to try several before you find the one that works best for you.

◆ The medicine may have side effects. Many of these are temporary and will go away as you get used to the medicine. If they continue, or if they bother you too much, talk to your doctor. You may need a different drug.

◆ Make sure to tell your doctor if you take any other medicines or herbal products. Tell your doctor about any other health problems you have.

◆ Once you start to feel better, you will need to keep taking your medicine for 6 months or longer to help prevent a relapse. Keep taking your medicine as prescribed, even after symptoms go away.

Do not stop taking the medicine on your own unless you have chest pain, hives, trouble breathing, trouble swallowing, or swelling of your lips. Call your doctor immediately if you have any of these serious side effects.

**More**

### Seasonal Affective Disorder

Some people feel more depressed during the winter months when there is less sunlight. This is sometimes called seasonal affective disorder (SAD).

It may help to:

◆ Go out in the sun as often as you can. (Remember to protect your skin.)

◆ Get regular exercise, either outdoors or indoors near a sunny window.

◆ Ask your doctor about light therapy. This involves sitting or working in front of special lights for up to several hours a day.

As with other forms of depression, medicine and counseling can also help.

## Depressed and Pregnant?

Some women get depressed during pregnancy. You are more likely to be depressed if you have had depression before. Your pregnancy can cause your symptoms to come back (relapse).

Managing your depression is important for your own health. It will also help you have a healthy baby. Work with your doctor to find a treatment you are comfortable with.

◆ If your depression is mild, your doctor may suggest that you try counseling first before you take medicine.

◆ If your depression is severe or counseling does not help enough, you may need medicine. You may also need medicine if you were depressed before and had a relapse when you stopped your medicine.

You may be worried about taking medicine while you're pregnant. But not treating your depression is also a risk to your baby. You may not take care of yourself as well if you're depressed. You may not bond well with your baby after birth. You may not eat or sleep well.

If you need an antidepressant, your doctor can prescribe one that's safe for you and your baby.

## While You Recover

Your mood will improve, but it takes time. In the meantime:

◆ Take your medicines as prescribed, and go to your counseling sessions. It may take several weeks before you notice a change.

◆ Take good care of yourself. Eat healthy meals. Get enough sleep. If you have problems sleeping, see the tips starting on page 237. Do not take sleeping pills.

◆ Stay active. Get outside and take walks. Go to a movie, concert, or ball game.

◆ Spend time with friends and family. Take part in social events or church.

◆ Do not drink alcohol or use illegal drugs. And don't take medicines that have not been prescribed for you.

◆ Break large tasks into smaller pieces that you can handle. Do what you can.

◆ If possible, put off major decisions like marriage, divorce, or a job change until you feel better. Talk over big changes with friends and loved ones who can offer other points of view.

◆ If you have another illness, like diabetes or heart disease, keep treating it.

Ask for help if you need it. And if you ever have thoughts of hurting yourself, call for help right away. You can call 911 or the national suicide hotline at 1-800-784-2433.

## Feeling Better?

If you are feeling better, you may think it's okay to stop going to counseling or to quit taking your medicine.

Wait! Talk to your doctor before you do this. To keep depression from coming back, you may need treatment for 6 months or longer after you feel better. Some people need to take medicines for years.

 For help deciding whether medicines are still right for you, go to the Web site on the back cover and enter **k616** in the search box.

### How to Prevent a Relapse

◆ Do not stop taking your medicine too early. It may help to keep taking it for another 6 to 12 months after you feel better (or longer in some cases). Some people need to take medicine for the rest of their lives to stay healthy.

◆ Do not stop taking your medicine suddenly. If you want to stop taking it, ask your doctor whether this is safe for you and how best to do it.

## When to Call a Doctor

◆ You feel hopeless and cannot stop yourself from thinking about hurting yourself or someone else. **Call 911 or the national suicide hotline at 1-800-784-2433.**

◆ You hear voices.

◆ You think you are depressed and have not talked to your doctor about it.

◆ Your depression gets worse even with treatment.

◆ You have any problems with your medicine.

◆ You are taking antidepressants and think that you're pregnant.

◆ Keep seeing your counselor after you stop the medicine. This helps some people avoid a relapse without medicine.

◆ Eat a healthy diet and get regular exercise. Stick to a regular sleep schedule.

◆ Avoid alcohol and illegal drugs.

◆ See your doctor right away if you have new symptoms or feel worse.

# Living Better With Diabetes

If you have diabetes, your body may not make enough of a hormone called **insulin** or may not use insulin properly. Insulin helps your body use sugar from your food as energy or store it for later use. When this doesn't happen, too much sugar stays in your blood.

Over time, high blood sugar can lead to serious problems.

◆ It can harm your eyes, nerves, and kidneys.

◆ It can damage your blood vessels, leading to heart disease and stroke.

◆ It can reduce blood flow to parts of your body, especially your feet. This can cause pain and slow healing.

How can you prevent these problems? The most important thing is to keep your blood sugar under control with these steps:

◆ Take your insulin or other medicine.

◆ Check your blood sugar often.

◆ Eat healthy, balanced meals and snacks.

◆ Exercise on most days of the week.

◆ See your doctor for checkups and tests on a regular schedule.

◆ If you have high blood pressure or high cholesterol, take medicines to control the problem.

Living with diabetes day after day can be a struggle. Watching what you eat, checking your blood sugar, taking your medicine on time—there will be times when you just can't do it all. Don't be too hard on yourself. Just try to get back on track.

And if you're already doing what you need to, keep it up!

## Medicines for Diabetes

Some people with type 2 diabetes need medicine to help their bodies make more insulin or use insulin properly. Pills for type 2 diabetes can also slow down how the body absorbs sugar. This can help keep your blood sugar at a safe level.

You may need to take one or more pills more than once a day. Some people need medicine for only a short time. Some have to take it for the rest of their lives. What you need will depend on how well your blood sugar stays in a safe range.

People with type 1 diabetes have to take insulin to control their blood sugar. If you have type 2 diabetes, you may be able to avoid or delay the need for insulin with careful eating, regular exercise, and proper use of other diabetes medicines. Many people with type 2 diabetes do wind up needing to take insulin at some point.

### Cost tips for medicines

Your diabetes medicine helps keep you healthy and avoid more serious, costly problems. While the costs of the medicine can add up, there may be ways to get your diabetes medicine for less.

You can buy most diabetes medicines either by their brand names or as generic drugs. (For example, many people with diabetes take the drug metformin. You may know it by its brand name, Glucophage.) There can be a big cost difference between these. If you are taking a brand-name drug, you might ask your doctor whether the generic one would work just as well for you.

See page 3 for other suggestions on how to save money on your medicines—like buying in bulk and using online drugstores.

## What About Carbohydrate and Sugar?

When you have diabetes, you have to be careful about how much carbohydrate you eat at one time. If you eat too much at once, your blood sugar will quickly rise (and then later may drop sharply).

Carbohydrate is an important nutrient you get from food. It is a great source of energy for your body and helps your brain and nervous system work at their best.

It comes in two forms:

◆ Starch (complex carbohydrate). Starch is in foods such as breads, cereals, grains, pasta, rice, flour, beans, and vegetables.

◆ Sugar (simple carbohydrate). Sugar is in foods such as fruits, juices, milk, honey, desserts, and candy.

All forms of carbohydrate raise your blood sugar, depending on how much carbohydrate is in the food.

The goal is to keep your blood sugar steady and avoid high blood sugar after meals. You can help by spreading your carbohydrate through the day, rather than eating a lot at once. This will also keep you from getting too hungry. See Meal Planning: What Does Your Plate Look Like? on page 286 to learn more about this.

Unlike what you may have heard, you can eat foods that have sugar when you have diabetes. But if foods that are high in sugar make up a large part of your diet, you are probably not eating enough of other, healthier foods. And your blood sugar levels may be too unsteady.

## Five Things to Do Today

1. Take an aspirin (if you have talked to your doctor about it). An aspirin a day may help you avoid a heart attack or stroke. If you have not discussed this with your doctor, ask about it at your next visit to make sure it's safe for you.

2. Order a medical alert bracelet or necklace online or at your local drugstore. If you have a health emergency and cannot speak, this ID will let medical staff know you have diabetes. This is even more important if you take insulin or often have problems with low blood sugar.

3. Check your feet for small cuts, sores, or toenail problems. Small problems can become big ones if you do not notice and take care of them. To learn how to take great care of your  feet, go to the Web site on the back cover and enter **y813** in the search box.

4. Take a walk. Regular exercise can help you control your blood sugar and reduce your need for medicine. Make sure you wear sturdy shoes.

5. Call your local hospital and ask if it has a support group or education program for people with diabetes. Or visit the Web site of the American Diabetes Association, www.diabetes.org. It has recipes, exercise tips, and all kinds of information that can help you.

**More**

# Meal Planning: What Does Your Plate Look Like?

Eating right helps keep your blood sugar in a safe range. For some people, healthy eating and regular exercise are enough to keep their diabetes under control without medicines. If you take medicine, eating right can help the medicine work better.

Meal planning for diabetes includes eating certain amounts and kinds of foods at regular meals and snacks. You may have heard about the need to count your carbohydrate grams and use diabetic exchange lists and food guides. It may seem overwhelming.

But there's an easy way to get started: the **plate format**. The plate format is a great way to learn about meal planning and get used to measuring how much you eat.

Using a plate format lets you picture what a meal should look like and how much space each food should take up on your plate. This can help you eat balanced meals. It also can stop you from eating too much carbohydrate at once.

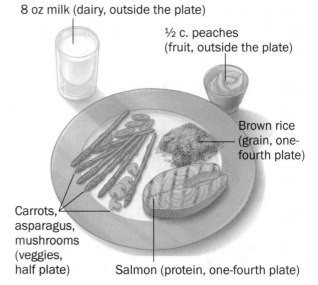

8 oz milk (dairy, outside the plate)

½ c. peaches (fruit, outside the plate)

Brown rice (grain, one-fourth plate)

Carrots, asparagus, mushrooms (veggies, half plate)

Salmon (protein, one-fourth plate)

Sample plate for dinner

A typical healthy plate for lunch or dinner will have:

◆ Bread, starchy foods, or grain on one-fourth of the plate.

◆ Meat or another form of protein (like beans or an egg) on one-fourth of the plate.

◆ Vegetables on half the plate.

◆ 1 small piece of fruit outside the plate.

◆ 1 cup of milk or yogurt or ½ cup of pudding or ice cream outside the plate.

Post a sample plate format on your refrigerator until you get used to what a healthy plate looks like. Once you can picture your plate, you can use the method anywhere, even when you eat out.

To learn how to use the plate format for all your meals and snacks, go to the Web site on the back cover and enter **f643** in the search box. And when you are ready to learn more about meal planning, talk with a registered dietitian or diabetes educator about other methods.

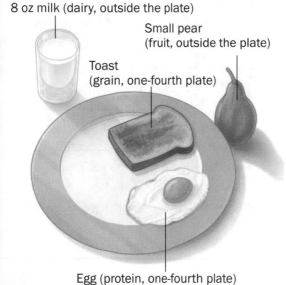

8 oz milk (dairy, outside the plate)

Small pear (fruit, outside the plate)

Toast (grain, one-fourth plate)

Egg (protein, one-fourth plate)

Sample plate for breakfast

## If You Have Prediabetes

Prediabetes (impaired glucose tolerance) is a warning sign for type 2 diabetes. Think of it as a wake-up call. Most people who get type 2 diabetes have prediabetes first.

If you have prediabetes, you may be able to avoid or delay type 2 diabetes (and the problems it can cause) by making some changes in your lifestyle.

◆ Eat a balanced, healthy diet. Try to eat an even amount of carbohydrate all through the day. This can help you avoid sudden peaks in blood sugar.

◆ Get at least 30 minutes of exercise on most days of the week. Exercise helps control your blood sugar. It also helps you control your weight. Walking is a good choice for many people. You also may want to try swimming, cycling, or other activities. See page 311.

◆ Try to stay at a healthy weight. If you need to lose weight, keep in mind that even a small loss of 5 to 10 pounds can help. See page 300.

◆ If you smoke, quit. Smoking can make prediabetes worse. If you need help quitting, see page 316.

## Check Your Blood Sugar

You may not like having to check your blood sugar every day and keep track of the results over time. But it can really help you keep your diabetes under control.

◆ Knowing how your blood sugar rises or falls in response to certain foods, exercise, and other things can help you reduce symptoms and prevent blood sugar emergencies.

◆ Having a record of your blood sugar over time can help you and your doctor know how well your treatment is working and whether you need to make any changes.

Simply put, you have a better chance of keeping your blood sugar in a safe range if you know what it is from day to day. Controlling your blood sugar will help you feel better and will slow down the long-term damage to your eyes, kidneys, and heart that can result when your blood sugar is not controlled.

 Many people are able to do a good job of tracking their blood sugar once they get in the habit. It helps to:

◆ Know how and when to check your blood sugar.

◆ Have the right supplies and know how to use them.

◆ Have an easy way to keep track of your results.

For help setting up a routine that works for you, go to the Web site on the back cover and enter **p039** in the search box.

## Safe Exercise

Exercise helps control your blood sugar. It also helps you stay at a healthy weight, reduce "bad" cholesterol, raise "good" cholesterol, and lower high blood pressure. These benefits help prevent heart disease, the main cause of death in people who have diabetes.

Aim for at least 30 minutes of exercise on most days. You may need to slowly work up to this if you are not used to being active. Even small amounts of exercise can help.

**More**

# If Your Child Has Diabetes

If your child has diabetes, he or she needs your help to feel better and to avoid emergencies and long-term problems.

Healthy eating and safe exercise are vital to controlling your child's blood sugar. Some kids also need insulin or other diabetes medicines. There are lots of ways you can help:

◆ Work out a plan for giving medicines on time and in the right amounts every day. Your doctor can help with this.

◆ Offer healthy choices for meals and snacks. A dietitian can help you design a meal plan that fits your child's needs. If your child eats the school lunch, find out what kinds of foods are offered.

◆ Cut down on junk food, especially soda. Soda has lots of sugar and calories and no health benefits.

◆ Take walks or bike rides with your child. Help your child find ways to be more active. (Check with your doctor if you're not sure whether an activity is safe for your child.)

◆ Set and enforce time limits on TV and video and computer games.

◆ Make sure your child's school knows he or she has diabetes. Meet with your child's teachers (including the gym teacher) to talk about what happens when your child's blood sugar drops. You may even want to give the school nurse special instructions for treating high or low blood sugar.

◆ Be a good role model. Your child will have the most success if the whole family chooses the same healthy foods and exercise habits.

◆ Make sure that your child always wears or carries ID showing that he or she has diabetes.

You will also need to help check and keep track of your child's blood sugar. Many older children and teens can do this on their own, but they still need support.

Talk to your doctor about what your child's blood sugar should be. And ask how to spot signs that your child's blood sugar is too low or too high before it becomes an emergency.

Walking, running, bike riding, and swimming are great for most people with diabetes. But some activities may not be safe. For instance, if you have diabetic eye disease (retinopathy), it may not be safe to lift weights. If you have nerve disease (neuropathy), running may cause foot problems.

Before you start a new exercise program, check with your doctor to find out what activities are best for you.

Here are some other safety tips:

◆ Check your blood sugar before you exercise, and be careful about what you eat. This is especially true if you take insulin or other medicines for diabetes. Do not exercise when your blood sugar is too low (less than 60 mg/dL).

◆ Try to exercise at about the same time each day to keep your blood sugar steady. If you want to exercise more, slowly increase how hard or long you exercise.

- Have someone with you when you exercise, or exercise at a gym. You may need help if your blood sugar drops too low.

- Keep some type of quick-sugar food with you. You may get symptoms of low blood sugar during exercise or up to 24 hours later.

- Pay attention to your body. If you are used to exercise and notice that you cannot do as much as usual, talk to your doctor.

## Tests That Can Help You

Seeing your doctor and having certain tests on a regular schedule can help you watch for and avoid many of the problems caused by diabetes. Diabetes can damage many different parts of your body, but you may not have symptoms of the damage until it's too late to do much about it. Tests give you and your doctor a chance to find problems early, when they are easier to treat.

The table below lists some of the tests a typical person with diabetes may need. Talk with your doctor about what test schedule is right for you.

## Schedule for Tests and Exams

| Test | Why you need it | How often to get it |
|------|-----------------|---------------------|
| Hemoglobin A1c blood test | Checks average blood sugar over past 3 months; best way to see how well treatment and self-care are working | Every 3 to 6 months |
| Blood pressure test | Need to monitor blood pressure; high blood pressure increases risk of blood vessel and nerve damage | Every 3 to 6 months |
| Sensory foot exam | Reduced feeling in feet can be sign of nerve damage (neuropathy) | At least every year |
| Eye exam by an ophthalmologist | Diabetes can damage vision (retinopathy); does not cause symptoms until severe | Every year. (Your main doctor may also check your eyes at each visit.) |
| Fasting cholesterol test | Diabetes puts you at risk for high cholesterol and heart disease | Every year (more often if you take medicine for high cholesterol) |
| Urine test for protein | Protein in urine may be the only sign of early kidney damage (nephropathy) | Every year |
| Dental exam and cleaning | Diabetes increases risk of gum problems and infection | Every 6 months |

**More**

# When to Call a Doctor

**Call 911 if:**

◆ Your blood sugar stays below 60 mg/dL after you treat low blood sugar, or you are getting more sleepy or confused.

◆ Your blood sugar is very high, you are becoming less alert, and your breathing is fast and deep.

◆ You have chest pain or pressure, especially if it occurs with other signs of a heart attack. See page 38.

**Call your doctor if:**

◆ You often have problems with your blood sugar being too high or too low. Your doctor may need to change your medicine.

◆ You have burning pain, tingling, numbness, or swelling in your feet or hands.

◆ You have vision changes or pain in your eyes.

◆ A wound looks infected or will not heal.

◆ You often have a lot of bloating, belching, constipation, nausea and vomiting, or belly pain after you eat.

◆ You have a hard time knowing when your blood sugar is low.

# Living Better With Heart Failure

When you have heart failure, your heart does not pump as much blood as your body needs. Failure does not mean your heart has stopped pumping. It means your heart is not pumping as well as it should.

Your body has an amazing ability to make up for heart failure. It may do such a good job at first that you may not feel like you have a disease.

But at some point, your body will not be able to keep up. Then fluid will slowly build up in your body and cause symptoms like weakness and shortness of breath. This fluid buildup is called congestion.

### What You Can Do

Heart failure usually gets worse over time. But there are many steps you can take to feel better and stay healthy longer. These are the most important:

- Take your medicines as prescribed. This gives them the best chance of helping you. See Take Your Medicines on this page.

- Limit salt (sodium). This helps keep fluid from building up and makes it easier for your heart to pump. See page 292.

- Watch for signs that you're getting worse so that your doctor can help you. Weighing yourself every day is one of the best ways to do this. Weight gain may be a sign that your body is holding on to too much fluid. See page 292.

- Try to exercise most days of the week. Exercise makes your heart stronger and can help you avoid symptoms. See page 293.

- Find out what your triggers are, and learn to avoid them. Triggers are things that make your heart failure worse, often suddenly. A trigger may be eating too much salt, missing a dose of your medicine, or exercising too hard.

There are other things you can do to help too, like eating right, not smoking, not drinking much alcohol, controlling your blood pressure, and staying at a healthy weight. These things make it easier for your heart to keep pumping. They will also reduce your risk of heart attack and stroke.

## Take Your Medicines

You will probably take several medicines for heart failure. You may also need medicine to treat the problem that caused your heart failure, such as high blood pressure, heart disease, or a heart attack.

- Take your medicines exactly as your doctor tells you to. If you can't do this, or if you think you need to stop or change your medicine, talk to your doctor about it.

- If you have any problems with the medicines, tell your doctor. Ask your doctor what side effects you may have and what problems to watch for.

- See your doctor regularly so that he or she can check whether your medicine is working or needs to be changed.

- Always ask your doctor before you take any new medicines, including those you can buy without a prescription. Some medicines can make heart failure worse.

**More**

To get the best results from your medicines, be sure to take them properly. This can be tricky when you have to take more than one. For tips that can help, go to the Web site on the back cover and enter **m817** in the search box.

### Cost tips for medicines

You will need medicine for the rest of your life to control your heart failure. This can get very expensive. But there may be ways you can reduce the cost—using generic instead of brand-name drugs and shopping for the best prices, for example. For help controlling costs, see page 3.

## Cut the Salt

Eating less salt (sodium) can help you feel better and stay out of the hospital. Salt makes your body retain water, makes your legs swell, and makes it harder for your heart to pump.

Your doctor may want you to eat less than 2,000 mg (2 g) of salt each day. That's less than 1 teaspoon. You can stay under this number by limiting the salt you eat at home and by watching for "hidden" sodium when you eat out or shop for food.

Write down what you eat and how much salt it has. That way you will know when you are close to (or over) your limit.

### Five ways to reduce salt

◆ Read labels on food before you buy it. Buy foods labeled "unsalted" (no salt used to process), "sodium-free" (less than 5 mg per serving), or "low-sodium" (less than 140 mg per serving).

◆ Eat lots of fresh or frozen fruits and vegetables. They have very little salt, and they're good for you.

◆ If you use canned vegetables or beans, rinse them before you cook with them. They are very high in salt unless you buy low-sodium or sodium-free kinds.

◆ Flavor your food with garlic, lemon juice, onion, vinegar, healthy oils (olive, walnut), herbs, and spices instead of salt. Do not use soy sauce, steak sauce, onion salt, garlic salt, mustard, or ketchup on your food. They all have a lot of salt.

◆ Eat fewer processed foods. These include anything that's not fresh, such as canned foods, packaged lunch meats and hot dogs, bottled sauces, boxed frozen meals, chips and pretzels, and pizza. Eat less often at restaurants, especially fast-food ones.

Eating less salt can be hard, but it has a big reward: feeling better and staying out of the hospital. The tips above can help you get started. If you are ready for even more ideas—or want an easy way to keep track of  what you eat—go to the Web site on the back cover and enter **b532** in the search box.

## Check Your Weight Every Day

Get in the habit of weighing yourself every day and writing down your weight. Sudden weight gain may mean that fluid is building up in your body and your heart failure is getting worse.

◆ Weigh yourself at the same time each day, using the same scale on a hard, flat surface. The best time is in the morning after you go to the bathroom and before you eat or drink anything.

◆ Wear the same thing each time you weigh yourself, or always wear nothing. Do not wear shoes.

◆ Keep a calendar by the scale. Write your weight on it each day, and take it with you when you see your doctor.

◆ Keep notes on how you feel each day. Is your shortness of breath worse? Are your feet and ankles swollen? Do your legs seem puffy?

Call your doctor if you gain more than 2 to 3 pounds over 2 days. Also tell your doctor if you are gaining weight slowly.

## Exercise Your Heart

If you are not active right now, starting to exercise may seem hard. But it's worth it. Regular exercise:

◆ Makes your heart stronger.

◆ Makes it easier to breathe.

◆ Helps you feel better and have more energy.

◆ Helps control your weight, blood pressure, and cholesterol.

See your doctor before you start exercising. He or she may want to do a test to see how much activity your heart can handle so you don't push too hard.

Walking is a great way to get exercise. If your doctor says it's safe, start out by walking a few minutes at a time. Slowly extend your walks until you are walking 20 to 30 minutes at a time. Swimming, cycling, or water aerobics might be other good choices. Your doctor can help you make a plan.

The important thing is to exercise regularly (3 to 5 times a week) and not to overdo it. There are many ways you can exercise safely with heart failure. For some ideas that might  work for you, go to the Web site on the back cover and enter **r291** in the search box.

### What about cardiac rehab?

You might ask your doctor about joining a cardiac rehab program. In this type of program, a team of people, such as a doctor, a nurse specialist, a dietitian, and a physical therapist, works with you to help you learn how to stay healthier and feel better.

 Many people with heart failure find cardiac rehab helpful. For help deciding whether this might be a good idea for you, go to the Web site on the back cover and enter **x867** in the search box.

## If You Have to Limit Fluids

Your doctor may give you pills called diuretics to help get fluid out of your body. For many people, taking this medicine and reducing salt is enough.

If you have advanced heart failure, you may also need to limit how much fluid you drink. This can reduce symptoms and help you stay out of the hospital.

Your doctor will tell you how much fluid you can have each day. Usually, it will range from 4 to 8 cups (32 to 64 fl oz), which is about 1 to 2 liters. You will need to keep track of your fluids so you do not take in more than your body can handle.

◆ Find a method that works for you. You might simply write down how much you drink every time you do. Some people keep a container (like a pitcher or large plastic bottle) filled with the amount of fluid they can have for the day. If they drink from a source other than the container, then they pour out that amount. Once the container is empty, they stop drinking.

**More** ➤

◆ Measure how much fluid your regular drinking glasses hold. Once you know this, you will not have to measure every time.

◆ Count any food that will melt or that has a lot of liquid as part of your fluid for the day. That means you need to measure and count ice cream, gelatin, ice, juicy fruits, and soup.

◆ If you feel thirsty, try chewing gum or sucking on hard candy, breath mints, or frozen grapes or berries. If your lips feel dry, use lip balm.

## When to Call a Doctor

### Call 911 if:

◆ You have chest pain or pressure that has not gone away with rest or within 5 minutes after you have taken one nitroglycerin, especially if the pain occurs with shortness of breath, sweating, and nausea.

◆ You have symptoms of a stroke (see page 53). These may include:

  ❖ Sudden tingling, numbness, or weakness on one side of your body.

  ❖ Sudden, severe headache.

  ❖ Sudden changes in vision or speech.

  ❖ Stumbling or clumsiness.

◆ You have severe trouble breathing.

◆ You cough up foamy, pink mucus.

◆ Your heart suddenly starts to beat very fast or unevenly and you feel dizzy, nauseated, or like you are going to faint.

**Call your doctor if** you have signs that your heart failure is getting worse. For example:

◆ You gain more than 2 to 3 pounds over 2 days.

◆ You have new or worse swelling in your feet, ankles, or legs.

◆ Your breathing gets worse. Activities that did not make you short of breath before are now hard for you.

◆ Your breathing when you lie down is worse than usual, or you wake up at night needing to catch your breath.

# Planning for the Future

Even if you are doing well now, it's a good idea to prepare for a time when your health might get worse. It can be hard to think and talk about these issues. But planning for the future while you are still active and able to communicate can:

◆ Bring you peace of mind.

◆ Help make sure your wishes are followed later.

◆ Save your loved ones the stress of making hard decisions for you.

## Advance Directives

The best way to make sure your wishes are followed is to put them in writing. A written plan for your health care is called an advance care plan or **advance directive**. It is used only if you become so sick that you can't make choices for yourself.

There are two main types of advance directives.

◆ A **living will** tells what treatment you want at the end of your life. For example, it tells when you would or would not want to be on a breathing machine or be fed through a tube.

◆ A **durable power of attorney** lets you choose someone now who can make health care choices for you if a time comes when you can't make them yourself. This person is called your health care agent or health care proxy.

Do not assume that your doctor and family will know what you want if you don't have a written plan. Without one, choices about your care may be made by a doctor who

doesn't know you, or by the courts. In some states, hospital staff must keep you alive as long as possible if they don't know your wishes. This may or may not be what you want.

### How to Write an Advance Directive

1. Get living will and durable power of attorney forms for your state. You can usually get them from a doctor's office, hospital, law office, or senior center. You also can find them online at www.caringinfo.org.

2. Choose someone to be your health care agent, the person you want to speak for you if and when you can't speak for yourself.

3. Fill out the forms. If you don't understand them, ask a doctor, nurse, lawyer, or family member to help. Get them notarized or witnessed if your state requires it (many states don't).

4. Make sure your doctor, your family, and your health care agent have copies.

 For help writing an advance directive, go to the Web site on the back cover and enter **q652** in the search box.

### Deciding About Life Support Treatment

When you create an advance directive, you can answer questions like:

◆ Do you want CPR if your heart stops?

◆ Do you want to be given liquids or food through a vein (IV) or stomach tube if you can no longer eat or drink?

**More**

◆ Do you want to have a tube in your windpipe and use a breathing machine (ventilator) if you cannot breathe on your own?

◆ Do you want kidney dialysis if your kidneys stop working?

Think about what you would want depending on things like how sick or hurt you were, how good your chances for recovery were, and what your life would be like if you chose treatment to keep you alive.

If you have an illness that can't be cured, a time may come when you decide not to have treatment that might keep you alive. This can be a hard decision. But if you are very ill, it may be the right choice for you and your family. Sometimes, using treatment to keep a dying person alive can cause unnecessary suffering.

 For many people, these are hard choices. If you want help thinking through them, go to the Web site on the back cover and enter **y609** in the search box.

Don't wait for your doctor to bring up the subject of an advance directive. Even if you are healthy right now, talk with your doctor about the kinds of treatment you would want or would not want. Try to get a clear idea of your wishes. And involve your family members so they know what you want.

## Estate Planning

Along with planning for future health decisions, it's a good idea to get your business and personal affairs in order.

◆ Write or update your will. If you don't have a will, your state's laws may decide what happens to your money and property (your "estate") when you die. Consider naming a person to oversee your estate after your death. This person is called an executor.

◆ Appoint someone to make financial decisions for you in case a time comes when you can't make them for yourself.

◆ If you have young children (or someone else you take care of), choose someone to take care of them. This person is called a guardian.

◆ Make sure your will and other records (life insurance policies, pension and retirement account records, real estate deeds, stocks) are in a safe place. Close family members, the executor of your estate, and your lawyer should know how to access these records in case something happens to you.

A lawyer can advise you on how best to organize your estate so your family can handle your affairs after your death. A financial planner or social worker can also help. These resources may be available in your community or through a local hospital or hospice program.

## If Your Health Gets Worse

### Palliative Care

Palliative care is a kind of care for people who have illnesses that don't go away and often get worse over time. It is different than care to cure your illness. It focuses on improving your quality of life—not just your body, but also your mind and spirit.

Palliative care is not just for people who are near death. You can have palliative care at the same time that you are getting treatment for your health problem.

Palliative care can help reduce pain or treatment side effects. The doctors, nurses, and others on a palliative care team can help you and your loved ones talk more openly about your feelings and make future plans. They can also make sure the rest of your health care team and your family and friends understand your goals.

Many people like palliative care because it can focus on what's most important to them. If you think it could help you, talk to your doctor.

### Hospice Care

Hospice provides medical care, emotional help, and spiritual support as you near the end of your life. It can also help your family and friends care for you and deal with their grief.

You can get hospice care when your doctor says that you have a limited time left to live. Medicare pays for hospice care when a person has 6 months or less to live if the disease runs its natural course. (Sometimes people getting hospice care wind up living much longer than 6 months.)

You may want to choose hospice care if:

◆ Treatment for your disease has become more of a burden than a benefit.

◆ You want to choose where to spend the time you have left (such as in your home).

◆ You want family and friends to be involved in your care.

The goals of hospice are to keep you comfortable and help you get the most out of life in the time you have left.

◆ Hospice focuses on relieving pain and other symptoms. It does not try to cure your illness.

◆ It does not speed up or lengthen dying.

◆ Hospice includes counseling and support for you and your loved ones; respite care, which gives some time off to those who take care of you; and help with things like meals and errands.

◆ Hospice programs can help 24 hours a day, 7 days a week in your own home or in a hospice center. Some hospices also go to nursing homes or hospitals.

Don't wait for your doctor or family to bring up your end-of-life care. Sometimes it's hard for a doctor to admit that a patient is nearing the final stages of an illness. And it can be hard for you and your family to accept.

 For help working through your decisions about end-of-life care, go to the Web site on the back cover and enter **w249** in the search box.

# Staying Healthy

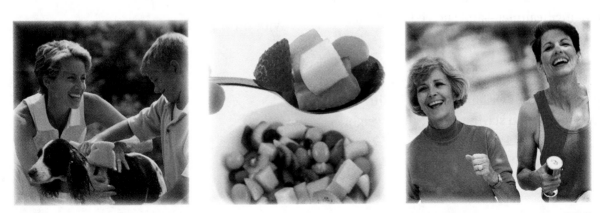

# Reaching a Healthy Weight

A healthy weight is a weight at which you feel good about yourself and have energy for work and play. It's also one that does not put you at risk for weight-related problems like heart disease, diabetes, stroke, arthritis, and cancer.

Many people are not at a healthy weight but want to get there. Does this describe you? If it does, there are things you can do today to move toward your goal.

Here are the big ideas to keep in mind as you get started:

◆ Focus on health first.

◆ Choose healthier foods.

◆ Be careful about how much you eat.

◆ Be more active.

◆ Decide not to gain any more weight.

◆ When you're ready, try to lose weight.

## Focus on Health First

Eating healthier and being more active will probably help you lose weight. Even if you don't lose much weight, these changes can help you feel better, have more energy, and prevent disease.

Focus on these healthy changes rather than weight loss. Losing weight is very hard for most people. But you can take steps to start living healthier—and succeed—right now.

## Eat Healthier Foods

The kinds of foods you eat have a big impact on both your weight and your health. Reaching and staying at a healthy weight is not about going on a diet. It's about making healthier food choices every day and changing your diet for good.

Pages 305 to 310 have information that can help you make healthier food choices at home and when you eat out. In general, fruits and vegetables, whole grains, lean protein (lean meats, fish, beans), and low-fat dairy foods should be most of what you eat.

But there's also room for a few sugary and high-fat foods in most people's diets. Most foods can be part of a healthy diet as long as you don't eat too much of them.

## Watch How Much You Eat

Many people eat more than their bodies need. Part of controlling your weight means learning how much food you really need from day to day and not eating more than that. Even with healthy foods, eating too much can lead to weight gain.

◆ Pay attention to how much food is on your plate.

◆ Read food labels to learn what a serving size is.

◆ Don't go back for seconds.

◆ If you eat out a lot, know that most restaurants serve much bigger portions than most people need.

With time, you can get used to eating less.

## Start With Small Changes in Your Diet

Changing your diet is a big step. But you can break it into lots of small ones like these.

◆ Eat a healthy breakfast every day. Try whole-grain cereal with milk and fruit, or whole wheat toast with an egg and a small glass of juice.

◆ Use a smaller dinner plate.

◆ Avoid buffets. If you go to a buffet, make one trip only. Forget about "getting your money's worth."

◆ Make a healthy lunch instead of eating out.

◆ Save money and calories when you eat out. Split an entrée with someone, or ask for half of it in a to-go box. Order a lunch portion instead of a dinner one.

◆ Bring a healthy snack to work: fruit, carrot or celery sticks with low-fat dip, or whole-grain crackers with string cheese. A good snack may keep you from overeating later.

◆ Drink water or nonfat milk with dinner instead of soda.

With time, these small changes may become routine. Look at every step you take as a success.

## Be More Active

When people think of losing weight, they most often think of food or diets. But a big part of weight control is exercise. When you change what you eat *and* you exercise, you increase your chances for success.

Exercise helps in three ways:

1. It burns calories. This makes it easier to lose weight and keep it off. To see how many calories you can burn when  you exercise, go to the Web site on the back cover and enter **q448** in the search box.

2. It reduces your risk for health problems like heart disease, high blood pressure, stroke, and diabetes.

3. It gives you more energy, makes you stronger, and lets you do more with less effort. For most people, the more active they are, the better they feel.

Pages 311 to 315 are all about how to be more active. For those who can't picture themselves "working out," there are tips on how to be more active that don't involve traditional exercise. You'll also find ideas for how to work around some of the things that may keep you from being active: having a busy schedule, feeling too out of shape, or not knowing how to get started.

Just being a little more active can make a difference. You can do it. Lots of people have.

## Avoid Weight Gain

You may not be ready to try to lose weight. But if you are like many people, you can take a great step toward better health by making sure your weight stays right where it is.

Unlike losing weight, most people can gain weight without thinking much about it.

◆ They often do it so slowly that they don't even notice.

More

◆ Most people tend to put on weight as they get older unless they are very careful. And as their weight creeps up, so does their risk for health problems.

How can you avoid this? Start by weighing yourself today. Use that as your weight limit, and then make sure you stay within a few pounds of that number.

If you start to put on weight, cut back on calories a bit or get a little more exercise so you can get back under your weight limit.

(Do not weigh yourself every day. Weight can go up and down a little from day to day without meaning that you are gaining or losing weight.)

## Try to Lose Weight

Weight loss seems like it should be simple. Burn more calories than you eat, and you will lose weight. But for most people, it's not simple at all.

There is some good news, though:

◆ You don't have to reach an "ideal" weight to be healthier.

◆ Losing as little as 5 to 10 percent of your weight can make a difference. For someone who weighs 200 pounds, that's only 10 to 20 pounds.

You may want and need to lose more than that. But for most people, setting small goals and building on small successes is easier than trying to reach one big goal. Feel good about all your efforts, big and small, to take better care of yourself.

## Which Diet Is Best?

By themselves, formal "diets" are not usually enough to lose weight and keep it off over the long run. The key is to make healthy food choices, not eat more than your body needs, and get regular exercise. If you stick with this approach most of the time, you will have the best chance of reaching a healthy weight and staying there.

Formal diets may help some people get started. If you think this might work for you, be sure to choose a sensible, healthy one. Look for diets that:

◆ Rely on normal, everyday foods. If you have to eat special foods while you're on the diet, it may be hard to keep weight off once you go back to "regular" food.

◆ Do not cut out entire food groups. Most foods can be—and should be—part of a healthy eating plan, even when you are trying to lose weight.

◆ Work on changing your eating habits for good.

◆ Focus on slow, steady weight loss. Fast, extreme weight loss is not good for your body. And most people can't keep the weight off when they lose it that way.

 To make sure you are on a safe path to weight loss, go to the Web site on the back cover and enter **a895** in the search box.

# Plan to Succeed

**1. Think about what stops you, and look for solutions.** Do you feel too busy to exercise or cook healthier meals? Are you afraid you are too out of shape and will feel foolish or hurt yourself? Do you not have the support you need? There are ways to get around all of these barriers.

**2. Start small.** For most people, it's easier to tackle a series of small changes than one or two big changes. Small successes add up. And if you don't succeed with a small change, it will be only a small setback—one that's easy to get past so you can try again.

**3. Be specific.** Simply planning to work out more and eat better is too general and too hard to follow. Instead, set specific goals you can measure (and reach). At the end of the day or the week or the month, you should be able to say "Yes, I met my goal" or "No, I did not meet my goal." For example:

◆ Make a plan to walk 2 days a week for 20 minutes each time.

◆ Replace your lunchtime soda with water or a low-calorie drink every day.

◆ Twice a week, bring a healthy lunch to work instead of eating out.

◆ Eat a piece of fruit in place of your regular dessert 3 nights each week.

Set goals like these that are right for you. When you have met them, set new ones.

**4. Track your progress.** It may help to write down what you eat and when and how long you exercise, at least in the beginning. This helps you do two things: feel good when you reach a goal, and know where you went wrong when you don't. Be sure to reward yourself when you succeed—perhaps with new clothes or new exercise gear.

**5. Make new habits part of your daily life.** Schedule exercise time on your calendar. Have your family eat the same healthy foods you do. It will be easier to stick to exercise and healthy eating when you think of them as part of a normal day rather than as extras.

Controlling your weight takes daily effort. Some days you just won't feel like exercising. Some days you'll want a cheeseburger, not lean turkey on whole wheat. That's okay. Just don't let those days add up.

**More** ▶

## Why Weight Isn't the Only Thing That Matters

Weight is only one measure of your health.

◆ You can be a little overweight and still be healthy if you eat right and are active.

◆ If you do not eat right or exercise, you may not be healthy no matter what you weigh.

Healthy bodies come in lots of shapes and sizes. Everyone can get healthier by eating better and being more active. Most of us will never look like fashion models or world-class athletes. But when you treat your body well—feed it healthy food and move it in the ways it's built to move—you can feel good about it.

## Are You at a Healthy Weight?

There are two measurements that can tell you whether your weight is healthy. Neither is perfect, but they can gauge whether your weight is putting you at risk for disease. They are:

◆ Your BMI (body mass index).

◆ Your waist size (circumference).

### BMI

BMI is a measure of your weight compared to your height. Your risk of weight-related disease may be higher if you are above or below a healthy BMI range. For adults, the healthy range is from 18.5 to 24.9.

Use the chart on this page to find your height and weight and find your BMI.

BMI is not always an accurate sign of your health risk. For example, athletes with a lot of muscle may have a high BMI but still be at a very healthy weight. A frail person with little muscle may have a low BMI but still have too much body fat.

But for the average person, BMI is a good guide, especially when you look at it with waist size.

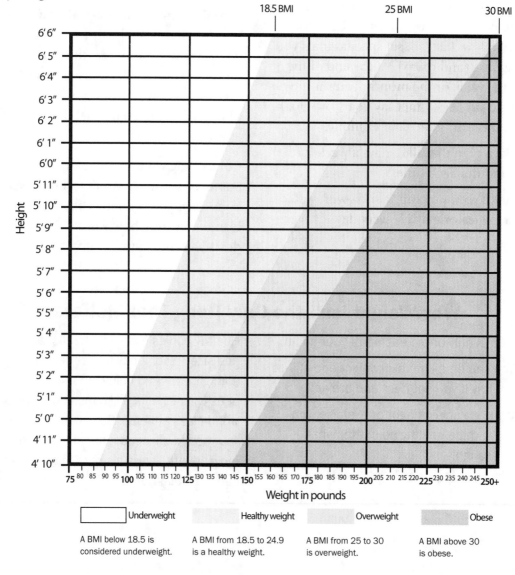

| | |
|---|---|
| Underweight — A BMI below 18.5 is considered underweight. | Healthy weight — A BMI from 18.5 to 24.9 is a healthy weight. |
| Overweight — A BMI from 25 to 30 is overweight. | Obese — A BMI above 30 is obese. |

## Waist Size: Apple or Pear?

Where you store fat in your body makes a difference.

◆ Some people store most of their fat around their hips; these folks are sometimes called "pear-shaped."

◆ Others store their fat around their belly, so they are "apple-shaped."

Of these two shapes, "apples" are more likely to have weight-related diseases.

One way to find out whether your body fat is putting you at risk is to measure the size of your waist. Place a tape measure around your body at the top of your hipbone. This is usually at the level of your belly button.

You have a higher risk of disease if you are:

◆ A man with a waist larger than 40 inches.

◆ A woman with a waist larger than 35 inches.

### How to Use These Results

◆ If your BMI is from 18.5 to 24.9 and your waist size is lower than the cutoff (40 for men, 35 for women), you are probably at a healthy weight. Eat right and exercise so that your weight stays in a healthy range.

◆ If your BMI is over 25, or if your waist size is above the cutoff, you may need to lose some weight. Even a small weight loss can help.

Also talk to your doctor about any other risk factors for disease, such as smoking, high blood pressure, and high cholesterol. If you have these in addition to being overweight, you are at higher risk.

# Eating Healthier

Eating healthy means eating a variety of foods from the basic food groups in reasonable amounts. It's not about "going on a diet." Food is one of life's great pleasures. All foods can be part of a healthy eating plan when eaten in sensible amounts.

There are lots of ways to eat healthier. Start with a few of the basics:

◆ Eat more fruits and vegetables.

◆ Learn which fats are good for you and which ones to avoid.

◆ Add whole grains and fiber to your diet.

◆ Choose lean sources of protein.

◆ Be careful about how much sugar you eat.

When you're ready to learn more, go to the Web site on the back cover and enter **h844** in the search box.

## Eat More Fruits and Vegetables

A healthy diet includes plenty of fruits and vegetables. Nearly everyone could benefit from eating more of them. They're full of vitamins, minerals, and fiber, and most are very low in fat and calories. They also have substances that may help prevent heart disease, high blood pressure, and some types of cancer.

**More** ▶

## Easy Ways to Add Fruits and Veggies to Your Diet

◆ Add fresh or frozen berries or a sliced banana to breakfast cereal or yogurt. Put apple slices in oatmeal.

◆ Have a glass of juice with breakfast. One 6-ounce glass is a serving. (Don't depend on juice for all of your fruit servings, though. Most juices have a lot more sugar and calories than plain fruits.)

◆ Add lettuce, tomato, cucumber, and bell peppers to sandwiches. Get pizza with veggies—try mushrooms, peppers, spinach, or broccoli.

◆ Add vegetables to soups, stews, and stir-fries. Purée them in a blender or food processor first if it makes them easier to use.

◆ Keep carrots, celery, and other veggies handy for snacks. Buy them already sliced and ready to eat if it makes you more likely to eat them.

◆ Have a salad with dinner every night. Make sure it's mostly vegetables, rather than mostly cheese, croutons, and salad dressing.

◆ Have fruit for dessert. If a piece of fruit doesn't seem like dessert to you, try baked apples or pears with cinnamon, or have fresh berries or melon with some vanilla yogurt.

◆ Make a fruit smoothie. Blend bananas, berries, or oranges with fat-free or low-fat yogurt or milk.

## Healthy Ways to Cook

How you cook affects how you eat. For many people, "cooking" means frying. This often means using lard, shortening, butter, or lots of oil to make food taste good. But there are healthier methods you can use and still have great-tasting food. Here are some low-fat ways to cook. Try one for your next meal.

◆ Bake in aluminum foil. This keeps food juicy and full of flavor. Wrap meat or fish in foil with some herbs for seasoning and even a little wine or broth. Add some vegetables too.

◆ Poach. Put chicken or fish in one layer in a pan. Cover it with water or broth, and add herbs or a little wine for flavor. Bring the liquid to a boil. Then lower the heat and simmer for 10 to 12 minutes until the food is done.

◆ Stir-fry. When you stir-fry, you cut meat, chicken, or vegetables into small pieces so they cook fast. Use a nonstick pan or a wok over medium-high heat. Add the food and constantly stir and turn it. If the food sticks, add a little canola, olive, or sesame oil; cooking spray; or water, wine, or broth.

◆ Try fat-free or low-fat yogurt, sour cream, or cottage cheese in place of full-fat cream and sour cream.

◆ Before you eat chicken or meat, cut off the fat. If you eat red meat, choose the leanest cuts. Lean cuts usually have the word "round" or "loin" in them.

## Understanding Fats

| Type of fats | What foods are they in? |
|---|---|
| **Healthy fats:** monounsaturated, polyunsaturated | Fish (salmon, mackerel)<br>Most nuts and seeds, soybeans<br>Vegetable oils (canola, olive, peanut, corn, safflower, sunflower, walnut, flaxseed)<br>Avocados, olives |
| **Unhealthy fats:** saturated fats, trans fats, cholesterol | **Saturated fats and cholesterol:**<br>Whole milk, whole-milk cheese, whole-milk yogurt<br>Butter, margarine, shortening, lard (and foods cooked in these)<br>Red meat (such as beef), chicken skin<br><br>**Trans fats:**<br>Packaged cookies, crackers, and chips<br>Processed foods<br>Nondairy whipped topping and creamer |

## Understanding Fats

Except for some fruits and vegetables, almost everything you eat has some kind of fat. Your body needs some fat to work properly.

But there are healthy "good" fats and unhealthy "bad" ones. For many people, the least healthy types of fats—saturated and trans fats—make up too much of their diet.

A healthy eating plan can and should include good fats in reasonable amounts. They are high in calories, but they can help lower your cholesterol and may reduce your risk of some diseases.

With unhealthy fats, it's best to avoid them as much as you can. Not only are they high in calories, but they also raise your cholesterol and increase your risk of heart disease.

Use the chart on this page to learn which fats to enjoy and which ones to avoid.

How much fat should you eat? If you're eating an average diet of about 2,000 calories a day:

◆ Aim for about 60 grams of fat each day. Most of that should be monounsaturated and polyunsaturated fats.

◆ Eat less than 20 grams of saturated fats a day.

◆ Eat as few trans fats as possible. Check food labels for trans fats.

## Get More Whole Grains

**Whole grains** like whole wheat, oats, and brown rice are full of B vitamins, minerals, and fiber and are a great source of energy. They're also very filling. **Refined grains**, which include white flour, white rice, and pasta, have fewer vitamins and minerals. They're not as filling because they don't have much fiber.

**More**

307

How do you know if it's whole grain?

◆ Read the food label. The first ingredient should be whole wheat, whole grain, or whole oats. "Enriched wheat flour" is a refined grain, not a whole grain. Multi-grain breads and crackers are not always whole grains.

◆ Don't go by color alone. Brown bread does not equal whole-grain or whole wheat bread.

You can add whole grains to your diet by choosing whole wheat bread instead of white bread; whole-grain crackers and cereals; oatmeal; brown rice instead of white rice; and whole wheat pasta. Don't be afraid to try other whole grains like bulgur, barley, and quinoa.

## Add Fiber to Your Diet

Fiber is the part of fruits, vegetables, and grains that your body cannot digest. It is found only in plants. Foods that come from animals (meats, milk and dairy foods, eggs) do not have fiber.

Eating plenty of fiber helps keep your digestive tract healthy. If you are often constipated, eating more fiber will help. People who eat a lot of fiber have fewer problems with the colon (large intestine).

A high-fiber diet may also help keep your blood sugar steady, lower your cholesterol, and reduce your chance of heart disease.

### How to Get More Fiber

Most people need 20 to 35 grams of fiber each day. To reach that amount:

◆ Choose whole-grain breads and cereals that have at least 2 grams of fiber in each serving. Read the label on the package.

◆ Buy bread that lists whole wheat, stone-ground wheat, or cracked wheat first in the ingredient list.

| High-Fiber Foods ||
| --- | --- |
| **Type of food** | **Examples** |
| Breads and grain products (especially whole-grain foods) | Bran (wheat bran, oat bran) <br> Oatmeal <br> Whole wheat breads, tortillas, and cereals <br> Brown rice <br> Barley, bulgur, and millet |
| Vegetables | Beans and peas <br> Cabbage, brussels sprouts <br> Broccoli, cauliflower <br> Beets, turnips, carrots <br> Baked potato skin |
| Fruits | Fruits with skin or seeds that you eat (apples, pears, strawberries, kiwifruit, figs, blueberries) <br> Oranges, grapefruit |

◆ Eat brown rice, bulgur, or millet instead of white rice.

◆ Eat more fresh fruits every day. See the list of high-fiber fruits on page 308.

◆ Eat more raw or lightly cooked vegetables every day.

◆ Eat cooked beans, peas, and lentils in place of meat sometimes.

## Choose Lean Protein

Protein is vital to your health. It helps keep your muscles, bones, skin, hair, blood, and internal organs healthy. But some forms of protein tend to have too much cholesterol and unhealthy fats. So it's best to choose lean sources of protein, such as:

◆ Fish, skinless chicken, and only the leanest cuts of beef.

◆ Beans, peas, and lentils.

◆ Tofu and other soy products.

◆ Fat-free or low-fat dairy products.

◆ Eggs (in moderation).

Most adults in North America get all the protein they need in their diets. If you eat animal products, your diet probably has plenty of protein. If you are a vegetarian, make sure you get protein from plant sources like beans, grains, and soy.

## Don't Eat Too Much Sugar

A little sugar is fine. It tastes good, and it's not harmful for most people. But most sweets also have a lot of "empty" calories—that means they're high in calories but do not fill you up or have much nutritional value. If too many of your calories come from sugar, you may not be getting enough of the healthy foods you need. (You may also gain weight.)

## Using the USDA's MyPyramid

- Activity
- Moderation
- Personalization
- Proportionality
- Variety
- Gradual improvement

GRAINS   VEGETABLES   FRUITS   OIL  MILK   MEAT & BEANS

**MyPyramid.gov**
STEPS TO A HEALTHIER YOU

The USDA's MyPyramid aims to help you make healthy food choices and be active every day. It is based on the idea that your calorie and nutrient needs depend on your age, sex, and activity level.

For example, a 40-year-old woman who gets more than 60 minutes of physical activity on most days may need about 2,200 calories a day. A 40-year-old woman who gets less than 30 minutes of daily exercise may need only about 1,800 calories a day. Both women need to eat a variety of healthy foods from all the food groups—grains, vegetables, fruits, milk, meat and beans, and healthy fats. But they don't need the same amounts of those foods.

Want to know what's right for you? Go to www.MyPyramid.gov. There you can:

◆ Figure out what kinds and amounts of food you should eat each day.

◆ Get help with meal plans and serving sizes.

◆ Track your progress toward healthier eating.

**More** ▶

Many people need to cut down on sugar. Here are a few things that can make a big difference:

◆ Drink fewer sugar-sweetened drinks, such as soft drinks, lemonade, and fruit juices. These are a major source of sugar for some people, especially kids. Try sparkling water or sugar-free soda instead. Or stick to plain water and milk.

◆ Make it a habit to eat fruit instead of sugary desserts and snacks most of the time. Have a bowl of strawberries instead of a bowl of ice cream. Grab an apple instead of a candy bar.

◆ Check the labels on food packages before you buy things. Yogurt, cereal, and canned fruits often have sugar added. Look for cereals that have 6 grams or less of sugar in each serving. Be careful with dried fruits—they have a lot of sugar.

## Nutrition for Your Family

Healthy eating habits are good for the whole family. If you're trying to eat healthier, it will be easier if the rest of the family eats healthier too. The same foods that are good for adults are good for children. A healthy diet can help your children feel good, stay at a healthy weight, and have lots of energy for school and play.

Get started by setting up a regular schedule for meals and snacks. Expect everyone to come to the table to eat. Offer healthy foods, but let your child decide how much to eat. This lets your child tune in to whether he or she is hungry. Meal times are important for learning about new foods and how to behave at the table. Make them a pleasant family time.

Childhood is a great time to learn healthy eating habits that can last a lifetime. Children learn by example: They will learn to eat the foods they see you eating, and they will learn what makes a good meal by what you serve them.

## Should You Take Dietary Supplements?

For most people, the best way to get all the nutrients they need is to eat a healthy, balanced diet that includes a variety of foods.

Supplements can't make up for a poor diet. But they can help fill in the nutrition gap for people who have special needs. For example, older adults tend to have trouble absorbing enough vitamin D and calcium from their diets, so they may need a supplement. Some women need to take calcium or folic acid.

Talk to your doctor or a dietitian about whether you need to take vitamin or mineral supplements. If you do:

◆ Unless your doctor recommends a specific vitamin or mineral, choose a balanced multivitamin-mineral supplement that has close to 100 percent of the Daily Values (DVs).

◆ Do not take a specific trace mineral unless your doctor recommends it. Taking some trace minerals as supplements can upset the way your body absorbs other minerals.

# Exercise and Health

Being more active is one of the best things you can do to improve your health and your quality of life. It helps you to:

◆ Feel stronger and have more energy. (And you will look better too!)

◆ Lower your risk for heart disease, stroke, certain cancers, diabetes, and high blood pressure.

◆ Reach and stay at a healthy weight.

◆ Keep your bones, muscles, and joints strong, and relieve arthritis pain.

◆ Deal with stress and anxiety.

◆ Make daily tasks easier—moving around, carrying bags of groceries, climbing stairs, taking care of your children.

◆ Keep your mind sharp as you get older.

If you are already in good health, regular exercise can help you stay that way. But if you are not in good health, or if you have a long-term health problem, just a little more exercise every day can make a big difference.

It's never too late to become more active. And it's never too late to get the benefits that exercise can bring. No matter how old you are, how fit you are, or what health problems you have, there is a form of exercise that will work for you. You just have to find it.

## Attitude Counts

Starting or changing an exercise routine doesn't have to be hard. Lots of people find ways to be more active that work for them. Success starts with the right attitude.

## What if I have a long-term health problem?

You may think that because you have a health problem like high blood pressure, arthritis, or diabetes, exercise is not for you. But exercise can help almost everyone. It may even be part of the treatment for your health problem.

You may not be able to do certain kinds of exercise. But there are dozens of ways to be more active. You only need to find a few. Talk to your doctor about what exercises are safe for you and how much exercise you should get.

### "I know I can find time for a little more exercise."

Even the busiest people can find time. If you're worried about not having enough time:

◆ Focus on being more active. You don't have to do formal "exercise" to improve your fitness. You just need to move more.

◆ Spread your workout throughout the day. You don't have to do all your exercise at once. For example, walk for 10 minutes 3 times a day.

◆ Get up early to walk, do a workout video, or go to a class at your local health club. It may seem hard at first, but you'll get used to it. You might even start to like it.

◆ Look for ways to be more active in your everyday life. Take the stairs instead of the elevator. Park farther away from work or the mall. Move faster through chores like cleaning, yard work, or vacuuming.

More ▶

You can get a good workout by doing daily tasks at a pace that gets your heart beating and gets you breathing hard.

◆ Be creative. Instead of e-mailing or phoning a coworker or neighbor, walk over. When meeting with someone, suggest that you take a walk instead of staying inside.

### "I'll have more energy if I exercise."

At first, exercise may make you feel tired because you're not used to it. Start by doing a little bit at a time, and stick with it. You may be surprised at how much more energetic you'll start to feel.

### "Exercise doesn't have to hurt."

Even gentle exercise can improve your health. If you are new to exercise, at first your muscles may ache and your lungs may "burn" a little when you are breathing hard. Start slowly, and your body will adapt. Talk with your doctor if you have chest pain or if your joints hurt.

### "Exercise is for big people too."

No matter what your size, exercise can make you healthier and happier. At first you may get tired quickly and not be able to move or bend very well if you are overweight. You might feel self-conscious. Just remember to take one small step at a time. Those steps will quickly start to add up.

### "Exercise doesn't have to cost much."

You do not need to spend a lot to stay fit.

◆ Start walking. It's free.

◆ Get home workout videos from the library or a used bookstore.

◆ Apply for a reduced-cost membership at your local YMCA.

◆ Shop for used exercise equipment in the newspaper or at yard sales. Make sure it's in safe condition.

### "I'll never be too old to exercise."

Exercise helps at any age. In fact, being active can help you avoid some of the problems that often come as we get older. Talk to your doctor about what kinds of activity might be best for you.

### "Exercise can help me avoid a heart attack."

If you have a heart problem, you may worry that you could have a heart attack or stroke while exercising. You are probably more likely to have one if you do not exercise. There may be some limits on what you should do, but regular, safe workouts will strengthen your heart, blood vessels, and lungs. See your doctor before you get started.

### "Exercise can be fun!"

◆ Look for something you enjoy. Try new things until you find something you like. If you like what you're doing, you are much more likely to stick with it. Ride a bike. Take a dance class. Go hiking.

◆ Don't do the same thing every day. Variety can keep you motivated, and it's good for your body. Swim one day, and take a walk the next. Try a yoga class.

◆ Get a partner, or join a group or class. For many people, the social aspect makes their workout more fun.

### "It never hurts to try."

Don't worry about failing, no matter what your past experience with exercise has been. Just go slowly, and set small goals. When you meet them, set new ones. And if you don't meet a goal, think about what might have helped you meet it, and try again.

## Make Your Heart Stronger

When exercise gets your heart beating and gets you breathing hard, it makes your heart stronger. Whether you call it aerobic exercise, cardio exercise, or just "exercising your heart," it all means the same thing. And just a little more every day can reduce your risk for heart attack, stroke, and other problems.

What kinds of workouts are good for your heart? Anything that raises your heart rate and keeps it there counts.

◆ Walking, hiking, and running

◆ Biking (outside or indoors)

◆ Swimming and water aerobics

◆ Dancing

◆ Doing household chores or yard work at a fast pace

◆ Climbing stairs

A simple way to tell if you are working your heart is the "talk-sing" test. If you are too short of breath to talk while you exercise, you may be pushing too hard. If you can sing while you exercise, you may do more for your heart by working just a bit harder. If you are in the "talking" range, your heart is getting a good workout no matter what you're doing.

 Getting started can be as simple as taking a walk a few times a week. If you want more help planning an exercise routine, go to the Web site on the back cover and enter **a481** in the search box.

---

## Walking Works

Want to start making your heart stronger today? Take a walk. Walking is one of the easiest ways to be more active and improve your health.

◆ Start with small, short-term goals you can reach. For example, if you have not been active in a long time, start with 15-minute walks 3 times a week. The next week, increase your walks to 20 minutes.

◆ Start each walk with a warm-up. Pick up your pace in the middle of the walk, and then slow down at the end.

◆ Walk fast enough to raise your heart rate and make you breathe harder. But do not walk so fast that you can't talk.

◆ Wear comfortable shoes with good arch support.

There are three tips that have helped lots of people stick to their walking routines. They can help you too.

◆ Find a friend, family member, or coworker to walk with. You will be less likely to skip your walk if you know someone is expecting you.

◆ Get a pedometer, a small device that counts your steps. Set a daily step goal, and wear your pedometer all day. You may be surprised how fast the steps add up when you park your car a little farther away, use the stairs instead of the elevator, or walk to the store instead of driving there.

◆ Get a dog. Dogs love to walk, and taking your dog for a walk once or twice a day is a great way to fit walking into your life.

**More** ▶

## Make Your Body Stronger

You do not have to lift heavy weights or grow big, bulky muscles to get stronger. Doing a few simple strength exercises twice a week can make a difference.

◆ You can do push-ups or sit-ups, use weights, or use machines. You can even do strength exercises with a piece of rubber tubing. For a guide to some basic  exercises, go to the Web site on the back cover and enter **s462** in the search box.

◆ Do exercises that include all of the different muscle groups: chest, arms, stomach, back, and legs.

◆ Give muscles at least a full day's rest between strength workouts.

Your goal may be to strengthen your knees or back or to be able to get around better. You may want to reduce body fat and stay trim. Or you may want to protect your bones as you get older. Strength training helps with all of these.

## Stretch

Stretching keeps you flexible and helps with sore or tense muscles. It improves your balance and posture and can also be a great way to relax. And you can do it for free.

There are lots of ways to bring stretching into your life.

◆ Stretch at home when you first get up in the morning or before you go to bed (or both). If you need help, get a video you can follow, or find a good fitness book or magazine that explains some stretches.

◆ Take a stretching class at a gym or health club.

◆ Try yoga or tai chi. These are great ways to stay flexible and reduce stress.

Basic stretches are easy to learn. The pictures on the next page show some simple stretches you can do on your own. The shaded area in each shows where you should feel the stretch. Here are a few tips to get you started:

◆ Ease into each stretch. Stretching is not about going fast or making sudden movements.

◆ Hold each stretch for at least 20 to 30 seconds. You should feel a pull in the area you are stretching, but you should not feel sharp pain.

◆ Do not hold your breath during a stretch.

### Should I see my doctor before I get started?

Talk with your doctor before you start an exercise program if:

◆ You have heart trouble, frequent chest pain or pressure, or high blood pressure.

◆ You often feel faint or dizzy.

◆ You have arthritis or other bone or joint problems.

◆ You have diabetes (you may need to adjust your medicine).

◆ You are older than 60 and are not used to exercise.

◆ You have two or more risk factors for heart disease. These include high cholesterol, high blood pressure, smoking, obesity, an inactive lifestyle, and a family history of heart disease before age 50.

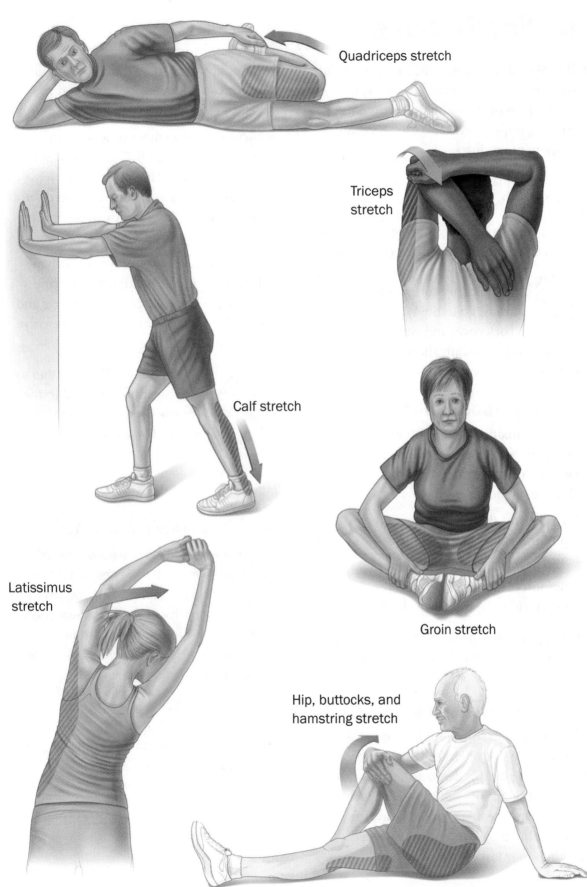

Quadriceps stretch

Triceps stretch

Calf stretch

Latissimus stretch

Groin stretch

Hip, buttocks, and hamstring stretch

# Quitting Smoking

Millions of people have quit smoking. Some have quit on their own. Some have quit with the help of stop-smoking programs or support groups. Some have used nicotine replacement products.

The point is that people find ways to quit for good. So can you.

But you have to be ready. Giving up tobacco is a big change, and the process of deciding  that you will quit may take time. If you aren't sure whether you're ready, go to the Web site on the back cover and enter **b373** in the search box. The quiz there can help you figure out where you are in the process.

## Thinking About Quitting?

If you're thinking about quitting, you're already on your way. It may help to know that you don't have to quit smoking through willpower alone. There are:

- ◆ Treatments that can help with the physical effects of giving up smoking and nicotine.
- ◆ Resources that can help with the emotional side of quitting smoking.

These approaches have helped many people stop smoking for good. They can help you too.

### Nicotine Replacement and Medicines

When you try to stop smoking, you may have trouble sleeping, strongly crave nicotine, or feel grumpy, depressed, or restless. These symptoms of withdrawal are at their worst during the first couple of days after you quit but may last up to a few weeks. Cravings may last even longer.

Treatment can reduce withdrawal symptoms and help you beat your body's nicotine addiction. You can try:

- ◆ Nicotine replacement products, such as gums, patches, inhalers, sprays, and lozenges. They help your body slowly get used to less nicotine until you do not need it at all. You can buy these products without a prescription.
- ◆ Medicine, such as buproprion (Zyban). This medicine does not have nicotine but can help you cope with cravings and mood swings. Your doctor can prescribe it for you.

 For help in deciding whether to try these approaches, go to the Web site on the back cover and enter **b169** in the search box.

## It's Never Too Late

Anyone who smokes has good reason to stop—even if you have smoked for decades. No matter how long you've smoked, your risk of a heart attack and other health problems will start to go down once you quit. You will start to feel better and breathe easier.

It can be hard to break a long-time habit. But you can do it, just like thousands of other smokers who have quit.

## It's Not Just the Nicotine

If you are like many smokers, smoking is part of your daily routine. You enjoy it. It's relaxing. When you quit smoking, you have to give all that up (or at least find something to replace it).

The good news is that you don't have to do it alone. Lots of ex-smokers have found support in:

◆ Stop-smoking programs. Call your health plan, your local hospital, or the American Lung Association to find out what programs are offered in your area.

◆ Telephone "quitlines," such as 1-800-QUITNOW (1-800-784-8669).

These connect you to trained counselors who can help you make a plan for how to quit.

◆ Online quit groups. Like quitlines, these are convenient for lots of people since you can get help from home at nearly any hour.

◆ Support groups, such as Nicotine Anonymous.

◆ Counseling from doctors, nurses, or therapists.

This kind of support can help you change your habits. Think about whether any of these options appeal to you, and give one a try. If it's not for you, try something else.

## 10 Reasons to Quit

1. Live longer and better. On average, people who smoke die nearly 7 years earlier than people who do not smoke. But it is not as simple as just dying a little younger. Smoking can affect the quality of your life as well. Having chronic lung disease is not an easy or pleasant way to live or die.

2. Breathe easier and cough less. You may have more energy and stamina after you stop smoking.

3. Reduce your risk of erection problems. Smoking can damage your blood vessels, including those that bring blood to the penis.

4. Cut your risk of heart attack in half within 1 year. Five years after quitting, your risk will be about the same as that of someone who never smoked.

5. Reduce your risk for lung cancer, mouth and throat cancer, gum disease, and dental problems.

6. Get fewer colds and be less likely to get the flu or pneumonia. If you have asthma, you will have fewer and less severe asthma attacks.

7. Set a good example. Children whose parents do not smoke are less likely to use tobacco than those whose parents are smokers.

8. Stop having to find places to smoke at work or in public and exposing others to secondhand smoke.

9. Have a brighter smile, better sense of taste and smell, and fewer wrinkles.

10. Save money by not buying cigarettes. (Also, as a nonsmoker, you may pay less for health insurance.)

**More** ▶

## Once You've Decided to Quit

No one approach works for every smoker, but for many people it helps to:

◆ **Set a quit date.** Pick a date within the next month. Give yourself time to get ready (but not too much time).

◆ **Plan.** Will you go to a class or use nicotine replacement? Make sure you have low-calorie snacks on hand. Clean your clothes, carpet, furniture, and car to get rid of the smoke smell. If you know you tend to smoke in certain situations, plan for ways to avoid them.

◆ **Quit!** Stick to your quit date. That day, get rid of cigarettes, ashtrays, and lighters.

*Go to Web* For more tips and techniques that can help you get ready to quit and then stop smoking for good, go to the Web site on the back cover and enter **p811** in the search box.

### Started Smoking Again?

You're not alone. Many people who have quit smoking had to try several times before they were able to quit for good. The good news is that each time you try to quit—whether it's your second attempt or your tenth—you can get closer to quitting for good.

Think about why you started smoking again. Was it stress? Were you with a certain group of people or in a certain situation? What might have triggered you to smoke? Learn from what worked for you and what didn't.

Knowing what went wrong can help you when you are ready to quit again. The important thing is to keep trying.

# Dealing With Stress

Some stress is normal and even healthy. Stress releases hormones that speed up your heart, make you breathe faster, and give you a burst of energy. This can be useful when you need to focus or act quickly. It can help you win a race, or finish a big job, or get to the airport on time.

But too much stress or being under stress for too long is not good for you.

◆ It can make you moody, anxious, and depressed. You may find it hard to concentrate and may lose your temper more easily.

◆ It can cause headaches, back pain, and muscle tension.

◆ It can make health problems like heart disease, diabetes, and asthma worse.

◆ It can hurt your relationships. You may not do as well at work or school.

You may not have these problems right away. Most people can get through short periods of stress without long-term effects. But over time, continued stress will take its toll on you.

The good news is that you can learn ways to reduce and cope with stress that will help you avoid stress-related health problems.

## Ways to Reduce Stress

1. Decide what is most important and what can wait. (Maybe there are things you don't need to do at all.) At work, ask your boss if you're not sure what the priorities are.

2. Learn to say no. Don't commit to things that don't matter to you.

3. Do one thing at a time. When you try to do too many things at once, each usually takes more time than it would if you focused on it alone.

4. Get organized. Make lists, or use an appointment book. Keep track of deadlines.

5. Don't put things off. Use a schedule planner to plan your day or week. Just seeing on paper that there is a time to get each task done can help you get to work. Break a large project into small pieces and set a deadline for each one.

6. Save some time for yourself. Leave your job at the office, even if your office is a room in your home. If you give up free time to get more work done, you may pay for it with stress-related symptoms. If your employer offers a flexible work schedule, use it to fit your work style. Come in earlier so you have time for a longer lunch or a workout.

7. "Unplug" when you leave work. Leave your work cell phone behind or turn it off. Don't check work e-mail at home.

8. Get enough sleep. Stress can seem worse than it is when you're tired all the time. And you may not get as much done when you're too tired.

## How to Cope Better With Stress

For most people, there's just no way to totally avoid stress. It's part of life. But you can control how you react to stress.

| Healthy Ways to De-Stress |
| --- |
| Listen to music |
| Exercise |
| Go outdoors |
| Play with a pet |
| Laugh or cry |
| Spend time with someone you love |
| Write, draw, or paint |
| Pray or go to church |
| Take a bath or shower |
| Work in the yard or do home repairs |
| Do yoga, meditation, or muscle relaxation |

| Unhealthy Ways to De-Stress |
| --- |
| Drive fast |
| Eat too much or too little |
| Bite your fingernails |
| Drink too much coffee |
| Criticize yourself |
| Avoid people |
| Yell at your spouse, children, or friends |
| Smoke |
| Drink alcohol |
| Take drugs |
| Get violent or aggressive |

People don't always realize that they feel bad because of stress. Classic signs of stress include headache, stiff neck, or a nagging backache. You may lose your temper more often. You may feel jumpy or exhausted all the time.

**More**

Just knowing why you're feeling the way you do may help you cope with the problem. For a tool that can help you gauge your stress level now or anytime, go to the Web site on the back cover and enter **r030** in the search box.

## Are You Stress-Hardy?

Some people seem to stand up to or bounce back from stress better than others. They adjust to change more easily. They are more "stress-hardy."

 How stress-hardy are you? There is a short quiz that can tell you. Go to the Web site on the back cover and enter **d856** in the search box.

If you would like to be more stress-hardy, here are a few things that may help:

◆ Know what's important to you, whether it's your family, your work, or something else. When you are under a lot of stress, it can help to remember what matters most.

◆ Try to have a sense of control over your life. You cannot control every detail, but look for areas where you can make a difference. Not everything is out of your hands.

◆ Try to look at change as a challenge or opportunity rather than a threat.

◆ Do things that let you be creative and let you be yourself. Some people can do this through their work. But sometimes activities outside of your job—hobbies, sports, social groups, volunteer work, travel—are better chances to "do your own thing."

◆ Stay in touch with friends and family. Knowing that you are not alone in the world makes stress easier to bear.

## Learn to Relax

There are many techniques you can learn to help you relax. Progressive muscle relaxation and the relaxation response are two that seem to work well.

To learn these skills, practice them in a time and place where nothing will interrupt you. Do them once or twice a day until you can do them easily.

### Progressive Muscle Relaxation

Relaxing your muscles can reduce tension and anxiety. It can help reduce stress-related health problems and often helps people sleep better.

You can buy a tape or CD that takes you through all the muscle groups, or you can do it by just tensing and relaxing each muscle group on your own.

◆ Choose a place where you can lie down on your back and stretch out.

◆ Tense each muscle group (hard, but not to the point of cramping) for 4 to 10 seconds. Then give yourself 10 to 20 seconds to release it and relax.

◆ At various points, check the muscle groups you've already done and relax each one a little more each time.

### Muscle Groups

Remember to relax between each muscle group.

**Hands:** Clench them.

**Wrists and forearms:** Extend them and bend the hands back at the wrist.

**Biceps and upper arms:** Clench your hands into fists, bend your arms at the elbows, and flex your biceps (the muscles in your upper arms).

**Shoulders:** Shrug them. Check your arms and shoulders for tension.

**Forehead:** Wrinkle it into a deep frown.

**Around the eyes and bridge of the nose:** Close your eyes as tightly as you can. (Take out your contact lenses before you do this.)

**Cheeks and jaws:** Grin from ear to ear.

**Around the mouth:** Press your lips together tightly. (Check your face for tension.)

**Back of the neck:** Press the back of your head against the floor.

**Front of the neck:** Touch your chin to your chest. (Check your neck and head for tension.)

**Chest:** Take a deep breath and hold it. Then let it go.

**Back:** Arch your back up and away from the floor.

**Belly:** Suck it into a tight knot. (Check your chest and belly for tension.)

**Hips and buttocks:** Squeeze your buttocks together tightly.

**Thighs:** Clench them.

**Lower legs:** Point your toes toward your face, as if trying to bring your toes up to touch your shins. Then point your toes away and curl them under at the same time. (Check the area from your waist down for tension.)

When you are finished, return to alertness by counting backward from 5 to 1.

## Relaxation Response

The relaxation response is the opposite of the stress response. It slows your heart rate and breathing, lowers your blood pressure, and helps relieve muscle tension.

1. Lie down in a place where you can stretch out. Close your eyes.

2. Begin progressive muscle relaxation. See page 320.

3. Tune in to your breathing for 10 to 20 minutes. Focus on breathing from your belly, not from your chest. Each time you breathe out, say the word "one" (or any other word) silently or out loud. Or, instead of saying a word, fix your gaze on an object in the room. As thoughts enter your mind, don't dwell on them. Let them drift away.

4. Sit quietly for several minutes, until you're ready to open your eyes.

5. Notice the difference in your breathing and your pulse.

Don't worry about trying to become deeply relaxed. The key to this exercise is to stay passive and let distracting thoughts go without thinking about them.

*(Technique adapted from Herbert Benson, MD)*

# Safe Sex

Safe sex is all about avoiding sexually transmitted diseases, also called STDs. STDs can cause a lot of problems in your body. Some of them can even kill you. It's up to you to protect yourself and your sex partner from them. The good news is that you can.

To learn about the symptoms of STDs and what to do if you think you have one, see page 229.

## Who Gets STDs?

Anyone who has sex can get an STD. It does not matter how old you are, whether you're male or female, what race you are, or whether you're gay, straight, or bisexual.

You can get an STD from any kind of sexual contact, not just intercourse. STDs are spread through skin-to-skin contact between the genitals and through contact with body fluids such as semen, vaginal fluids, and blood (including menstrual blood). This means you can get an STD from:

- Vaginal sex.
- Anal sex.
- Oral sex.

## How You Can Stay Safer

Only two things completely get rid of the risk of STDs and HIV infection:

1. Not having sex at all (abstinence). This means not having vaginal, anal, or oral sex.

2. Total monogamy between uninfected partners. This means you and your partner have sex only with each other and you are absolutely sure that neither of you has a disease.

If you do not choose one of those two options, you can still greatly reduce your risk if you follow the guidelines below.

- Have safe sex every time you have sex. This means using condoms correctly every time. Use latex condoms from the beginning to the end of sexual contact. "Natural" or lambskin condoms do not protect against HIV infection or other STDs.

- Do not rely on spermicides or a diaphragm to protect against STDs. If spermicide irritates your genital area, it may increase your risk of infection.

- Before you have sex with a new partner, ask about his or her sexual history. Keep in mind that a person can have HIV or an STD and not know it.

- Do not have sex without a condom with anyone who has symptoms of an STD or whose behavior puts him or her at risk for HIV infection or an STD.

- Agree with your partner that neither of you will have sex with anyone else.

- Do not have sex if you or your partner has symptoms of an STD, such as sores on the genitals or mouth.

- Do not have sex while you or your partner is being treated for an STD.

- If you or your partner has genital herpes, do not have sex when either of you has a blister or an open sore or feels tingling or pain in the genital area. These may be signs of an outbreak. At other times, use latex condoms. You can spread genital herpes even when no sores are present.

## How to Use a Condom

Condoms work best if you follow these steps:

- Use a new condom each time you have sex.

- When you open the wrapper, be careful not to poke a hole in the condom with your nails, teeth, or other sharp objects.

- Put the condom on as soon as your penis is hard (erect) and before any sexual contact.

- Before putting the condom on, hold the tip of it and squeeze out the air to leave room for the semen.

- If you are not circumcised, pull down the loose skin from the head of the penis (foreskin) before you put on the condom.

- While holding onto the tip, unroll the condom all the way down to the base of your penis.

- If you want to use a lubricant, never use petroleum jelly (such as Vaseline), grease, hand lotion, baby oil, or anything with oil in it. Oil or petroleum can make the condom break. Instead, use a personal lubricant such as Astroglide or K-Y Jelly.

- After you ejaculate, hold onto the condom at the base of your penis and pull out from your partner while your penis is still hard. This will keep semen from spilling out of the condom.

- Wash your hands after handling a used condom.

Buy latex condoms made in the United States. These condoms meet strict safety standards and are less likely to break or leak.

Keep the condom in its original package until you are ready to use it. Store it in a cool, dry place out of direct sun. Do not keep it in your wallet, car, or other hot places for a long time. The heat weakens the latex.

## Allergic to Latex?

Some people are allergic to latex. If you have a skin reaction after using a latex condom, think about whether it could have been something else (lubricant, spermicide) that caused the problem. If you are sure it was the latex, do not use latex condoms again. Use polyurethane ones instead.

Polyurethane condoms may not prevent STDs as well as latex condoms do. But they are much safer than not using a condom at all.

# Get Immunized

Immunizations help protect the body from diseases. When you get a vaccine, your body learns to find and attack the virus or bacteria that causes the disease before it can cause problems.

Immunizations save lives. They help prevent serious illness in children as well as adults. They cost less than treating the diseases they protect against. And the risk of serious side effects from the vaccines is much lower than the risk of serious illness if you do not get the vaccines.

 Make sure to get your child (and yourself) immunized. If you need more information than you find here, go to the Web site on the back cover and enter **w921** in the search box.

Keep good records. You may need to show proof of immunizations when you enroll your child in day care or school. You may need them for travel too.

## Immunizations for Children

The chart on page 325 is a basic guide to which vaccines children need and when. Talk to your doctor about what schedule is best for your child.

◆ If your child is at higher risk because of a long-term (chronic) illness or weakened immune system or because of where you live or travel, he or she may need a different schedule.

◆ If your child has missed any vaccines, he or she may need a "catch-up" schedule.

◆ If there is a disease outbreak (such as measles) and your child has not been vaccinated yet, call your doctor to see if your child should get the vaccine early.

◆ Even the basic schedule changes from time to time. Make sure you have the most current information.

You do not need to delay immunizations because your child has a cold or other minor illness. If you have concerns, talk with your doctor.

### Reactions to Immunizations

Brief, mild reactions are common.

◆ If your child gets a slight fever, acetaminophen (Tylenol) or ibuprofen (Advil, Motrin) can help. Do not give your child aspirin. Also see Fever on page 158.

◆ The area around the shot may swell and hurt a little. Put ice or a cold pack on it for 10 to 15 minutes.

◆ A mild skin rash may appear a week or two after the chickenpox or MMR vaccine. The rash does not need treatment and should go away within a few days.

Call your doctor right away if your child has more than just a mild reaction.

## Immunizations for Teens and Adults

The need for immunizations does not end with childhood.

◆ Thousands of adults are hospitalized, and many die, because of flu and other diseases that vaccines can prevent.

◆ Illnesses like chickenpox and measles can be quite serious if you get them as a teen or adult. They are especially dangerous for pregnant women.

◆ Having rubella or chickenpox while you are pregnant increases the risk of miscarriage, stillbirth, and severe birth defects.

◆ Hepatitis B can lead to serious, sometimes fatal liver disease.

If you are in any of the groups for whom a vaccine is recommended, make sure you get immunized. Use the chart on page 326 as a guide, and then talk to your doctor. The recommendations change from time to time.

## Other Immunizations

If you are in close contact with people who have contagious diseases or you are planning to travel to places where malaria, typhoid, cholera, yellow fever, or other illnesses are common, call your local health department. You may need to get other shots.

| Childhood Immunizations | | |
|---|---|---|
| **Immunization** | **Who should have it** | **Comments** |
| Diphtheria, tetanus, pertussis vaccine (DTaP) | All children | 5 shots: First shot at age 2 months, last at 4–6 years<br><br>Booster shot every 10 years starting at age 11–12 years |
| Polio vaccine (IPV) | All children | 4 shots: First shot at age 2 months, last at 4–6 years |
| Pneumococcal vaccine(PCV) | All children under 2 years | 4 shots: First shot at age 2 months, last at 12–15 months |
| *Haemophilus influenzae* type b (Hib) vaccine | All children | 3 or 4 shots: First shot at age 2 months, last at 12–15 months |
| Measles, mumps, rubella vaccine (MMR) | All children | 2 shots: First shot at age 12–15 months, second at 4–6 years |
| Hepatitis B vaccine (HBV) | All children | 3 shots: First shot at birth, last by age 6 months |
| Flu shot | All children 6–23 months | 1 shot each year; cannot be given before age 6 months |
| Chickenpox vaccine | All children 12 months and older who haven't had chickenpox | 1 shot at age 12–18 months |
| Hepatitis A vaccine (HAV) | All children 12 months and older | 2 shots: First shot at age 12 months, second at least 6 months later |
| Meningococcal vaccine | All children 11–12 years | 1 shot at age 11–12 years |

**More**

## Teen and Adult Immunizations

| Immunization | Who should have it (if not already immunized) |
|---|---|
| Flu shot (once a year) | ◆ All adults 50 years and older<br>◆ Pregnant women<br>◆ People with chronic health problems (asthma, heart or lung problems, weakened immune system)<br>◆ Caregivers of children 0–23 months<br>◆ Anyone who lives or works with people at high risk |
| Chickenpox | ◆ All teens and adults who have not had chickenpox (pregnant women cannot have the vaccine) |
| Meningococcal vaccine | ◆ All teens by age 15 (advised at age 11–12)<br>◆ All college freshmen living in dorms<br>◆ People who live in or travel to areas where disease is common<br>◆ People with weakened immune systems (HIV, damaged or missing spleen) |
| Hepatitis A vaccine | ◆ Anyone who lives in or travels to areas where outbreaks have occurred (includes parts of United States)<br>◆ People who inject illegal drugs<br>◆ Men who have sex with men<br>◆ People with chronic liver disease<br>◆ People with blood-clotting problems |
| Hepatitis B vaccine | ◆ Anyone 18 years or younger who has not been vaccinated<br>◆ Adults whose travel or work puts them at risk<br>◆ Health care and public safety workers<br>◆ People who inject illegal drugs<br>◆ Men who have sex with men<br>◆ People who have had more than one sex partner in the past 6 months or who have a history of sexually transmitted disease<br>◆ Household contacts and sex partners of hepatitis B carriers<br>◆ People with chronic liver disease<br>◆ Prison inmates |
| Measles, mumps, and rubella (MMR) | ◆ Health care workers, college students, and international travelers<br>◆ Adults born after 1956<br>◆ Women of childbearing age |
| Pneumococcal vaccine (PPV) | ◆ All adults over 65<br>◆ Anyone under 65 who has a chronic disease (such as heart or lung disease) or has a damaged or missing spleen |
| Polio vaccine (IPV) | ◆ People whose travel or work puts them at risk |
| Tetanus, diphtheria, and pertussis booster (once every 10 years) | ◆ All teens and adults, starting at age 11–12 years<br>◆ Anyone who gets a deep, dirty wound and hasn't had a booster in the past 5 years |

# Wellness Exams and Screening Tests

One way to protect your health is to watch for changes in your body and find problems early, when they may be easier to treat.

**Preventive health care** can help you do this. This type of care includes:

◆ Wellness exams. These are checkups you have when you are healthy. They are focused on your overall health.

◆ Screening tests. Screening tests look for signs of disease before you have symptoms. Pap tests, mammograms, and PSA (prostate-specific antigen) tests are examples of screening tests for cancer.

◆ Immunizations. See page 324.

The recommendations for wellness exams and screening tests here are for mostly healthy people at average risk for health problems. Some of the things that affect your level of risk include your overall health, your family history (whether your close relatives have had certain diseases), and lifestyle factors, such as tobacco use, exercise habits, and sexual history.

Children and adults who have a chronic illness or other problems may need checkups and tests more often. Work with your doctor to decide on the best schedule for you.

## For Children

Up to age 2 years:

◆ Well-baby visits: A good schedule for visits is at age 2 weeks and at 2, 4, 6, 9, 12, 15, 18, and 24 months. Your doctor may suggest a slightly different schedule. The point is that babies need regular checkups during their first 2 years.

◆ Hearing tests: All babies should be tested for hearing problems by age 3 months.

Older than 2 years:

◆ Well-child visits: Talk to your child's doctor about how often to come in for a checkup. It's important to keep an eye on height, weight, blood pressure, and other measures of your child's growth and health.

◆ Vision tests: Have your child's vision checked between ages 3 and 4 years.

Don't forget immunizations! See page 324. These can be done at well-baby visits and regular checkups.

## For Adults

The right schedule of wellness exams and screenings is one you and your doctor agree on, based on your age, your risk factors for disease, how healthy you are, and how important preventive care is to you.

The schedule on page 328 lists some of the most common screening tests. Most adults need some or all of these tests.

### For Women: Pelvic Exams and Pap Tests

A pelvic exam looks for early signs of problems in the reproductive organs. The exam usually includes:

◆ An external genital exam. The doctor looks at the genital area for skin changes, sores, or other problems.

◆ A manual exam. The doctor inserts two gloved fingers into your vagina and presses on the lower belly with the other hand to check the shape and size of your ovaries and uterus.

◆ A Pap test.

**More**

## Sample Health Screening Schedule

| Screening | Who should have it? | How often? |
|-----------|---------------------|------------|
| Blood pressure | All adults | Every 1 to 2 years. More often if you are at risk for high blood pressure. See page 191. |
| Cholesterol | All adults | Every 5 years or as agreed on with your doctor. More often if you are at risk for heart disease. See page 193. |
| Vision problems, especially glaucoma (see page 172) | All adults | Talk to your doctor. Need for exams increases with age. |
| Colorectal cancer (colonoscopy, flexible sigmoidoscopy, fecal occult blood test, or barium enema) | All adults starting at age 50. Sooner if you are at increased risk. | Depends on which tests you have. See Colorectal Cancer on page 127. |
| Breast cancer (mammogram and clinical breast exam) | All women starting at age 40. Sooner if you are at increased risk. | **Mammogram**<br>Age 50 and up: Every 1 to 2 years<br>Age 40 to 49: Talk to your doctor.<br><br>**Clinical breast exam**<br>Age 40 and up: Every year |
| Pap test for cervical cancer | All women starting at age 21 or when they become sexually active, whichever comes first | Every 1 to 3 years for women at average risk. See page 327. |
| Chlamydia (see page 230) | All sexually active females 25 and younger<br><br>All females over 25 who are at risk | Whenever you have a pelvic exam and Pap test. See page 327. |
| Prostate cancer (PSA test or digital rectal exam) | Some men. See Should You Be Tested? on page 221. | Talk to your doctor. |

Other things you and your doctor may want to keep an eye on: height and weight; hearing; blood sugar level; thyroid level; HIV status (if you are at risk); and skin changes that could be cancerous.

## Pap tests

The Pap test is a screening test for cancer of the cervix, which is the lower part of the uterus that opens into the vagina. The test looks for early changes in the cells that could lead to cancer. When done regularly, Pap tests can find most cervical cancers.

To do the test, the doctor inserts an instrument called a speculum into your vagina to spread apart the vaginal walls. He or she then collects cell samples from your cervix with a wooden or plastic device that gently scrapes some cells off the surface. The cells are sent to a lab.

Your doctor should let you know the results of your Pap test when they return from the lab. If your results are abnormal, you may need to return for more tests. You may need another Pap test, or you may need a test called a colposcopy, which provides a more complete view of the cervix.

Abnormal Pap results can mean many things. Most of them are not cancer.

Women should have their first Pap test within 3 years of becoming sexually active or at age 21, whichever comes first. After that, Pap tests are recommended every 1 to 3 years, depending on your risk for cervical cancer.

You may not need yearly Pap tests if:

◆ You have had normal Pap results at least 3 years in a row.

◆ You have only one sex partner.

◆ You do not smoke.

◆ You do not have a history of abnormal Pap tests, cervical cancer, a sexually transmitted disease such as genital warts or HIV infection, or exposure to the drug diethylstilbestrol (DES).

◆ You have had a hysterectomy for a reason other than cancer.

◆ You are older than 65 and have had normal Pap tests over the past 10 years.

Talk to your doctor about the best schedule for you.

Arrange to have the test 1 to 2 weeks after your period ends. Do not douche, have sex, or use feminine hygiene products for at least 24 hours before a Pap test, because it may affect the test results.

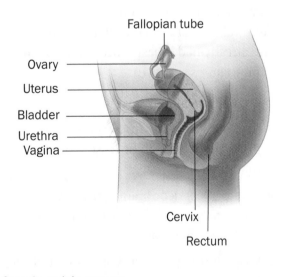

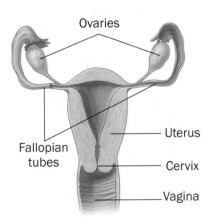

The female pelvic organs (front and side views)

## For Women: Mammograms and Clinical Breast Exams

Breast cancer can often be cured if it is found early. There are two ways to screen for early breast cancer: mammograms and clinical breast exams.

A **mammogram** is a breast X-ray that can find tumors while they are still too small to be felt in a breast exam.

Mammograms save lives. If you are not at high risk for breast cancer and you are:

◆ Age 50 or older, have a mammogram every 1 to 2 years.

◆ Age 40 to 49, have a mammogram every 1 to 2 years or agree on a different schedule with your doctor.

◆ Younger than 40, you probably do not need mammograms for routine screening.

If your mother, a sister, or another close female relative had breast cancer before menopause, you may need to start having mammograms sooner and have them more often. Talk to your doctor. Women who have already had breast cancer need to have mammograms every year.

To prepare for a mammogram:

◆ Arrange to have it 1 to 2 weeks after your period ends. (It will be least painful at that time.)

◆ Do not wear deodorant, perfume, powder, or lotion. They can affect the quality of the X-ray.

◆ Wear clothing that lets you easily undress from the waist up.

◆ If your last mammogram was at a different facility, have a copy sent before your test or bring a copy with you.

During a **clinical breast exam**, a doctor or nurse looks at your breasts and gently feels them for lumps or other changes. A clinical breast exam is recommended every year starting at age 40 (and anytime you have problems with your breasts).

No matter what your age, talk to your doctor if you find a lump or have a problem with your breasts. See Breast Problems on page 103. You may need a breast exam or a mammogram to help find the cause.

### What about breast self-exams?

Breast self-exams are a good way for you to learn what your breasts normally look and feel like. Once you know what's normal for you, you'll be better able to notice changes and know when to get help early instead of waiting for your next checkup. A self-exam is not a substitute for a mammogram or a clinical breast exam.

A breast self-exam is easy to do. It includes looking for changes in the shape of your breasts or nipples as you stand in front of a mirror and move your arms in different ways. For the second part of the test, you use your hands to examine all areas of each breast, nipple, and armpit.

If you do not know how to do a breast self-exam, ask your doctor or nurse for help. Your doctor's office may have the instructions printed on a sheet or card that you can take with you.

## Self-Exams

Watching for changes in your own body is an easy thing you can do to find problems early. Self-exams help you better understand your own body and what is normal for you.

Some of the self-exams you can do include:

◆ Breast self-exam for women. See page 330.

◆ Testicular self-exam for men. See page 246.

◆ Skin self-exam. Every month or so, look for changes in moles (changing color, size, or shape), sores that won't heal, or any other changes in your skin that could be early signs of skin cancer. See page 235.

In general, try to be a good observer of your body. If you notice a change from what's normal for you and the change does not go away, it may be a good idea to talk to your doctor about it.

## Dental Checkups

Regular visits to the dentist are an important part of your preventive care.

◆ Most experts recommend that your child see a dentist either by age 1 or within 6 months after the first tooth comes in.

◆ Children and adults should see the dentist twice a year. During a checkup:

❖ The dentist will examine your teeth and gums for cavities, tooth decay, and gum disease.

❖ You may have X-rays of your teeth (usually once a year).

❖ A dentist or dental hygienist will scrape hard buildup (tartar) off your teeth with a metal tool, floss your teeth well, and clean and polish your teeth.

For people who go to the dentist regularly and take good care of their teeth, cleanings are usually not painful. If you have not been to the dentist in a long time, or if you have problems with your teeth or gums, cleanings may be a little uncomfortable.

## Tuberculin Skin Test

A tuberculin test is done to find out if you have been infected with the bacteria that cause tuberculosis (TB). TB is a lung infection that spreads among people easily. It can be very serious in children and in people who have weak immune systems.

Whether you need to be tested depends on how common TB is in your area and how likely you are to come in contact with TB. If you think you may have been exposed to TB and want to be tested, call your doctor or the local health department.

# Be Safe

## Ten Steps to a Safer Home

1.  Install smoke detectors. Check the batteries once a month, and replace them every year.

2.  Keep a working fire extinguisher in your home. Make sure everyone in the house knows where it is and how to use it.

3.  Have an emergency plan in case of a fire. Include how everyone will get out of the house and where to meet outside. Practice the plan with your family. Don't forget your pets.

4.  Set your water heater to 120°F or lower to prevent burns. When you are cooking, turn pot handles toward the back of the stove. Never smoke in bed.

5.  Keep appliances away from water. Turn off or unplug appliances when you are done with them. Replace frayed electrical cords. Unplug appliances (including your computer) when you need to clean or repair them. Turn off power at the circuit breaker if you need to work on wall or ceiling fixtures.

6.  If you have children, plug bare electrical sockets with plastic inserts. Keep electrical cords out of the reach of small children and pets.

7.  Have your heating and cooling system checked at least once a year. Keep fireplaces and stoves in good working order. Think about installing a carbon monoxide detector.

8.  Store firearms unloaded and with the safety on in a secure, locked place. Lock ammunition in a separate place.

9.  Keep medicines, cleaning products, plant food, and other poisonous products (see page 44) where kids and pets cannot reach them. Keep products in their original containers. Never store poisons in food containers. Use childproof latches on your cabinets.

10. Make your home fall-proof. Use good lighting inside and out. Keep stairs and walking paths clear of electrical cords and clutter. Make sure carpets are firmly attached to the floor. Remove snow and ice from porches and sidewalks promptly.

## Prevent Serious Injuries

◆ Wear your seat belt every time you get in a car. Teach your children to do the same. Children under age 12 should ride in the backseat. Use car seats for babies and small children (see pages 333 to 334).

◆ Never drink and drive, and don't ride in a car with a drunk driver. Do not drive if you are taking medicine that makes you sleepy.

◆ Wear a helmet and other protective gear whenever you are biking, motorcycling, skating, kayaking, horseback riding, skiing, snowboarding, or rock climbing.

◆ If you keep a gun in your home:

❖ Make sure you know how to use the gun properly. Take a safety course.

❖ If there are children living in your home, store the gun unloaded, with the safety on, and locked in a secure spot. Do not store the ammunition with the gun.

◆ Do not dive into shallow or unfamiliar waters.

◆ Do not let young children play near water without a responsible person watching them.

◆ Wear safety glasses whenever you mow the lawn, use power tools, or work with chemicals. Closely follow the instructions on the label when you work with pesticides, fertilizers, strong cleaning products, and other chemicals. If it says to wear a mask and gloves, wear them.

◆ Use a sturdy step stool or ladder to reach objects that are up high. Do not stand on chairs or countertops. And be extra careful when you are up high on a ladder or on a roof. Don't take chances.

### Use Child Car Seats

Infant and child car seats save lives. Children who are not in car seats can be hurt or killed during crashes or even by sudden stops at low speeds.

Most states require car seats for all children under age 4 and those weighing less than 40 pounds. Find out what the laws are where you live. The guidelines below are a good rule of thumb:

◆ Babies under 20 pounds, regardless of age: Use an infant seat that reclines and faces the rear.

◆ Babies younger than 1 year, regardless of weight: Use an infant seat that reclines and faces the rear.

◆ Children over 20 pounds and older than 1 year: Use a toddler seat that faces the front of the car and has a shield or harness. Some infant seats can be converted to toddler seats.

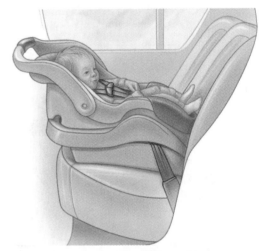

An infant seat that faces the rear

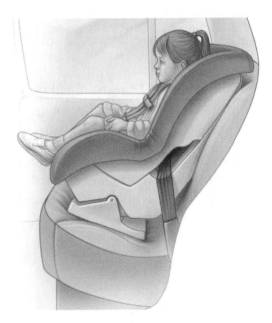

A toddler seat that faces the front

**More**

◆ Children over 40 pounds and older than 4 years: Use a booster seat that raises the child so that the regular lap and shoulder belts fit properly. Adjust the shoulder belt to fit across the shoulder, not the neck. Use the booster seat until your child is big enough to use the seat belt properly.

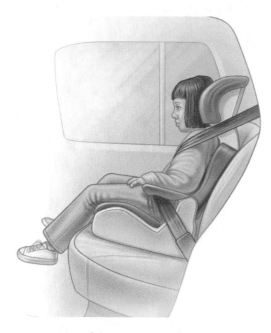

A booster seat

◆ Children under 12 years should ride in the backseat if the car has passenger side air bags that you cannot turn off.

For the safest use of a child car seat, follow the manufacturer's recommendations. They should include weight guidelines as well as how to install the seat and how to secure your child in it.

## Be Prepared for Emergencies

Natural disasters, chemical spills, disease outbreaks—these are dangers of modern life. They can affect air quality, cause shortages of safe water and food, and cut off access to electricity, gas, phones, and other services. Family members may be separated. Hospitals and clinics may not be able to handle everyone who needs help.

While these events are scary to think about, there are things you can do to be better prepared:

◆ Have a plan for you and your family. This can help in almost any kind of disaster.

◆ Keep an emergency kit with water, food, first-aid supplies, and other essentials. It's also a good idea to know how to purify water (see page 336).

◆ Learn what to do if you are exposed to chemicals (see page 27) or other hazards.

◆ Always follow the advice of local authorities and public health officials.

❖ During an emergency, tune in to a local radio or TV station. Don't try to call for instructions. Phone lines may be busy or out of order.

❖ If you are told to evacuate, do it. Follow the schedule and route for your area.

❖ If there is an outbreak of a contagious disease in your area, don't leave your community unless authorities tell you to. If you are already infected, you could spread the disease or miss getting treatment you need.

❖ For major public health crises, you can rely on information from the Centers for Disease Control and Prevention (www.cdc.gov) and the World Health Organization (www.who.int/en).

## Your Emergency Plan

It's easy to put together an emergency plan.

◆ Choose a contact person for family members to call or e-mail if they get separated. A friend or relative who lives out of state is best. Make sure everyone has the contact's phone number and e-mail address.

◆ Pick a place to meet outside your neighborhood in case you can't go home. Make sure everyone has the address and phone number.

◆ Pick a place to meet just outside your home, like a neighbor's front yard, in case there's a fire in your home.

◆ Write down where and how to turn off water, gas, and power. Make sure you have any tools this requires.

◆ Talk about what you would do if you had to leave. Include your pets in your plans. Shelters and health facilities may not let you bring your pets.

You may have other things you want to include in your plan, especially if you have children in school or if anyone in your household has special needs.

Review your plan once a year. Make sure that phone numbers, e-mail addresses, and other items are still correct.

## Your Emergency Supplies Kit

You need the same basic supplies no matter what the situation:

◆ Water. Store 1 gallon (4 quarts) for each person for each day. Most people need to drink about 2 quarts a day. Count on another 2 quarts for hygiene and cooking.

**Example:** A family of four that wanted to keep a 3-day supply of water on hand would need to store 12 gallons. That's 4 gallons a day (1 for each person) times 3 days. A 7-day supply for four people would be 28 gallons.

◆ Foods that you don't have to cook or keep cold, such as canned foods, peanut butter, crackers, granola bars, powdered milk, and staples like sugar, salt, and pepper. (Don't forget a manual can opener or utility knife.)

◆ First-aid supplies and medicines

◆ Blankets and clothing

◆ Soap, toilet paper, and other personal hygiene items

◆ Special needs items (such as baby formula, diapers, and contact lens supplies)

◆ Certain tools and household items, such as a battery-powered radio, a flashlight, extra batteries, matches, and tools needed to shut off the water, power, or gas.

◆ Cash or traveler's checks. ATM machines may not be working.

More

For a complete checklist to help you build your emergency kit, go to www.redcross.org.

Store everything in one place. Somewhere cool and dark is best. You also might want to keep a small version of your emergency kit on hand in case you ever have to leave your home.

Once you have your supplies, remember to check them from time to time. Replace water, food, batteries, expired medicines, outgrown clothing, and other items as needed. Even bottled water and "nonperishable" food need to be replaced after a while.

You should also know where your important documents are so that you can gather them quickly if you need to. These are things like passports, social security cards, wills, insurance policies, bank account and credit card information, and health records.

## Safe Drinking Water

Knowing how to purify water can help you if:

◆ Your normal water supply becomes unsafe. Never ignore a "boil order" issued by local officials.

◆ You are in a place where there is no clean water.

◆ You run out of the clean water you have stored for an emergency.

Purifying water can greatly reduce your chance of getting sick from the water. You can purify water with one of these methods:

◆ Boil the water for 3 to 5 minutes. This method works the best but may not be practical if you need a lot of water. It also requires a stove, fire, or other heat source, which you may not have.

◆ Use an eyedropper to add 16 drops of liquid bleach to a gallon of water. Stir, and let it stand for 30 minutes. If the water does not smell slightly like bleach after 30 minutes, add 16 more drops of bleach and let it stand for another 15 minutes. There should be a bleach smell.

◆ Use iodine or chlorine tablets or drops. You can buy these at stores that sell camping equipment and at some drugstores. Do what the label says. Tablets and drops don't work as well as boiling or bleach, but they do kill some types of organisms.

◆ Use a water filter. Filters can get rid of some harmful things in the water and can improve the taste. Some filters work better than others.

# Index